ENT

DO-HNS and MRCS (ENT) OSCE GUIDE

Revision notes for Otolaryngology

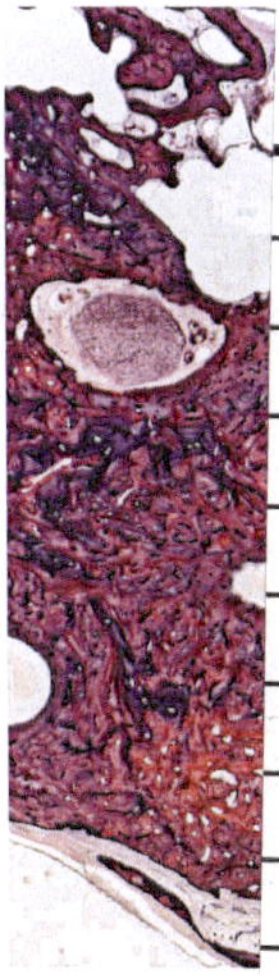

Fore

Ricardo Persaud
MBBS MSB CBiol MPhil MRCS (Gen) DO-HNS FRCS (ORL-HNS)
Locum Consultant ENT, Head and Neck Surgeon
Leicester Royal Infirmary
University Hospitals of Leicester
Examiner, Imperial College Medical School London, UK
Chartered Biologist (Europe).

Wai Sum Cho
BMedSci BMBS MRCS (ENT)
Core Surgical Trainee
East Midlands South Deanery, UK.

Antonia Tse
BSc (Hon) MBBS MRCS (ENT)
Core Surgical Trainee
Kent, Surrey and Sussex Deanery, UK.

Konstantinos Argiris
BSc MBBS MSc MRCS (ENT) DO-HNS
Specialist Registrar
Kent, Surrey and Sussex Deanery, UK.

Professor Henry Pau
MD FRCS (*ad eundem*) FRCSEd (ORL-HNS)
Consultant ENT Surgeon
Leicester Royal Infirmary
University Hospitals of Leicester
Visiting Professor, University of Loughborough
Honorary Senior Lecturer, Leicester University Medical School, UK.

First published 2013 by FASTPRINT PUBLISHING
Peterborough, England.
FastPrint Publishing
www.fast-print.net/store.php

DO-HNS and MRCS (ENT) OSCE GUIDE
Revision notes for Otolaryngology

A catalogue record for this book is available from the British Library

ISBN 978-178035-657-0

An environmentally friendly book printed and bound in England by www.printondemand-worldwide.com

Mixed Sources
Product group from well-managed forests, and other controlled sources
www.fsc.org Cert no. TT-COC-002641
© 1996 Forest Stewardship Council
FSC

PEFC Certified
This product is from sustainably managed forests and controlled sources
www.pefc.org
PEFC
PEFC/16-33-415

This book is made entirely of chain-of-custody materials

DO-HNS and MRCS (ENT) OSCE GUIDE

Revision notes for Otolaryngology

CONTENTS

Preface

The impetus for this book came from feedback received from candidates who attended ENTTZAR DO-HNS courses. We were asked to write a guide containing strategies and vital core ENT information relevant to every section of the examination. This book is therefore written as an examination revision tool covering all aspects of the examination, rather than an ENT textbook. It is laid out into two sections (unmanned and manned stations) to reflect the structure of the diploma examination. The first section comprises of practice questions, model answers and revision notes highlighting additional key information not covered in the questions or answers. The second section provides essential material pertaining to the interactive part of the examination.

We believe that we have succeeded in producing the most comprehensive up-to-date revision guide to optimize your chance of securing the DO-HNS or MRCS (ENT) diploma. However, whilst it should be emphasised that the tips, questions, answers and revision notes provided in this book will help you significantly to prepare, in order to succeed comfortably you will need to read a standard ENT textbook as well as attend at least one revision course which offers a full mock examination (see www.enttzar.co.uk). This is because the manned stations cannot be mastered adequately by studying any textbook or guide. It is very important to practice under examination conditions in order to overcome mistakes induced by nervousness. Finally, remember the more time, work and effort you put in early the more likely you will pass first time.

Ricardo Persaud, Wai Sum Cho, Antonia Tse,
Konstantinos Argiris & Henry Pau
May 2013

Foreword

It gives me great pleasure to write the foreword for *DO-HNS and MRCS (ENT) OSCE Guide: Revision notes for Otolaryngology*. The book contains an excellent set of questions, which accurately reflect key topics over the breadth of the syllabus. Some of the questions, eg temporal bone histology, congenital hearing loss and nystagmus, are challenging but this is necessary as the intercollegiate examination is becoming increasingly difficult probably because of its importance in the current ENT training system.

Within this revision guide, the authors have also highlighted essential information relevant to other sections of the OSCE examination. They have provided sound coping strategies, templates and advice, especially for the interactive stations. More importantly, the authors have addressed the needs of ENT trainees by providing clear succinct answers and well illustrated revision notes to optimize learning difficult concepts. Furthermore, the chapter on Fundamentals of Clinical Audiology fulfills the desperate needs of most, if not all, ENT trainees. I have no doubt that this book will succeed. I plan to have a copy in my office to grill trainees as they pass through the ENT Department.

Professor Antony Narula MA FRCS FRCS Ed
Consultant ENT Surgeon
St Mary's Hospital, Imperial College Healthcare NHS Trust,
Visiting Professor, Middlesex University,
Council Member, Royal College of Surgeons of England,
Past President of British Society of Otology,
President-Elect, ENT UK.

Contributors

Ashwin Algudkar
Locum Appointed Trainee (LAT)
London Deanery
OSCE for DOHNS and MRCS (ENT) Diploma

Bilal Anwar
ENT CT2
North Western Deanery
Chapter7

Sonna Ifeacho
ENT Specialist Registrar
London Deanery
Chapter 1

Hiten Joshi
Research Fellow
East Anglia Deanery
Chapters 4, 9

Muhammud Fadil Khoyratty
ENT CT2
Bristol
Chapter 6 & Editorial Assistant

Praneta Kulloo
Research Fellow
East of England Deanery
Chapter 4

Sridhayan Mahalingam
Foundation Year 2 Doctor
London Deanery
DO-HNS OSCE Examination 2013: A Candidate's Perspective

Fatima Mallick
Clinical Research Fellow
East Midlands (South)
Chapter 8

Phil Touska
ENT CT 2
London Deanery
Chapter 1

Gada Yassin
Surgery Education Fellow
West Midlands Deanery
Chapter 10

'Life affords no higher pleasure than that of surmounting difficulties, passing from one step of success to another, forming new wishes and seeing them gratified.'

- Samuel Johnson

Acknowledgements

Many thanks to all those who made this book a reality, especially the list of talented contributors. We are very grateful to all our patients, friends and colleagues who have kindly given permission to include their photographs in this book, eg Revatha Basnayake. Our gratitude also extends to Dr Reza Jarral for providing the outstanding line diagrams and Dr Matthew Piergies for taking some of the photographs. Many thanks to Mr Awad and Prof Narula for some of the clinical photographs. We are also thankful to all those who have kindly allowed us to use slides from their excellent presentations, especially Darren Cordon and Sally Wood. Finally, we are very grateful for the generous editorial help from Anusha Bala, Muhammud Fadil Khoyratty, Faiz Tanweer and Vadsala Baskaran.

Dedications

To all ENTTZAR Ambassadors:

Past, Present and Future

OSCEs for DO-HNS and MRCS (ENT Diplomas

Objective structured clinical examinations (OSCEs) consist of multiple stations (interactive and non-interactive) through which all candidates rotate on a timed basis. There is good evidence to show that OSCE examination has advantages over other forms of assessments, such as pure oral examinations, and that it can be used for competency assessment that is valid, reliable, feasible and defensible. In fact, the OSCE is considered the gold standard performance-based tool for evaluating postgraduate clinical performance, particularly in high-stakes settings such as certification examinations and maintenance of competency reviews.

In order to progress to higher training in ENT in the UK, trainees must be in possession of either DO-HNS and MRCS or MRCS (ENT). The latter has only been available since 1st August 2011. To be awarded the MRCS (ENT) diploma, candidates must have passed both the MRCS part A and the DO-HNS part 2. After obtaining a pass in the MRCS part A, current regulations state that a total of four attempts at any combination of the MRCS part B and the DO-HNS part 2 are permitted to be awarded the MRCS or the MRCS (ENT). Candidates need to take both MRCS part A and B as well as DO-HNS part 1 and 2 to be awarded MRCS and DO-HNS diplomas.

The DO-HNS examination has been available since 2003. It replaces the Diploma in Laryngology and Otology which had been available since 1923. The DO-HNS became "intercollegiate" in 2008 (London, Edinburgh and Glasgow) and since 2012 also includes Dublin. The part 1 examination is held simultaneously at all centres three times a year with the part 2 also being held three times a year but rotating through the 4 colleges. College regulations recommend at least 6 months experience in ENT before attempting the part 1 examination. At present there is no limit on the number of attempts that candidates have to pass the constituent parts of the DO-HNS examination.

The examination is made up of two parts. Part 1 is a two-hour written paper consisting of multiple true/false questions and extended matching questions (EMQs). There are approximately 140 questions in total. Once a candidate has passes the part 1 he/she will be eligible to take the second part. This takes the form of an OSCE with up to 30 stations of 7 minutes each (see Table 1), taking just over three hours in total (with rest stations). Usually 6 of the stations are interactive and involve performing an examination on a patient, taking a history, explaining a disease, consenting for an operation or performing a basic procedure (e.g. flexible nasendoscopy) (Table 1). There is an examiner present at the practical stations. The remainder of the stations are non-interactive and involve interpreting and answering questions related to photographs, scans, audiograms, data interpretation, instruments or anatomical specimens. No examiner is present at the non-interactive stations. During the part 2 examination the candidate writes his/her answers on a blank sheet and places them in a folder which the candidate takes to every station. At the end of the examination the folder of completed answer sheets is collected from candidates.

Table 1 - A typical DO-HNS/MRCS (ENT) OSCE consisting of 30 stations.

MANNED (interactive) STATIONS (x6)	UNMANNED (non-interactive) STATIONS (x24)
History taking (Information gathering)	Clinical cases (most with photographs)
Communication station (information giving): • Explaining the result of an investigation, procedure or breaking bad news. • Counselling a worried, angry, upset or distressed patient.	Anatomy questions: • Osteology - eg skull or temporal bone. • Wet specimen - eg laryngeal specimen.
Consent for a surgical procedure	Data interpretation (eg TFTs)
Examination of ear, +/- nose, neck or oral cavity	Clinical radiograph stations
Outpatient skills (eg FNE)	ENT instruments or device station
	Audiograms
	Histology photomicrograph
	Operation notes
	Discharge summary

Examination Revision Advice

As with all postgraduate examinations, failure can be frustrating and expensive. With this in mind preparation should begin early to get a good grounding in the areas commonly examined. No doubt a certain amount of 'cramming' will also be required so allocate time off to revise in advance and be aware of the importance of working towards a peak of knowledge for the exam. Everyone reading this will have their own approach to examinations 'hard-wired' having done many to get to this stage. A good knowledge of the syllabus as well as commonly examined topics (as presented in this book) is a good starting point. Writing notes on these areas is always worthwhile. Knowing the key points for presentation, diagnosis and management of a wide range of ENT conditions is vital. ENTTZAR team believes that the best way to prepare for any examination is to work through as many previous questions as possible and to learn in a retrograde fashion. With this in mind, we have provided not only commonly asked questions but also highly relevant revision notes on the subject that were not covered in the questions and answers. In addition, we have incorporated a few challenging questions to stimulate learning at a higher level. Although this book fulfils most of the requirements for passing the OSCE section of the DOHNS and MRCS (ENT), we strongly believe that each candidate still needs to practice, practice and practice before the real exam. This is particularly important for the manned stations because you cannot learn how to pass such stations purely from reading books. We, therefore, recommend attendance to any course which offers a full simulated mock examination, and ideally a review of all the past questions (for further information visit www.enttzar.co.uk).

Recommended reading

1. Ludman H, Bradley PJ. ABC of Ear Nose and Throat. 6th edn. Wiley-Blackwell, 2013.
2. Bull T, Almeyda J. Color Atlas of ENT Diagnosis. 5th edn, New York: Thieme, 2009.
3. Dhillon RS, East CA. Ear, Nose, Throat Head and Neck Surgery: An Illustrated Colour Text 3rd edn. London: Churchill Livingstone, 2006.
4. Gleeson M, Browning GG, Burton MJ, et al.(eds). Scott-Brown's Otorhinolaryngology, Head and Neck Surgery, 7th edn. Hodder Arnold, 2008.
5. Lee KJ. Essential Otolaryngology: Head and Neck Surgery, 9th edn. New York: McGraw-Hill Medical, 2008.
6. Roland NJ, McRae RD, McCombe AW. Key Topics in Otolaryngology, 2nd edn. Oxford: BIOS Scientific Publishers Ltd, 2001.
7. Ellis H, Mahadevan V. Clinical Anatomy: Applied Anatomy for Students and Junior Doctors, 12th edn. Wiley-Blackwell, 2010.

DO-HNS OSCE Examination 2013

A successful candidate's perspective

I had been interested in Head & Neck Anatomy and Surgery throughout medical school. Having successfully passed the DOHNS MCQ exam in my first year of foundation training, I thought it would be a real challenge to attempt the OSCE during my FY2 year.

By talking to those who had taken the exam I quickly realised that some clinical experience at the SHO level would be imperative. Hence I pursued a rotation involving 4 months of ENT surgery. It was during this 4-month period that I prepared for the OSCE.

In retrospect I believe somewhere between 3-6 months is advisable to prepare for the OSCE especially as many of us have to juggle exam preparation with day to day clinical work and on call commitments. I tried to make the most of my ENT job. Having read the syllabus, I took every opportunity to further my clinical experience by regularly observing and helping in consultant led subspecialty clinics: Head & Neck, Rhinology, Otology, Paediatric ENT and Audio-vestibular. I became accustomed to certain basic skills such as the Head & Neck examination, Flexible Nasoendoscopy and analysis of various Hearing Tests, all of which are common OSCE scenarios. I often used my own SHO Emergency Clinics to practice these routine examinations with patients as if in an OSCE style scenario, which I found extremely useful.

Furthermore, during my time in theatre, I learnt the names of various instruments and observed a range of procedures to study the anatomy involved – again common themes for the OSCE. Importantly, I actively observed how consultants and specialist registrars consented patients thereby learning about common complications and naturally picked up on good communication skills.

Out-of hours I carried out independent reading, focusing particularly on data interpretation. I used the common books (Key Topics in Otolaryngology, Oxford Handbook of ENT, Pastest: Total Revision - ENT) but particularly focused on data interpretation (Colour Atlas of ENT Diagnosis is a good book for this). I made the most of my friendly approachable Registrars and Consultants, whom I would relentlessly question on concepts that I just couldn't grasp from independent study.

There are an increasing number of courses available. Around a month before the exam itself, I went to the ENT Tzar OSCE Revision course. The morning was run in an OSCE format, where we were assessed on a range of clinical examinations and written stations. The afternoon was spent reviewing each station together, with previous candidates giving short presentations on common clinical stations and pitfalls they encountered. This course was particularly useful as it offered me a practice run-through, highlighting my strengths and weaknesses and I was able to gauge my standard compared to other candidates. During the day I realized that many of the candidates were much more experienced than me, which initially made me a little anxious, but this is what really encouraged me to work that extra bit harder and focus more on my revision goals in the last month prior to the exam. Perhaps most importantly from this course I met a few other candidates with whom I forged relationships and organised regular revision sessions with thereafter (we all worked together, helped each other out, and passed on the same sitting).

The exam itself took place at the Royal College of Surgeons of England, in a very well structured format. On the whole, examiners were polite in the clinical stations, probing me with relevant questions, and asking me to skip certain parts appropriately in order to save time. It is always important to address the patient first in the practical stations as a significant proportion of the marks are based on communication skills. The written stations included a huge variety of themes involving Head and Neck, Otology, Rhinology, Paediatric ENT and Clinical Audiology. There was a plethora of data interpretation questions including histology slides, radiology, pictures of instruments/patients and hearing test results. As with all OSCEs some stations were more rushed than others leaving me completely exhausted by the end of the almost 4 hour ordeal. Overall, however, the experience was a pleasant one.

Preparation for the DO-HNS OSCE should not be taken lightly, as it assesses a variety of Head & Neck conditions requiring candidates to have a wide breadth of knowledge in ENT. It is my belief that taking the exam towards the end of my ENT attachment facilitated my revision, since I felt completely immersed in the specialty. From my personal experience seeking guidance from peers who have just sat the exam is beneficial and starting preparation early gives one time to make and then correct mistakes. If you decide to take a course, go at a stage when you have done much of your preparation, but also leave enough time to spare before the exam to fine-tune your skills and learn the course materials (which are often quite extensive in themselves). Be aware that many people may be more experienced than you, but don't let that affect your performance and concentrate on your own revision goals. I cannot stress the importance of practicing common scenarios with colleagues who will actively critique you. With practice comes fluency, confidence, and in turn good communication will be more natural - this will be evident on the day of the exam.

In hindsight, I was fortunate to have passed the DO-HNS OSCE in my first attempt. Many would argue that perhaps taking the exam at such a junior level year is premature. However, with preparation for the DO-HNS OSCE, my clinical confidence in the management of common ENT conditions has significantly improved, and this was the general impression amongst my colleagues, whether they were Surgical or GP Trainees. The DO-HNS is definitely an exam worth sitting if you are interested in ENT related themes, so long as you have the motivation to conduct some out-of-hours study to pass the exam. Good luck!

Sridhayan Mahalingam
Academic FY2
London Deanery
May 2013

DO-HNS OSCE Examination

General tips and advice for success

I passed my DO-HNS Part 2 after 6 weeks of being an ENT SHO. It wasn't an easy task! Here is my guide for DO-HNS success, some useful tips that I would have appreciated at the time if someone had told me.

Format of the exam

The exam itself is around 3 hours 20 minutes long with approximately 30 stations in total, each of which last 7 minutes. There are usually 2 or 3 rest stations, making 28 active stations (of which 5 are manned/interactive and 23 are un-manned/non-interactive).

Manned stations (examiner +/- patient/actor present)

Designed to assess the following:

Clinical skills, Clinical examination, History taking, Communication skills

Unmanned stations (no examiner or patient/actor present)

These are written stations with questions designed to elicit short, succinct answers are designed to assess the following:

Anatomy/physiology, Pathology/histology, Audiometry, Otology, Rhinology, Laryngology, Neck conditions, Written communication skills, Radiology, ENT surgical/ medical instruments and Paediatric ENT surgery.

These can be in the form of picture/photo questions, labeling of pictures, interpretation of audiograms /tympanograms, radiological scans, instruments and equipment, anatomy – skull base, temporal bone, oncological neck levels and larynx.

Tips for the examination

As you read this book, you will find that we have given you tips/ advice where possible along the way. However, here is list of some of things that may be useful to remember:

Manned stations

- Remember **WIPER** (**W**ash hands, **I**ntroduce yourself, gain **P**ermission, **E**xpose patient, **R**eposition patient)
  "Hello, my name is Dr Smith. I am one of the ENT doctors. What is your name? I have been asked to examine your ears today – would that be ok? Do you have any pain anywhere? Can I ask you to remove your glasses for the purpose of the examination please? Thank you….."
- Have a system. It does not have to be the system we give you in the book (everyone has their own way of examining a patient or was taught a certain way – as long as you are confident and you cover the whole examination.
- Running commentary – talk to the examiner and patient as you go along so they know what you are doing and what you are looking for.
  "Looking at the ears there are no scars or obvious deformities. I will now proceed with otoscopy….."
- Summarise for the examiner.
  "In summary, this is a 45 year old lady ……
  "Webers lateralises to the …… and Rinnes Test …. This patient has …."
  "To complete my examination…."
  Speak up! Practice in the mirror and ask your friend to listen to you. If he/ she can pick up all the words you say, then you're on the right track.
- In some of these stations there is a 'hidden agenda' that you need to find out from the actor/actress to get more points!

- Don't straddle the patient! – If you are sitting down to examine your patient, for example when examining the nose, it is best not to have your legs either side of the patient!

Unmanned stations

At the start of the exam, you will be given a folder which you are to carry around with you to put your answers in for each station. There is usually plenty of time for these stations and usually, only short answers are required to gain the marks. During the rest stations, there is nothing to stop you from going through your answers in the folder so if you didn't have time to finish one of the stations, use the time you have in the rest station.

General advice

- The one piece of exam advice which you will hear time and time again is to read the question properly before answering. This is such crucial advice that I will repeat it for emphasis: TAKE YOUR TIME AND READ THE QUESTION PROPERLY!
- Time yourself, especially for the stations requiring you to write an operation note or discharge summary. There is a lot to cover and 7 minutes will go by all too quickly! As you work your way through this book, you should try and complete the exercises under timed conditions as it is always good exam practice.
- Have an OSCE 'buddy'. For those of you who trained in the UK, you will be familiar with the OSCE-style examinations. Have someone to practise with – it doesn't necessary have to be someone doing the same exam (though this may be better) as you only need to find yourself a 'patient' to practise on (one of my friends practised on a teddy bear propped up on the bed and yes, he passed!).
- Try not to use any abbreviations in your answers.

- Make sure your handwriting is legible! The questions are marked by human beings – it is unlikely that you will receive marks for correct answers if the examiner cannot read your writing!
- For instruments, the best way to learn is to go into theatres and ask your seniors or theatre nurses for the names of common ENT instruments.
- Apply what you have learnt on paper to your clinics/on-calls. For example, when doing a nasoendoscopy on a patient, explain the procedure to them in the same way that you would in your exam i.e. use thorough and detailed explanations. That way it becomes second nature to you.
- ENT.UK provides very good leaflets on common ENT conditions and explanations of operations in layman's terms.
- Sit in with your hospital's audiologist – it makes it easier to learn about the topic if you have seen how it is done.

Plan ahead

I would recommend that you take at least 3 months to prepare for this exam and to learn the topics thoroughly. There is a lot to cover but with careful revision-planning and hard work, your chances of success should be high. Write a timetable of what you are going to cover from the first day of revision up until the day of the exam. Start learning and practising the communication stations early on so you get sufficient practice before the real thing!

Antonia Tse
ENT CT 2
KSS Deanery
Faculty member
ENT Tzar DOHNS OSCE Course

May 2013

Section 1

Unmanned (Non-interactive) Stations

Chapter 1

Clinical Cases for OSCE Stations

1.1 Introduction

In this chapter, we present 62 OSCE stations. As one would expect, some of the questions will be more challenging than others. Each question is centred around one of the following: a clinical photograph, scenario, clinical audiology, imaging, skull anatomy, histology slide, surgical specimen, ENT apparatus or data interpretation. The answers are provided immediately after the questions. The legends for the clinical photographs are given at the beginning of the answers. Essential revision notes follow the answers. Where appropriate, Tables and Figures are included to avoid lengthy text and to enhance visual learning. The OSCE stations are presented in a random order to reflect the DO-HNS examination (an inventory of the cases is in the Appendix, along with the TNM classifications of all head and neck cancers).

1.2 OSCE Stations (Total 62)

Station 1

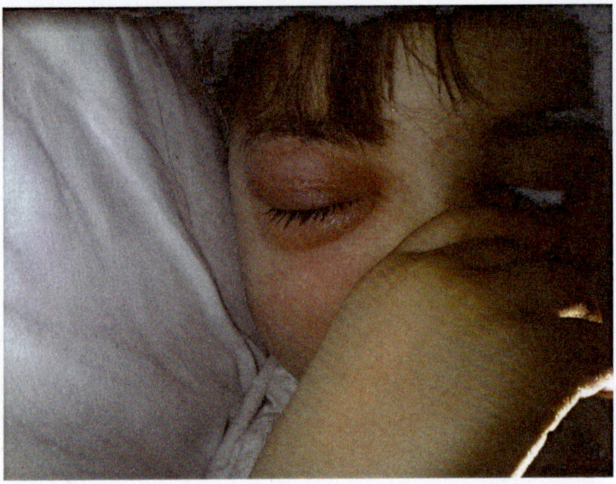

Questions

A. Which organism is commonly involved in the condition shown in the clinical photograph?

B. What should be assessed in the examination of the eyes?

C. What imaging may be required?

D. How is this condition graded?

E. List the treatment options.

F. What are 6 possible complications of surgery for this condition?

Answers (Station 1)

Clinical photograph showing a child with peri-orbital cellulitis.

A. *Streptococcus* spp.

B. EYES: colour vision, visual acuity, eye movements, pupillary reflexes.

C. Contrast CT of brain, nose and paranasal sinuses (especially axial sections through the orbit to check for an abscess).

D. Chandler's Grading System (Table 1.1)

Table 1.1 Chandler's grading system for periorbital cellulitis.

Grade	Description	Details
I	Pre-septal cellulitis	Eyelid swelling without proptosis, opthalmoplegia or loss of vision
II	Orbital cellulitis	Inflammation of orbital fat, connective tissue and skin
III	Sub-periosteal abscess	Pus collection between the ethmoid sinus and periosteal layer of the medial orbital wall (causing lateral displacement of the medial rectus muscle).
IV	Orbital abscess	Pus collection within the orbit
V	Cavernous sinus thrombosis	Clotting of blood within the cavernous sinus (fortunately this is rare as it is associated with a high mortality rate)

E. **Medical**: intravenous broad spectrum antibiotics (eg Co-amoxiclav) if no abscess is present.
Surgical: if an abscess is present (drainage either by an open approach via a modified Lynch Howarth incision or endoscopic drainage by removing the partially dehiscent lamina papyracea).

F. Complications of surgery:

- Immediate - surgical damage to orbital structures leading to bleeding or blindness.

- Early – Diplopia (commonly resolves)
    - Progressive swelling is normal 24 h post-op
    - Residual/recurrent disease
    - Intracranial sepsis or abscess

- Late – residual defect (diplopia, decreased acuity)
    - Scarring
    - Enophthalmos

Revision Notes

- Periorbital cellulitis is a disease of young children with an average of about 3.5 years.
- It is usually a complication of acute rhinosinusitis, whereby the infection spreads most commonly from the ethmoid sinuses into the orbit via lamina papyracea (Figure 1), which may be partially dehiscent.
- The presenting features are classical signs of inflammation: redness, pain and swelling; loss of function , i.e., colour vision and acuity may occur (red colour vision is usually affected first).
- Inflammation anterior to the tarsal plate of the eyelid is referred to as pre-septal cellulitis (Figure 1.2) and requires antibiotic treatment only (ideally intravenous broad-spectrum antibiotic).
- Post-septal periorbital cellulitis may require an urgent CT scan with contrast to rule out a sub-periosteal or intra-orbital abscess (Figures 1.3a and b).
- The presence of an abscess requires urgent surgical intervention to prevent blindness (which is thought to

be due to stretching of the intraorbital optic nerve and ischaemia).

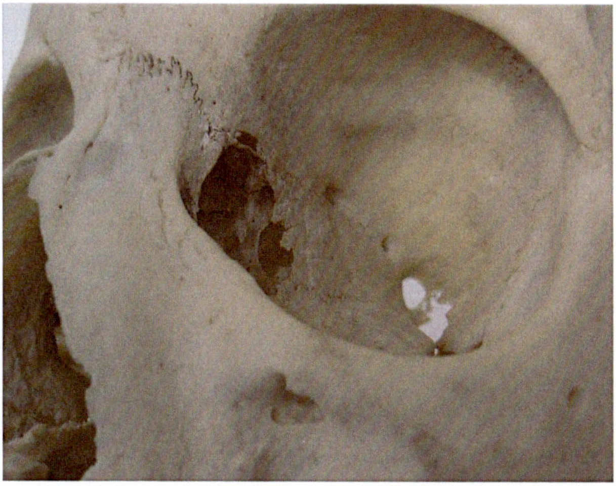

Figure 1.1 Photograph illustrating the thin remnants of the lamina papyracea separating the ethmoid sinus from the orbit (note the foramen for the anterior and posterior ethmoidal arteries and the rule of halves, ie, anterior ethmoidal artery is 24 mm from anterior edge of the lacrimal crest, the posterior ethmoidal artery is 12 mm behind the anterior ethmoidal artery and the optic nerve is 6 mm behind the posterior ethmoidal artery).

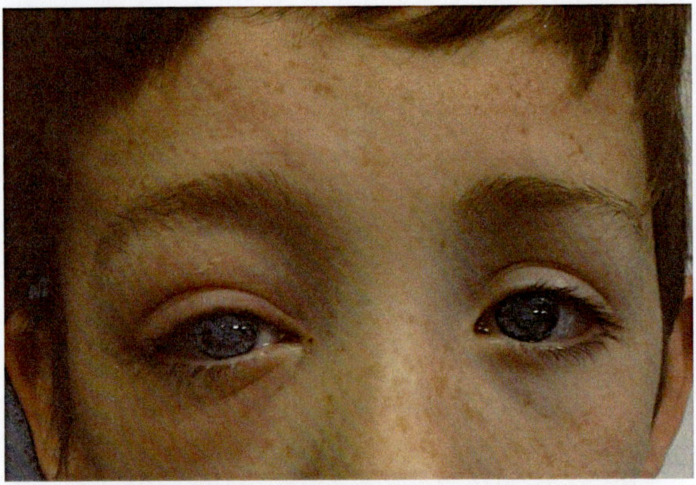

Figure 1.2 Right pre-septal cellulitis.

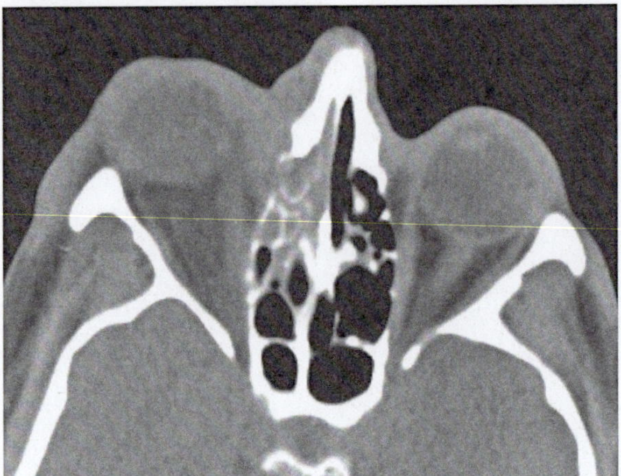

Figure 1.3a Axial CT scan showing right ethmoid sinusitis with proptosis and a small subperiosteal collection.

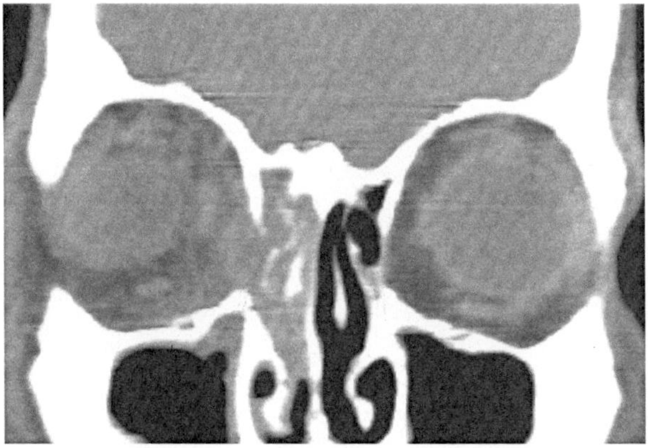

Figure 1.3b Coronal CT scan showing right ethmoid sinusitis with a breach in lamina papyracea and a small abscess.

Station 2

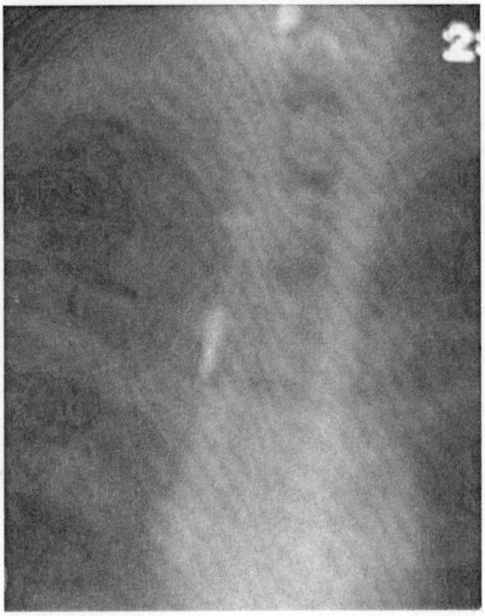

Questions

A. What abnormality is shown in the above chest x-ray?
B. How would you manage this patient on arrival in A&E?
C. List 3 differentials if a child presents with respiratory distress.
D. What investigations would you request?
E. Name 2 instruments which may be helpful in the management of the above case.
F. List 3 potential complications.

Answers (Station 2)

Chest X-ray showing an inhaled foreign body.

A. A foreign body within the respiratory tract at the level of the right main bronchus.
B. In accordance with the APLS protocol. If there is no evidence of hyperinflation of the lungs as a result of ball-valving by the foreign body, the patient should receive high-flow oxygen, as well as nebulised adrenaline and heliox. In addition, anaesthetic, paediatric and senior

ENT support should be sought.

C. Congenital (laryngomalacia in the infant)
Traumatic (vocal cord palsy, subglottic stenosis)
Infective [severe adenotonsillitis, acute epiglottitis, laryngotracheobronchitis (croup)]

D. AP and lateral radiographs of the chest and neck.

E. Rigid ventilating bronchoscope and optical forceps

F. Failure of removal
Bleeding (managed with topical adrenaline)
Tracheobronchial perforation
Dental injury
Hoarse voice due to trauma to vocal folds

Revision Notes

- Common foreign bodies in the aerodigestive tract are coins (Figure 2.2), toys and food.
- Incidence of foreign body inhalation is highest between the ages of 1 and 3 and has a male preponderance.
- Inhaled foreign bodies are a particular risk to young children whose airways are much narrower, particularly at the subglottis and even slight oedema, caused by the foreign body may lead to fatal airway compromise.
- Patients typically present with a history of choking and coughing. Less commonly, they may initially be asymptomatic following inhalation and present later with persistent cough or recurrent pneumonia.
- Foreign bodies enter the right main bronchus preferentially because it is less angled than the left.
- The investigation of choice includes lateral soft tissue neck radiograph and AP and lateral chest radiographs. AP chest radiographs may reveal 'obstructive emphysema', which results from a 'ball-valve' effect caused by the bronchi dilating slightly during inspiration and subsequently being constricted by increased intrathoracic pressure during expiration. This leads to

progressive air-trapping (hyperinflated lung) and mediastinal shift

- The main concern in the management of these patients is the patient's airway and they should be managed in conjunction with paediatric and anaesthetic teams. An experienced ENT surgeon should perform removal as soon as possible as a delay may lead to increased oedema, especially with organic foreign bodies.

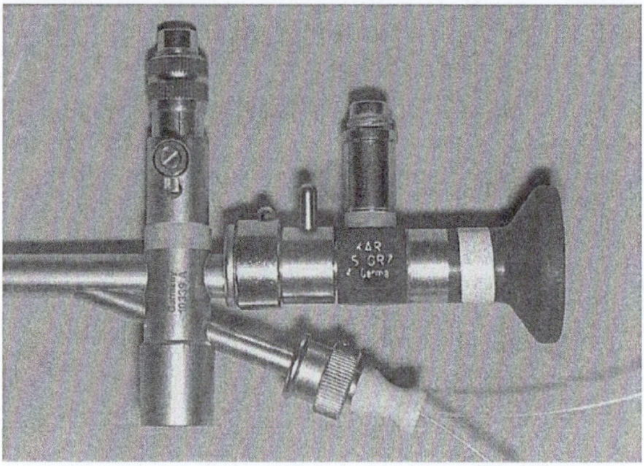

Figure 2.1a The top end of a rigid bronchoscope.

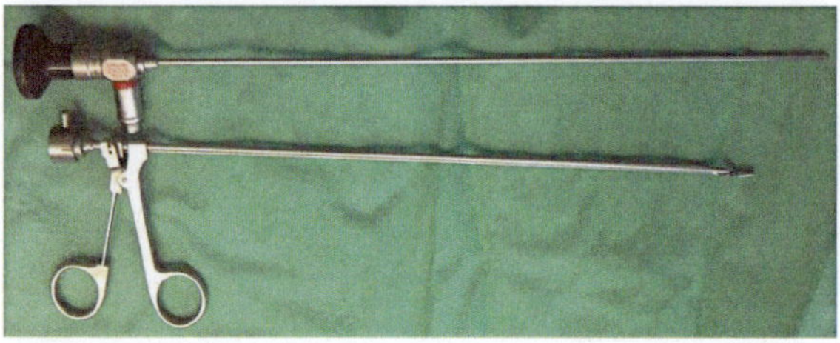

Figure 2.1b Optical forceps and rigid endoscopy un-united.

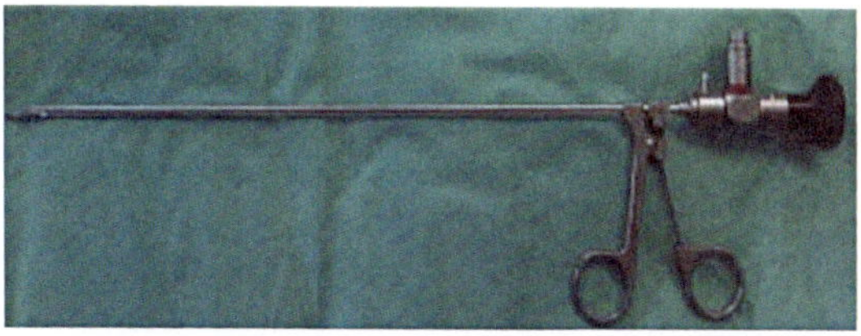

Figure 2.1c Optical forceps and rigid endoscopy united.

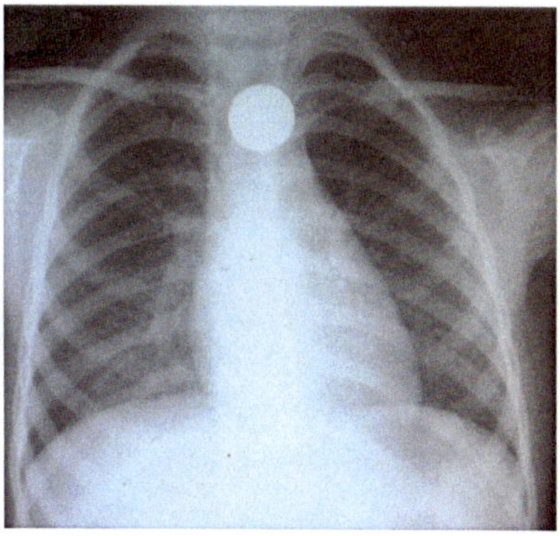

Figure 2.2 A coin stuck in the aerodigestive tract at the level of cricopharyngeus – a common presentation in children.

Station 3

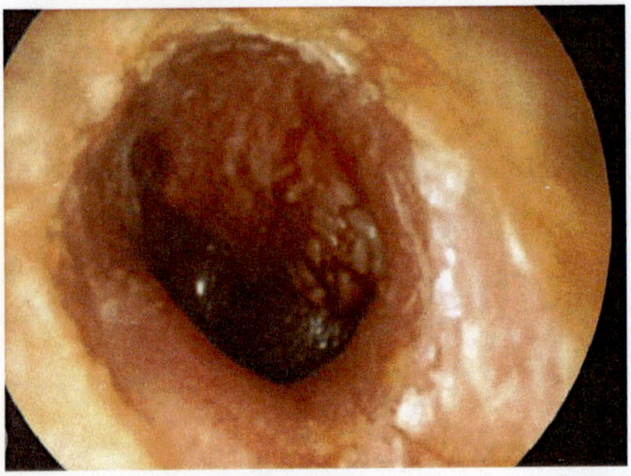

Questions

A. This is the tympanic membrane of a 2 year old boy who is unwell with fever, loss of appetite and irritability. What is the diagnosis?

B. List 3 symptoms associated with this condition.

C. Name 3 bacteria associated with this condition.

D. List 9 complications of this condition.

E. Briefly outline a treatment plan.

Answers (Station 3)

Clinical photograph showing a bulging inflamed tympanic membrane.

A. Acute otitis media.

B. Fever, otalgia, irritability, reduced feeding.

C. *Streptococcus pneumonia*
Haemophilus influenza
Moraxella catarrhalis
Streptococcus pyogenes
Staphylococcus aureus

D. **Intratemporal**: hearing loss, vertigo, facial nerve palsy, TM perforation, otitis externa, mastoiditis
Intracranial: brain abscess, sigmoid sinus thrombosis, meningism, subdural empyema, otic hydrocephalus.

Extracranial: Bezold, Citelli and Luc abscesses.

E. **Conservative**: All patients should rest in a warm, well-humidified room. Many will get better with analgesia and antipyretics.
Medical: If there is little or no improvement after 24-48 hours, consider intravenous broad-spectrum antibiotics. For recurrent AOM, some surgeons advocate low dose antibiotics, such as trimetroprim, for 3 months.
Surgical: grommet insertion after about 6 recurrent episodes.

Revision Notes

- Acute otitis media (AOM) may be defined as inflammation of the middle ear cleft associated with purulent discharge. In contrast, otitis media with effucsion (OME or glue ear) is associated with non-purulent discharge behind an intact tympanic membrane and is a silent condition.
- AOM is one of the most common infectious diseases of childhood, with its peak incidence at the age of 2 years. OME has a bimodal distribution at 2 and 5 years.
- In AOM, there is usually a history of coryzal symptoms with spread of the infection via the eustachian tube to the middle ear within 3-4 days.
- Symptoms may include otalgia, hearing loss, otorrhoea, fever, systemic upset, excessive crying, irritability, poor feeding and ear pulling.
- Classically the otalgia is relieved by rupture of the tympanic membrane with mucopurulent ear discharge.
- The tympanic membrane may be retracted or bulging and erytematous (Figure 3.1a).
- Within the acute setting surgery has a limited role. Myringotomy, with or without grommet insertion, is generally reserved for severe cases in the presence of or suspected complications or to relieve pain.

- Long-term sequelae of AOM include non-suppurative middle ear effusion, high frequency sensorineural hearing loss, tympanic membrane perforation (Figure 3.1b), adhesions, tympanosclerosis and erosion of the ossicular chain.

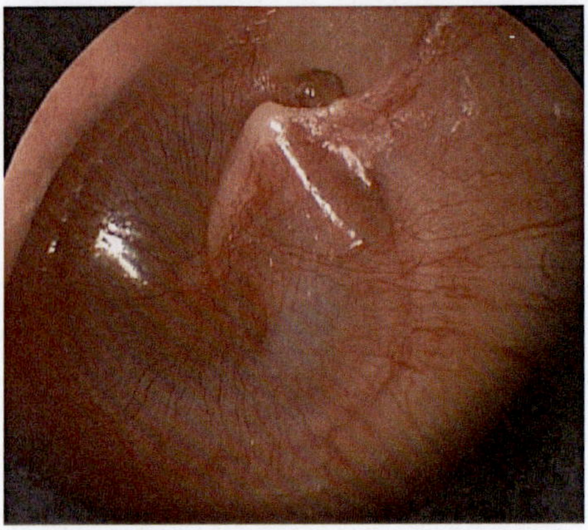

Figure 3.1a Resolving AOM in the left ear without perforation.

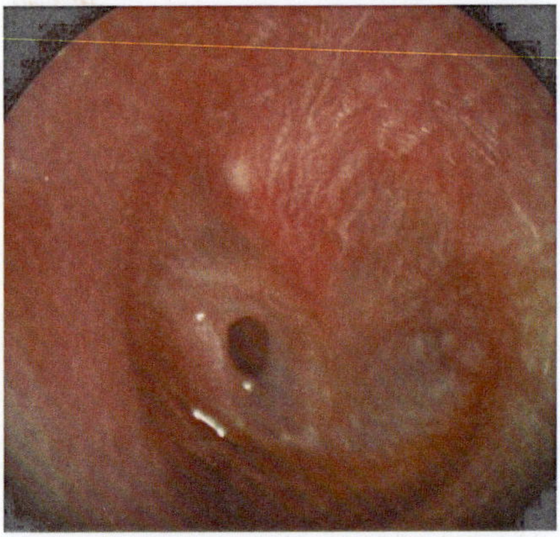

Figure 3.1b Resolving AOM associated with a perforation in the left ear.

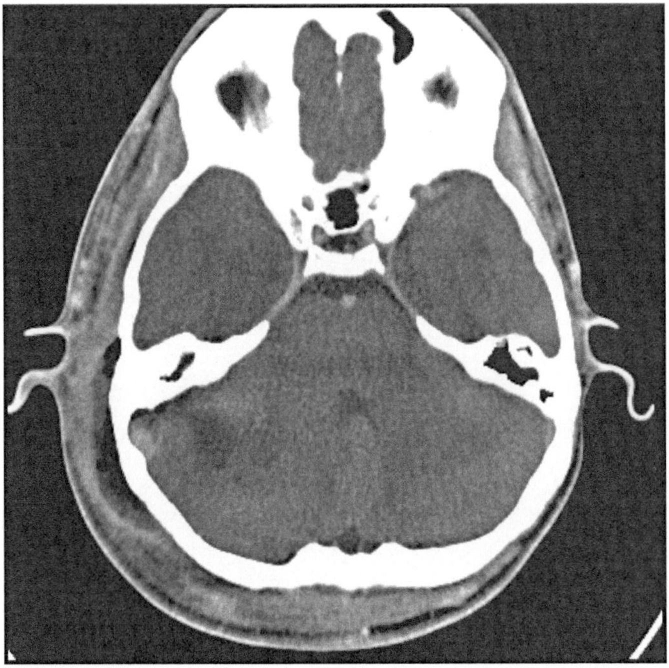

Figure 3.2 Axial CT scan (soft tissue window) showing a right subperiosteal abscess as well as an intracerebral abscess, both secondary to AOM.

Station 4

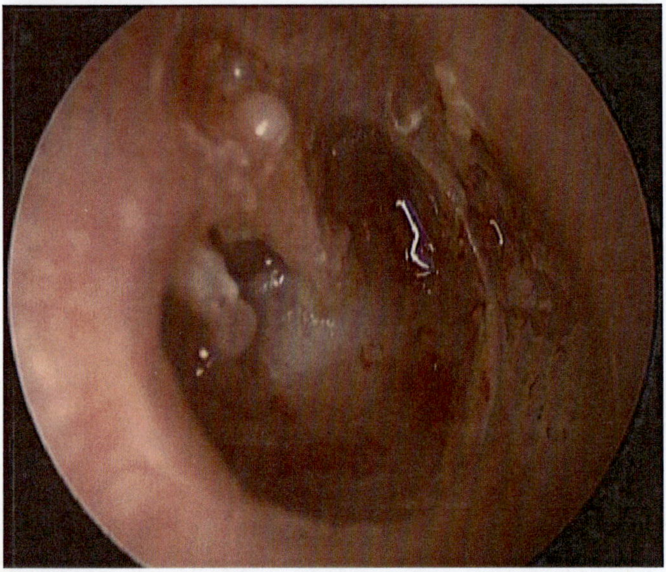

Questions

A. Is this a left or a right ear?

B. What abnormalities are present?

C. How are the abnormalities classified?

D. What type of hearing loss and how much would be present (give range)?

E. What are the treatment options?

Answers (Station 4)

Clinical photograph showing an otoscopic view of chronic otitis media.

A. Right ear (because the ***lateral*** process of the malleus is pointing to the right).

B. Severe retraction of the *pars tensa* and *pars flaccida.*

C. Sade's classification for *pars tensa* and Tos's classification for *pars flaccida.*

D. Conductive hearing loss (20-60dB).

E. Treatment options:

1. Conservative
   - Watch and wait
   - Hearing aid

2. Surgical (not evidence-based)
   - Ventilation tube such as a grommet or extra-annular t-tube
   - Resection of retracted tympanic membrane and reconstruction of neo-TM

Note that it is vitally important to know the status of the other ear when presented with pathology in one ear.

Revision Notes

- Chronic otitis media (COM) is a chronic inflammation of the middle ear and mastoid lasting more than 12 weeks.
- It is often a complication of acute otitis media (AOM), negative middle ear pressure or otitis media with effusion (OME).
- Three separate entities exist; active, inactive and healed. Active squamous COM is essentially a cholesteatoma, whilst inactive squamous COM is a retraction pocket (with potential to become active). Healed COM has a permanent tympanic membrane abnormality but the ear does not have the propensity to become active.
- Most patients would present with hearing loss of varying severity and recurrent ear discharge. Otalgia and vertigo are uncommon complaints.
- Retraction of the tympanic membrane could be classified into the Sade and Tos classifications:

Table 4.1 Classification proposed by Sade for *pars tensa* retraction pockets.

Grade	Description	Appearance
1	Retracted ear	Slight retraction of tympanic membrane
II	Severe retraction	Retracted tympanic membrand touching the incus or stapes
III	Atelectasis	Tympanic membrane touching the promontory
IV	Adhesive otitis	Tympanic membrane adherent to the promontory

Table 4.2 Classification proposed by Tos for *pars flaccida* (4 'Ds').

Grade	Description
I	Mild retraction, with air still present between the pocket and malleus neck (**D**imple)
II	Retraction pocket touches malleus neck +/- erosion of neck (**D**raping malleus neck)
III	Retraction pocket expands causing erosion of outer attic wall (**D**estruction of scutum)
IV	Depth of retraction pocket difficult to see (**D**eep)

- Pure tone audiogram and CT scan of temporal bone are useful to assess the degree of hearing loss and also ossicular continuity.

Section 5

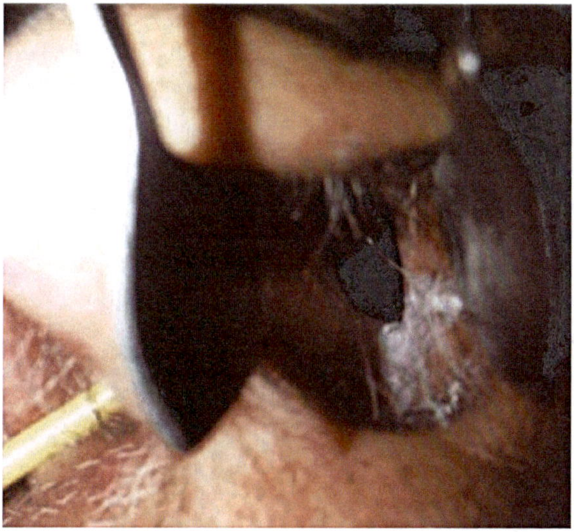

Questions

A. What is the diagnosis?
B. List 10 possible causes.
C. List 4 associated symptoms.
D. List 4 blood relevant blood tests.
E. What are the treatment options?

Answers (Station 5)

Clinical photograph showing an anterior septal perforation.

A. Septal perforation
B. **Trauma:** Nose picking nasal surgery or cautery
Infective: TB, syphilis, leprosy, septal abscess
Inflammatory: Wegeners, sarcoidosis
Neoplastic: Squamous cell carcinoma
Chemical irritants: Cocaine as a recreational drug
C. Bleeding, crusting, whistling, saddle nose deformity.
D. FBC, ESR, c-ANCA, p-ANCA, ACE
E. **Conservative** if asymptomatic.
Medical: Crusting may be managed with regular nasal

douching and nasal cream. Nose bleeds may be difficult to manage as cautery leads to excessive dead tissue crusting and osteitis. Sometimes it is better to remove the edge of bone so that the mucosa can seal over it. This would obviously make the perforation bigger but it will stop the bleeding.

Surgical: If whistling is the main issue with a small perforation one can solve the problem by making the hole bigger. Perforation could be closed with a septal button or a flap (septal or sublabial).

Revision Notes

- Most septal perforations involve the anterior quadrilateral cartilaginous septum (Figure 5.1a) apart from syphilis, which affects the bony septum (Figure 5.1b).
- Although trauma is the commonest cause of septal perforation, there are various other causes to consider prior to making the diagnosis as summarised in the table below (Table 1).
- Patients with septal perforation may complain of whistling, epistaxis, crusting and nasal obstruction although most patients are asymptomatic.
- Large crusts around perforations lead to symptoms of perceived blockage as nasal airflow is usually very good.
- Small perforations may cause a whistling noise or nasal breathing.
- Very large perforations produce rhinolalia (secondary nasal speech) and inability to clear secretions.
- Considering the aetiology shown in Table 5.1, investigations may include FBC, ESR, VDRL, cANCA, PR3, pANCA, MPO, ACE titres, U&Es, CXR, urine analysis and possibly a biopsy of the nasal septum.
- Conservative management is preferred if the patient is asymptomatic. Crusting and epistaxis could be medically

treated with nasal cautery, regular nasal douching and nasal cream. If needed, the perforation could be closed with a septal button or surgically with a graft or flap.

- Silver nitrate cautery should be avoided if possible as it leads to osteitis of the exposed bony septum.
- Small to medium holes can be closed surgically and the variety of repairs can be classified as:
    - Free grafts (simple or composite autografts, allografts, e.g. split skin graft or pinna)
    - Pedicled flaps (local nasal mucosa, buccal mucosa, composite septal cartilage and mucosa, composite skin cartilage)
    - Rotation/advancement of mucoperichondrial/mucoperiosteal flaps

Table 5.1 Aetiology of perforation of the nasal septum.

Trauma	Iatrogenic (septoplasty, bilateral cautery) Self-inflicted (nose picking, foreign body such as button batteries)
Infection	Septal abscess (especially following septal haematoma), Syphilis, TB, Aspergillosis
Inflammatory	Wegener's granulomatosis, Sarcoidosis, Relapsing polychondritis Systemic lupus erythematosus, Rheumatoid arthritis
Neoplastic	Squamous Cell Carcinoma, Adenocarcinoma, Melanoma
Surface irritants	Drugs and medications (cocaine inhalations, heroin inhalation, decongestant nasal sprays) Occupational (chrome, arsenic, alkaline dusts)
Idiopathic	Cause unknown

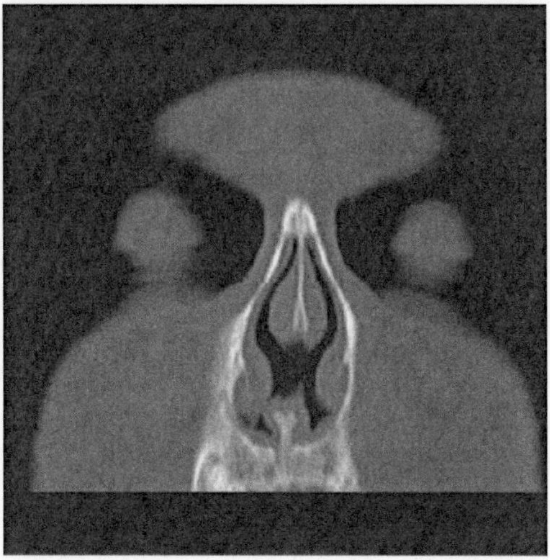

Figure 5.1a Axial CT scan showing septal perforation.

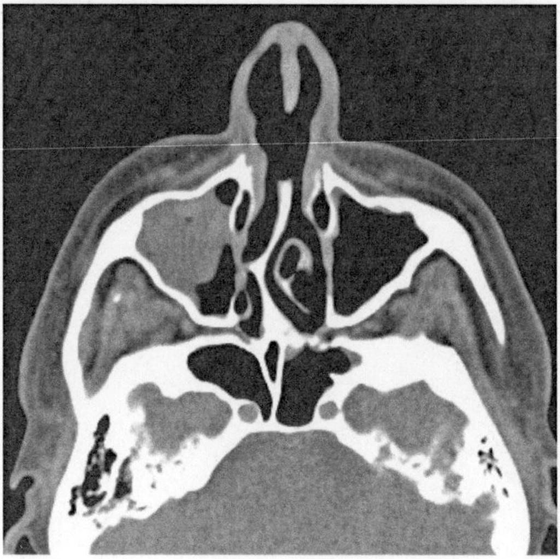

Figure 5.1b Axial CT scan showing septal perforation.

Station 6

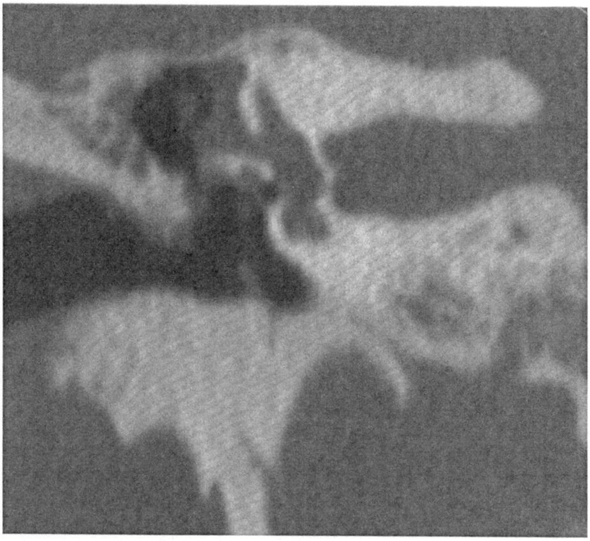

A CT image of the right temporal bone showing a fistula in lateral semicircular canal caused by a cholesteama.

Questions

A. What is the plane of the CT scan?

B. During the operation to remove the right sided cholesteatoma, clear fluid gushed from the fistula site. A graft over the fistula site failed to control the leak and the lateral canal was packed off with bone wax. The patient woke up feeling very dizzy. A Weber tuning fork test was referred to the left ear. What type and direction of nystagmus would you expect to find?

C. When performing a Caloric test on a normal person, what direction would we expect the nystagmus to be when warm water (44 degrees) is applied to the left ear?

D. What is meant by 3rd degree nystagmus?

Answers (STATION 6)

A. Coronal plane (note the 'rabbit ears'sign).

B. Horizontal nystagmus to the left.

Explanation: Paralysis or destruction of right lateral SCC (eg after right lateral semicircular fistula leak or iatrogenic right dead ear would result in *a relatively higher afferent activity from left lateral SCC* (see Figure 6).

C. Horizontal to the left.

Explanation: Warm caloric testing of LEFT lateral SCC (Warm Same, Cold Opposite cf: CO**WS**). This is due to induced convectional currents in the endolymph resulting in *relatively higher afferent activity from LEFT lateral SCC* (see Figure 6).

D. Most severe form of nystagmus, ie, nystagmus on gazing in all 3 directions (left, right and straight ahead).

Revision Notes

- Nystagmus is a sign not a disease
- Nystagmus may indicate a disorder or no disorder (physiological nystagmus)
- Horizontal nystagmus may be present with disorders afffecting the lateral SCCs
- 5 key physiological points worth noting:
- (1) The left and right horizontal (lateral) semicircular canals are orientated so that any movement in one canal always induces an antagonistic response in the other canal (similar to the wings of a plane – see Figure 6).

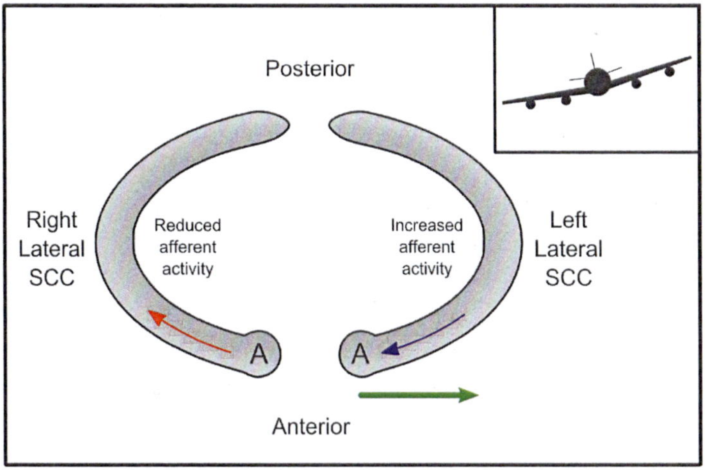

Figure 6 Schematic diagram of clockwise horizontal rotation showing the lateral semicircular canals (SCCs) with ampulla (A), ampullopetal endolymphatic flow on the left (blue arrow), ampullofugal endolymphatic flow on the right (red arrow) and direction of associated horizontal nystagmus (green arrow).

- (2) With the exception of pendular (see-saw) nystagmus, commonly seen in congenitally blind people, horizontal nystagmus has 2 phases: a slow phase due to slow eye movement (or smooth pursuit) and a fast corrective phase due to fast eye movement (or saccadic movement).
- (3) The slow or drift phase is always in the same direction as that canal which is inhibited (and which therefore sends a reduced afferent response to the brain), whilst the fast phase is in the same direction as that canal which is stimulated (and which therefore sends an increased afferent response to the brain).
- (4) Ampullopetal (towards ampulla) endolymph flow is stimulatory (i.e. ↑afferent activity) whilst ampullofugal (away from ampulla) endolymph flow is inhibitory (i.e. ↓ afferent activity).

- (5) The direction of nystagmus is traditionally given as the direction of the fast phase, and this is always in the direction of the higher afferent activity or opposite to the direction of endolymph flow.
- The severity of horizontal nystagmus is described in terms of 1st, 2nd and 3rd degrees (Table 6.1).
- First degree is the presence of nystagmus only on gaze in the direction of the fast phase (ie 1 direction only) whilst second degree is the presence of nystagmus on looking straight ahead and in the direction of the fast phase (ie 2 directions).

Table 6.1 Severity of nystagmus (**+** nystagmus present, – nystagmus abscent)

	Gaze in the direction of		
	Fast phase	**Straight ahead**	**Slow phase**
1st degree	+	-	-
2nd degree	+	+	-
3rd degree	+	+	+

Alexander's law: The amplitude of nystagmus increases as gaze increases in the direction of the fast phase and decreases with gaze in the direction of the slow phase.

Top tips for clinical practice

- Irritative (stimulatory) nystagmus is always towards the affected side.
- Paralytic (destructive or inhibitory) nystagmus is always opposite to the affected

Station 7

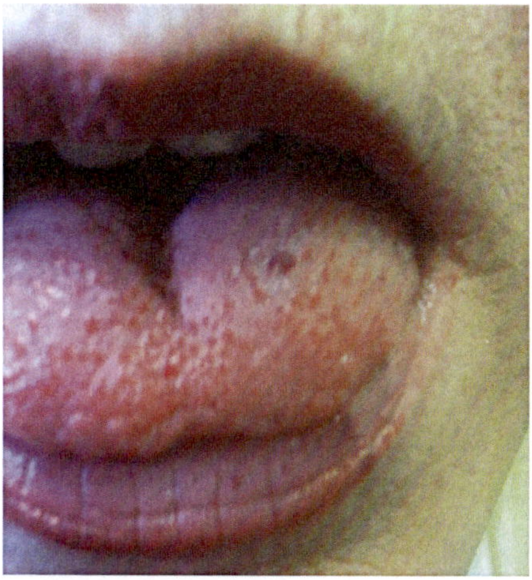

Questions

A. What is the name of the lesions seen on the tongue and lips of this patient?

B. What is the most likely diagnosis?

C. What is the inheritance pattern?

D. List 2 possible presenting features

E. List 2 associated abnormalities

F. What are the medical and surgical treatment options when this condition affects the nose?

Answers (Station7)

Clinical photograph showing hereditary haemorrhagic telangiectasias (HHTs)

A. Multiple small punctate telangiectases

B. Hereditary Haemorrhagic Telengiectasia (HHT) or Rendu-Osler-Weber disease

C. Autosomal dominant

D. Epistaxis
Gastro-intestinal bleeding *(also haemoptysis, CNS complications, cardiac and hepatic failure)*

E. Arteriovenous malformations, aneurysms

F. Conservative (monitoring, follow-up and surveillance)
Medical (oestrogens or progesterone)
Surgical (laser, septodermoplasty, modified Young's procedure,)

Revision Notes

- Hereditary haemorrhagic telangiectasia (HHT) is an autosomal dominant condition characterised by multiple vascular lesions, leaving the patient prone to haemorrhage. Telangiectases are tiny punctate, erythematous lesions which blanche on pressure and are usually clearly evident by the age of 40. They may affect any mucosal or cutaneous surface commonly affecting the nose and the upper GI tract.
- Mutations in three genes have been associated with the disease, namely *endoglin* (ENG), *activin-like receptor kinase* (ALK-1) and SMAD4. The mutated genes have a deleterious effect on the TGF-β signalling pathway, which is vital for normal angiogenesis.
- According to the location these patients may present with recurrent epistaxis, PR bleeding and iron deficiency anaemia due to chronic blood loss. Patients with HHT are also associated with arterioveneous malformations (AVM) in the lungs, liver, brain and spine.
- Investigations for HHT include FBC, CXR, echocardiography and an MRI brain to exclude AVMs. Genetic screenings in these patients are also extremely important.

Medical treatment

- Acute bleeds may be initially managed with adrenaline-soaked sponges and epistaxis balloons (cautery and conventional packing may exacerbate bleeding).

- Systemic oestrogen therapy (e.g. HRT or the oral contraceptive pill) has been shown to reduce bleeding and may be of particular use in female patients. Topical preparations are also available. Antifibrinolytic agents (e.g. tranexamic acid) may be considered and there is some evidence that anti-angiogenic agents such as bevacizumab and thalidomide may be beneficial in HHT.

Surgical treatment

- Laser photocoagulation of the nasal mucosa with telangectasia (Figure 7.1) using NdYAG, KTP532 or argon lasers is a useful initial therapy.
- Arterial ligation and embolisation have limited roles.
- Young's procedure (surgical closure of the nares, Figure 7.2).
- Septodermoplasty involves replacement of more heavily affected areas of nasal mocosa with a split skin graft. However, the technique is associated with crusting and recurrence.

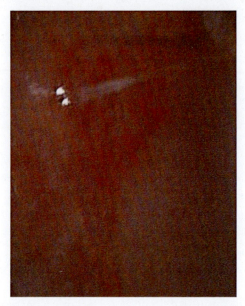

Figure 7.1 Nasal septal mucosa with multiple telangiectasias in a patient with HHT.

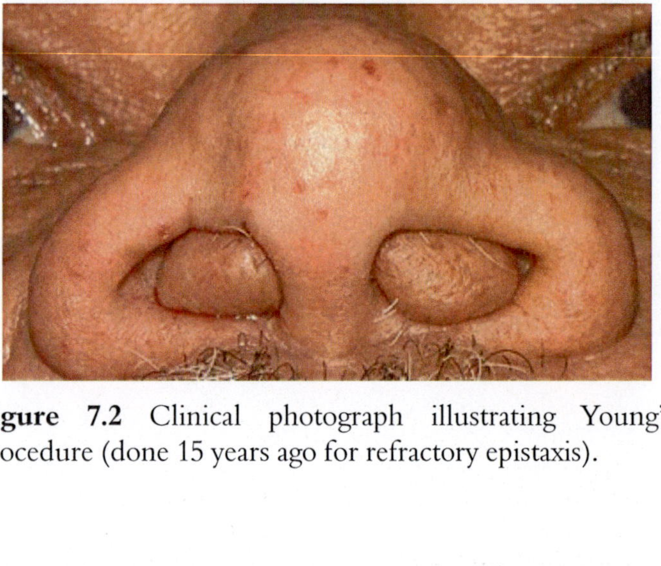

Figure 7.2 Clinical photograph illustrating Young's procedure (done 15 years ago for refractory epistaxis).

Station 8

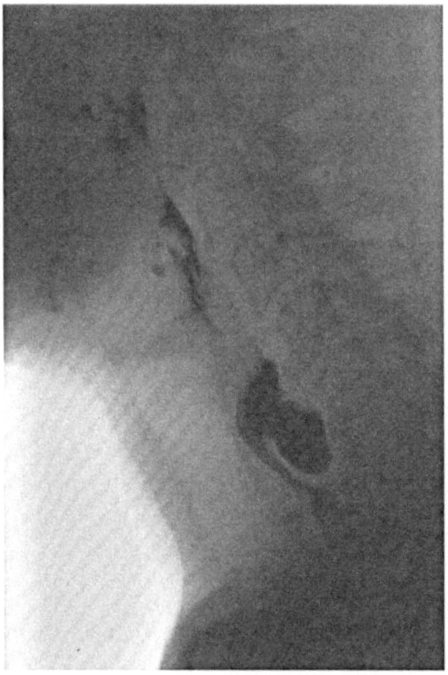

Questions

A. What test is the name of this investigation?
B. What is the diagnosis?
C. List 5 symptoms of this condition.
D. What are the treatment options?
E. List 5 complications of surgical treatment

Answers (Station 8)

Barium swallow showing a pharyngeal pouch (negative image).

A. Barium swallow
B. Pharyngeal pouch
C. Dysphagia
Regurgitation
Weight loss
Chest infections
Halitosis
D. Conservative (if pouch is small and asymptomatic)
Medical (botox injection to cricopharyngeus)
Surgical (endoscopic or open)

E. Oesophageal perforation
Hoarseness
Bleeding
Infection
Recurrence
Injury to teeth

Revision Notes

- A pharyngeal pouch refers to the herniation of pharyngeal mucosa through a weak area in the posterior pharyngeal wall that is known as Killian's dehiscence. This defective area lies between the two parts of the inferior constrictor muscle, between the thyropharyngeal and the cricopharyngeal fibres.
- A pharyngeal pouch is more common in Caucasian men and the most common age of presentation is between the sixth and ninth decades.
- These patients usually complain of regurgitation of undigested food, halitosis, dysphagia, recurrent aspiration pneumonia and weight loss due to dysphagia.
- The main differential diagnosis to exclude in these patients would be head and neck malignancy.
- If the pouch is large, the patient may have a neck mass which gurgles on palpation (Boyce's sign).
- The investigation of choice would be a barium swallow.
- The definitive treatment of pharyngeal pouch is surgical excision either endoscopically (by division of the bar separating the pouch) or an open excision (with cricopharyngeal myotomy). Table 8.1 summarises the complications associated with pharyngeal pouch surgery.

Table 8.1 Post-operative complications of pharyngeal pouch surgery.

Immediate	Early	Late
Primary haemorrhage	Secondary haemorrhage (infection)	Stricture (due to overzealous excision of mucosa when dividing sac)
Perforation and conversion to external surgery	Wound infection	Persistent hoarseness if recurrent laryngeal nerve is damaged directly or indirectly
Surgical emphysema	Hoarseness (due to direct or indirect recurrent laryngeal nerve injury)	Recurrence
Pneumothorax	Fistula (usually secondary to infection)	
	Mediastinitis (perforation with leak tracking inferiorly)	

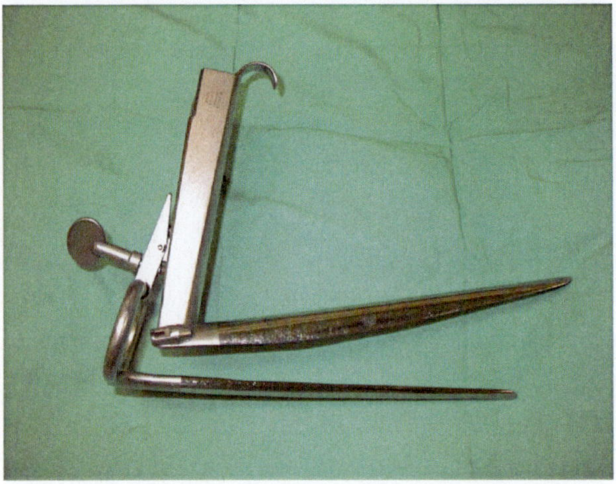

Figure 8.1a Weerda diverticuloscope used in endoscopic stapling of pharyngeal pouch.

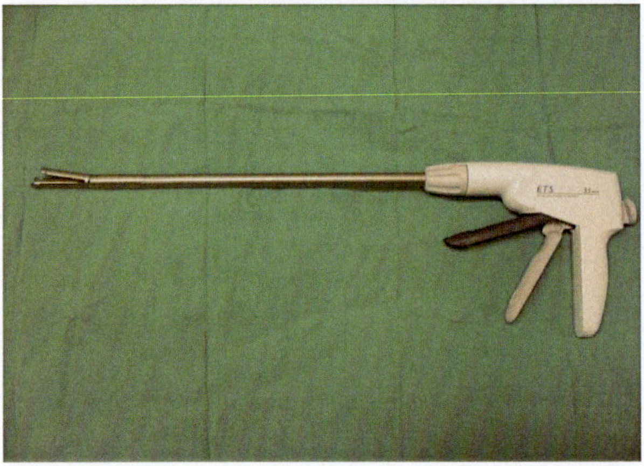

Figure 8.1b Endoscopic stapling gun for pharyngeal pouch.

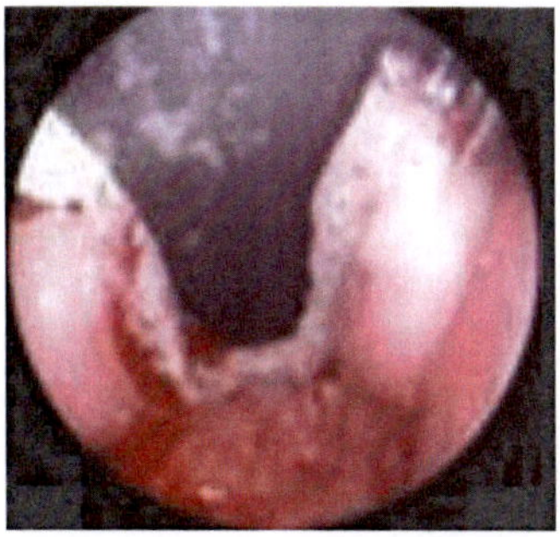

Figure 8.1c Endoscopically stapled pharyngeal pouch.

Station 9

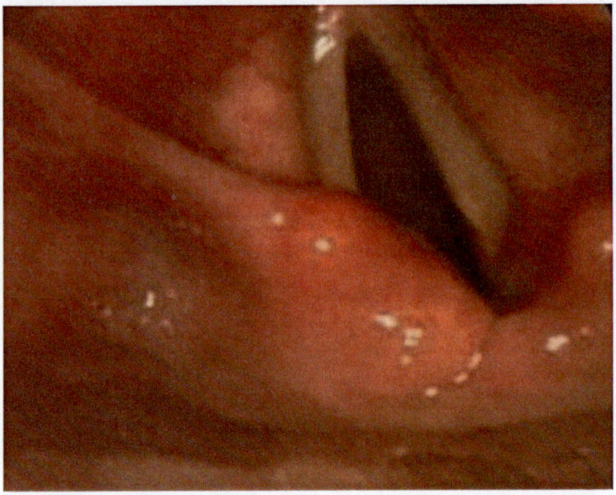

Questions

A. What is the diagnosis?

B. List 4 common causes?

C. List 4 symptoms this patient is most likely to complain of?

D. What is the principle of surgical treatment of this condition?

E. What is the length of time you would wait before surgery?

Answers (Station 9)

Clinical photograph showing a left vocal cord palsy.

A. Left vocal cord palsy (notice slight bowing of left vocal fold).

B. Iatrogenic – post thyroid surgery, post carotid endarterectomy, mediastinal surgery
Malignancy such as lung cancer, thyroid carcinoma
Traumatic
Viral infection
Idiopatic.

C. Hoarse voice

Inadequate voice projection
Breathy quality to voice
Difficulty swallowing.

D. The main aim is to medialise the affected vocal cord to allow approximation of the vocal cords.

E. Wait 6 months, as occasionally the contralateral cord could compensate for the palsy, and also to allow any viral cause to resolve.

Revision Notes

- During the examination there may be a video on a laptop of a patient's vocal cords with unilateral vocal cord palsy. These patients would present with a hoarse, weak and breathy quality to voice and coughing/choking on swallowing.
- It is important to know the course of the Vagus nerve (CN X). From the skull base, it gives rise to a branch that loops around the arch of aorta on the left and the subclavian artery on the right, which subsequently form the recurrent laryngeal nerves. Generally, these run in the tracheoesophageal grooves before finally inserting into the larynx to innervate the intrinsic muscles of the larynx, except cricothyroid muscle.
- Any lesions or operations along the course of the nerve may cause vocal cord palsy.
- Investigations would involve a CT scan from skull base to the mediastinum.
- A surgical sieve is a useful tool as there are other causes of vocal cord palsy such as inflammatory conditions (rheumatoid arthritis, Crohn's), granulomatous diseases (Sarcoidosis, Wegener's granulomatosis) and trauma.
- Management of this condition initially involves voice rehabilitation. However, if the patient has not improved after 6 months, surgical intervention is indicated.
- The principle of surgery is to medialise the affected vocal

cord to aid phonation. This could be achieved by injection of bulking agents to medialise the vocal cord.

- The vocal cord consists of both the vocal fold and the vocal process. The layers of the vocal fold are shown in Figure 9.1.
- Most pathologies occur in the cover which consists of the epithelial layer and superficial lamina propria (Figure 9.2). The ligament of the vocal fold is formed by the intermediate and deep lamina propria and forms the limit for laser resection of T1 SCC lesion.

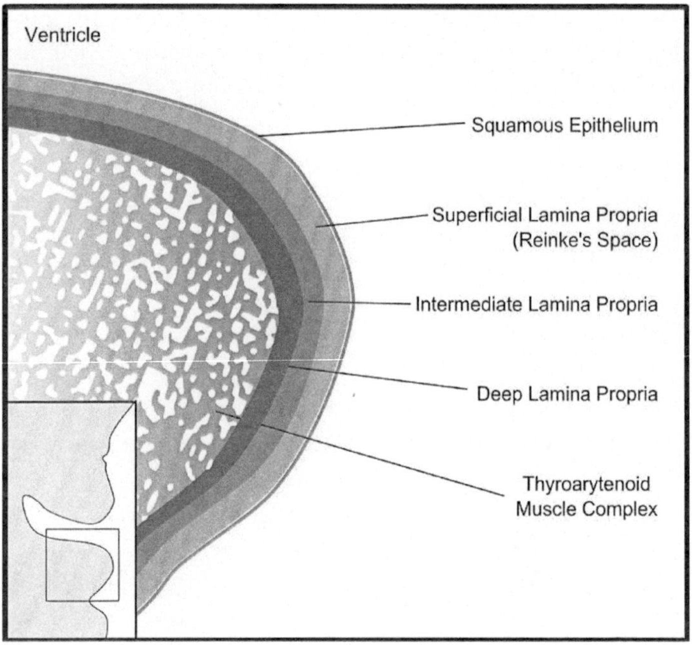

Figure 9.1 The layers of the vocal fold.

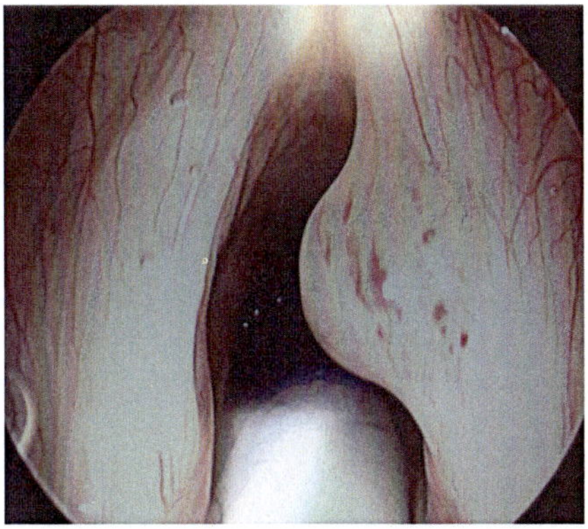

Figure 9.2 A cyst within the vocal fold cover (where most pathologies occur).

Station 10

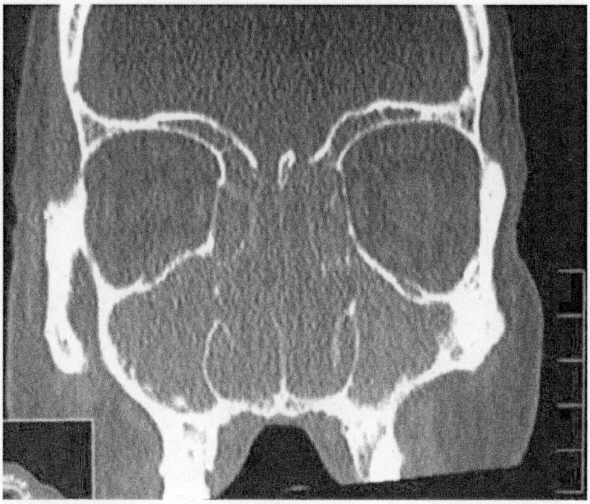

Questions

A. What is this CT scan view?
B. What is this investigation?
C. Describe the abnormality shown.
D. What artery causes increased intra-ocular pressure if damaged?
E. What are the complications of surgical treatment of this condition?

Answers (Station 10)

Coronal CT scan of the nose and paranasal sinuses showing pan-sinusitis.

A. Coronal view
B. Computerised tomography (CT) scan of the nose and paranasal sinuses
C. There is opacification of the maxillary sinuses and nasal airway bilaterally
D. Anterior ethmoidal artery
E. **Local complications**: bleeding, infection, hyposmia, anosmia, adhesions, facial pain, periorbital ecchymosis or emphysema, nasolacrimal duct injury, recurrence

Ocular complications: diplopia (due to injury to medial rectus muscle), blindness (injury to optic nerve and orbital heamatoma),
Intra-cranial complications: cerebrospinal fluid leak, pneumocephalus, meningitis, brain abscess, headache, intracranial bleed, stroke and carotid injury.

Revision Notes

- The aim of this question is to test the candidate's ability to differentiate between the different radiological views eg: axial, saggital and coronal and also the anatomy of the paranasal sinuses.
- Rhinosinusitis could be divided into acute and chronic. The acute form is usually secondary to an infective and inflammatory cause for example after an upper respiratory tract infection. The microorganisms involved include rhinovirus, parainfluenza virus, pneumococcus and haemophilus influenzae.
- The aetiology of chronic rhinosinusitis is, however, not as clear. It is believed to be multifactorial with bacterial biofilms playing a role in its refractory characteristics to medical therapy. Fungi may also play a role; the diagnostic criteria for allergic fungal rhinosinusitis is shown in Table 10.1.
- The European position paper on rhinosinusitis and nasal polyps defines rhinosinusitis as inflammation of the nose and the paranasal sinuses characterised by two or more symptoms, one of which should be either:
  - o Nasal blockage/obstruction/congestion, or
  - o Nasal discharge (anterior/posterior nasal drip)
    ± Facial pain/pressure
    ± Reduction or loss of smell
  - o **And either endoscopic signs of:**
  - o Polyps and/or mucopurulent discharge primarily from middle meatus (see Figure 10.1)
  - o And/or oedema/mucosal obstruction primarily in

middle meatus
  - And/or CT changes: mucosal changes within the osteomeatal complex and/or sinuses
  - **Duration**:
  - Acute: <12 weeks complete resolution of symptoms
  - Chronic: >12 weeks symptoms without complete resolution of symptoms may also be subject to exacerbations
- An interesting 'tell-tale' sign of chronic rhinosinusitis, especially in children, is the transverse nasal line caused by repeated upward wiping of the nose (Figure 10.2).
- Initial treatment includes decongestants, topical nasal steroids, systemic steroids and broad-spectrum antibiotics.
- If medical treatment fails, surgical treatment is indicated, such as Functional Endoscopic Sinus Surgery (FESS).

Table 10.1 Diagnostic criteria for allergic fungal rhinosinusitis.

Features	Findings
Clinical	Nasal polyps
Radiological	Heterogenous areas of hyperdense material
Histological	Positive fungal staining on surgical specimen and eosinophilic mucus without fungal invasion of the tissue
Immunological	Type 1 hypersensitivity reaction to fungi

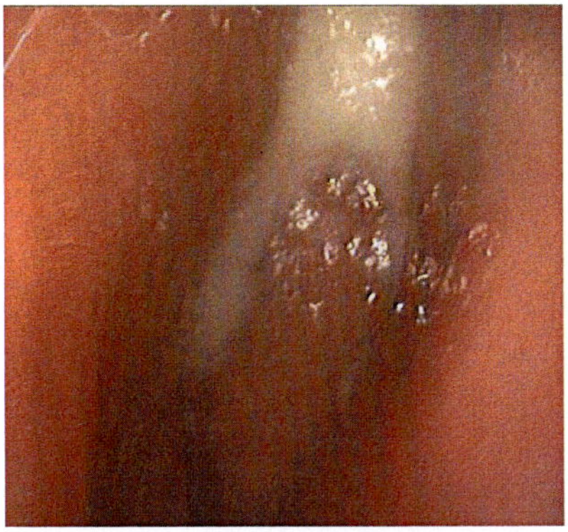

Figure 10.1 Chronic rhinosinusitis associated with mucopus around the middle turbinate.

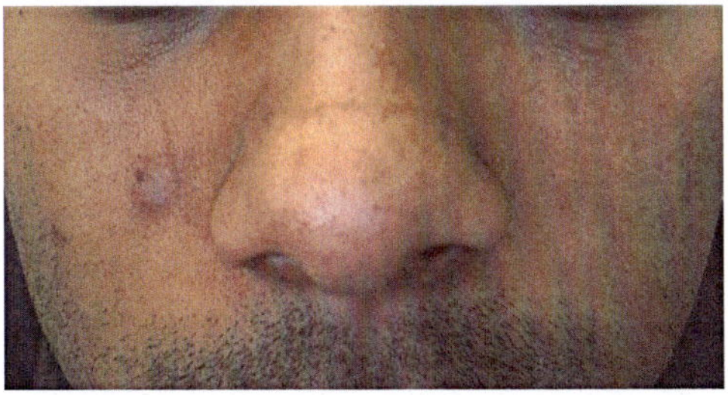

Figure 10.2 Transverse nasal line of chronic rhinosinusitis (caused by repeated wiping upwards).

Station 11

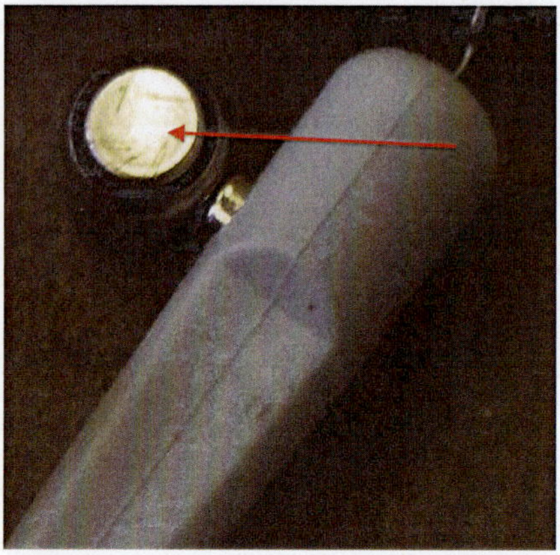

Questions

A. What is the arrow pointing to?

B. List two complications occurring if this object was placed in the nose.

C. List two complications occurring if this object was placed in the ear.

D. If an adult patient with learning difficulties presented after swallowing this object, what would be your first line investigation?

Answers (Station 11)

Photograph of a button battery (attached to a cleaning brush for a white noise masker).

A. Button battery

B. Septal perforation
Erosion of nasal mucosa
Aspiration

C. Erosion into bony ear canal wall
Tympanic membrane perforation

D. Plain radiograph imaging of chest, abdomen
Lateral soft tissue of neck

Revision Notes

- Button batteries in ENT practice are used mainly for hearing aids and also white noise maskers for tinnitus.
- When in contact with mucosal surfaces, the battery causes electrolysis to the surrounding tissues leading to erosion and inflammation.
- When placed in the nose, it can also lead to adhesions and sinusitis.
- If the battery were ingested, investigations would be a lateral soft tissue x-ray, chest x-ray and an abdominal x-ray.
- A lateral chest x-ray would be useful to determine if the battery is in the trachea or the oesophagus.
- Most of the batteries would pass through the GI tract without any complications.
- However, if the battery is lodged in the oesophagus, it could cause oesophageal perforation, strictures, tracheoesophageal fistulae, vocal cord paralysis and bleeding.
- The battery shown above is part of the kit of a white noise masker used to treat tinnitus

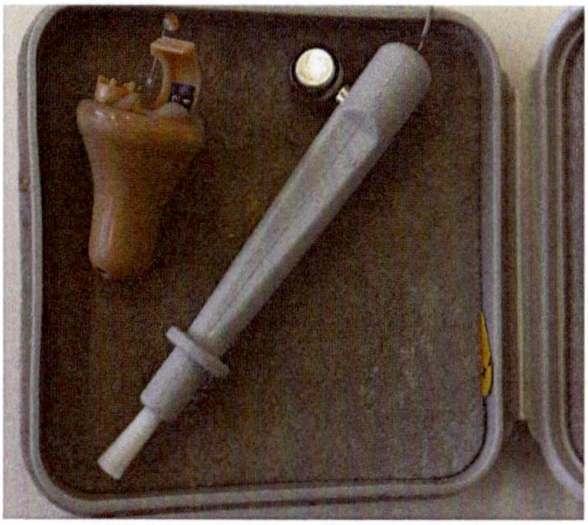

Figure 11.1 A white noise masker for the management of tinnitus (note the battery is kept safe on a magnet of the cleaning brush).

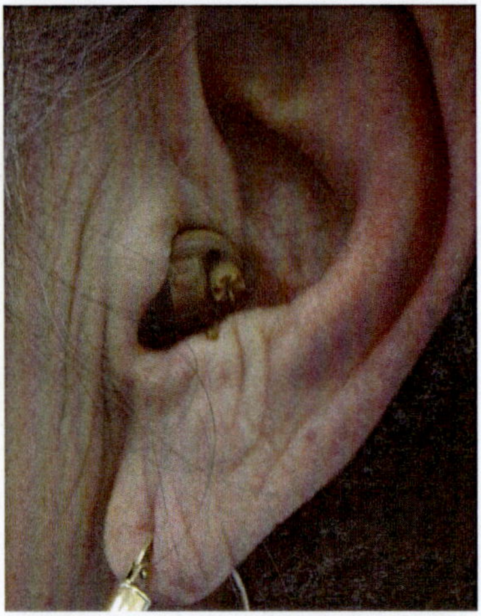

Figure 11.2 A white noise masker *in situ* for the treatment of persistent tinnitus.

Station 12

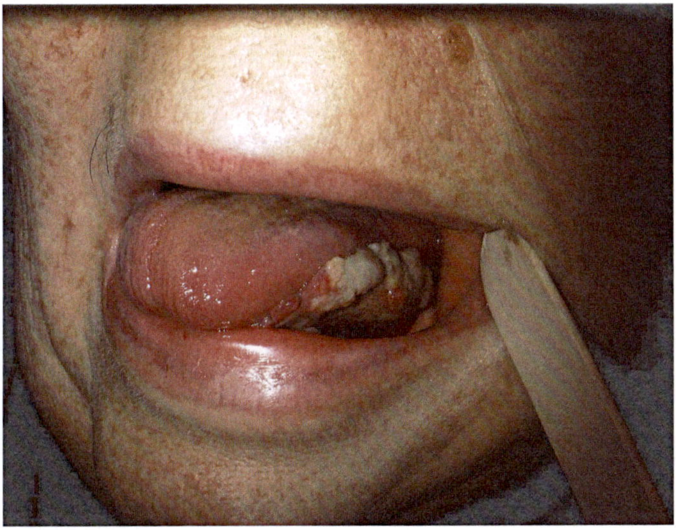

Questions

A. Describe the lesion.
B. What is the likely histology of this lesion?
C. List 5 risk factors for this condition.
D. What are the treatment options?
E. List 3 factors (excluding histology) which affect which treatment option is used.

Answers (Station 12)

Clinical photograph showing squamous cell carcinoma of the tongue.

A. A large exophytic lesion with irregular edges on the left lateral surface of the tongue and extending towards the tongue base (this lesion is involving the anterior 2/3 and posterior 1/3 of the tongue).
B. Squamous cell carcinoma.
C. Alcohol, smoking, Human Papilloma Virus (HPV) infection (for tonsil and tongue base mainly), previous

radiotherapy, betel nut chewing, sharp teeth and spicy food.

D. Conservative (if patient terminally ill with other co-morbidity)
Chemoradiotherapy
Surgical excision with neck dissection if indicated
Palliative treatment.

E. Tumour, Nodal, Metastasis (TNM) classification
Patient's fitness for surgery
Patient's consent for treatment
Local expertise.

Revision Notes

- Tongue cancer is the second most common oral cancer.
- Patients would present with a non-healing ulcer, pain, dysphagia, odynophagia or even trismus.
- The differential diagnoses for this presentation includes apthous ulcers, trauma, infective (Herpes Simplex virus), Crohns's disease or malnutrition such as iron deficiency. However, the main diagnosis to exclude is cancer.
- The commonest histology for tongue cancer is SCC, which accounts for more than 90% of oral cancers.
- The TNM classification for oral cavity cancer is provided in the Appendix (Table 4) and Oropharyngeal (Table 6).
- Oral cancer is mainly treated with surgery, occasionally radiotherapy may be used. Defect may be reconstructed with a free flap such as radial forearm, anterior thigh or rectus abdominis if bulk is needed. Work up usually involves OPG, MRI oral cavity and neck, CT chest as well as EUA and biopsy.
- Panendoscopy and CT chest are important for possible synchronous lesions.

Station 13

Figure 13a

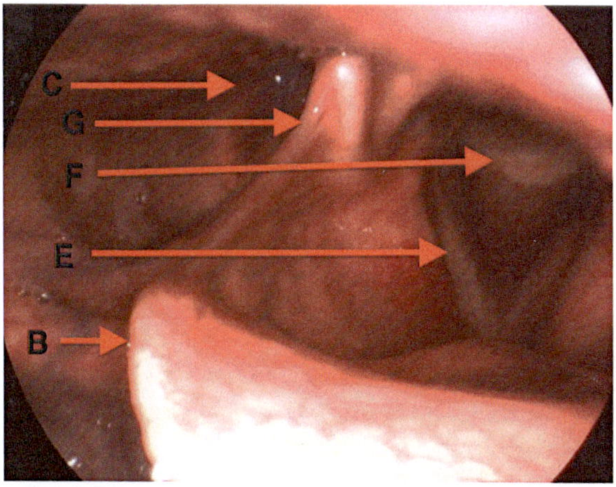

Figure 13b

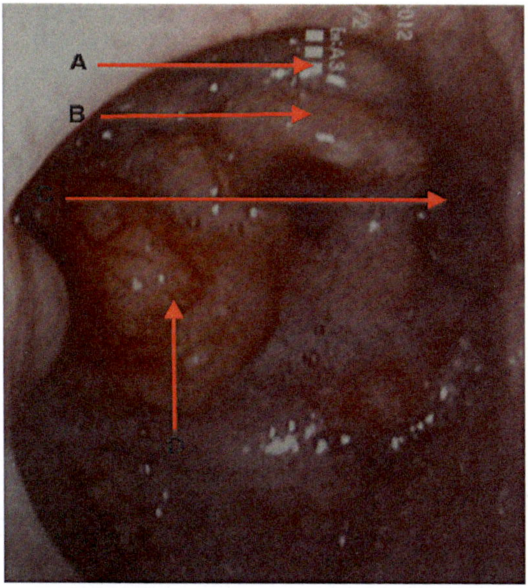

Questions

A. Name the structures labelled (A to G) in Figures 13a – b).

B. Describe the abnormality shown in Figure 13b.

C. What is the histology of the lesion shown in Figure 13b likely to be?

D. List 3 risk factors.

E. List 4 signs or symptoms that this patient is likely to complain of.

F. Explain why the patient might complain of otalgia.

G. What classification system is used for the condition present in 13b?

H. List 3 treatment options.

Answers (Station 13)

A picture of larynx for labelling and a picture of a hypopharynx tumour.

A. A. Valeculla
B. Epiglottis
C. Piriform fossa
D. Tumour
E. Vocal fold (right)
F. Trachea
G. Aryepiglottic fold (right)

B. An exophytic soft tissue mass arising from the left hypopharynx.

C. Squamous cell carcinoma.

D. Smoking
Alcohol
Human papilloma virus 16 and 18 (16 mainly, surrogate marker is p16 detected by immunocytochemistry).

E. Sensation of lump on swallowing
Dysphagia
Dysphonia
Weight loss.

F. Stimulation of the auricular branch of the vagus nerve (Arnold's nerve) when the sensory branches of the vagus nerve supplying the larynx (internal branch of superior laryngeal nerve) are stimulated by laryngeal malignancy.

G. The TNM (tumour, nodes, metastases) classification system that takes into account the extent of the tumour, lymph node spread and presence of distant metastases.

H. Depends on **Stage Grouping** of disease - options are:
- Transoral laser microsurgery (TLM)
- Chemoradiotherapy
- Laryngopharyngectomy
- Palliative therapy

Revision Notes

- Laryngeal carcinoma is among the top 20 most common cancers affecting men in the UK and the incidence is rising in women. Squamous cell carcinoma (SCC) accounts for >90% of cases.
- For the purposes of the exam, only SCC will be considered in this section. However, it is important not to forget that other tumours can arise in the larynx and a histological diagnosis is essential prior to carrying out major laryngeal surgery e.g. laryngectomy.
- Laryngeal cancer is divided into glottic, supraglottic or subglottic. The glottis is anatomically 1 cm from the apex of the ventricle.

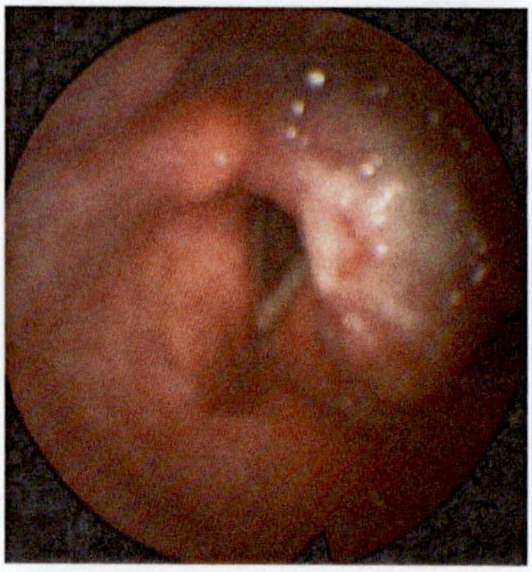

Figure 13.1 Left supraglottic carcinoma

- Glottic carcinoma spreads more slowly than other subtypes due to the relative lack of lymphatic drainage of the vocal cords.
- Risk factors for laryngeal carcinoma include smoking, alcohol, human papilloma virus infection subtypes 16 and 18, previous radiotherapy, positive family history and occupational exposure to nickel and asbestos.
- Table 13.1 shows the typical symptoms caused by the tumours of the three anatomical locations. It must be noted that the list below is not exhaustive and there is a huge amount of cross-over.
- Large laryngeal tumours that have spread locally often cause similar symptoms, regardless of their anatomical origins. Also, symptoms play an extremely important part indicating whether patients present early or late.
- Vocal cord (glottic) tumours often present early as patients notice a change in their voice and most physicians see this symptom as a potentially ominous sign. However, vague feelings of globus etc. (as seen in supra- or subglottic tumours) contribute to delayed presentation and diagnosis.

Table 13.1 Typical symptoms of tumours of the laryngeal subsites and timeliness of diagnosis.

	Typical Symptoms	Timeliness of diagnosis
Supraglottic	**Globus** **FOSIT*** Otalgia Haemoptysis Dysphonia Neck mass	Usually late (often with palpable neck nodes at diagnosis)
Glottic	**Dysphonia** Recurrent aspiration Stridor	Early
Subglottic	**Globus** **FOSIT*** Dysphonia Stridor Neck mass	Usually late

**FOSIT = feeling of something in the throat*

- Otalgia is an important symptom of both pharyngeal and laryngeal cancers. Otalgia arises as a consequence of stimulation of the sensory branches of the pharynx and larynx (glossopharyngeal and vagus nerves), both of which subsequently unite with tympanic afferents (Jacobson's and Arnold's nerves). The term 'referred otalgia' is used in such cases.
- The TNM classification system is used for cancers of the head and neck, including laryngeal SCC (see Appendix). It enables clinicians to gather several pieces of data regarding a patient's tumour and convey them in a standardised manner.

- It is important to understand the difference between the **TNM classification** and the **STAGE** of the disease. For instance, a **T1N1M0** hypopharyngeal cancer is **Stage III** disease which obviously has a poorer prognosis than Stage I disease (T1N0M0).

Stage Grouping

1. Once the T, N, and M have been assigned, this information is combined to assign an overall stage for the cancer. This process is called **stage grouping.**
2. Stage grouping rules are the same for all cancers of the hypopharynx and the supraglottic, glottic, and subglottic areas of the larynx.
3. In general, patients with lower stage cancers tend to have a better outlook for a cure or long-term survival.

Table 13.2 Relationship of TNM classification with stage grouping.

STAGE GROUPING	TNM CLASSIFICATION
STAGE 0	Tis, N0, M0
STAGE I	T1, N0, M0
STAGE II	T2, N0, M0
STAGE III	T3, N0, M0 **OR** T1 to T3, N1, M0
STAGE IVA	T4a, N0 or N1, M0 **OR** T1 to T4a, N2, M0
STAGE IVB	T4b, Any N, M0, **OR** Any T, N3, M0
STAGE IV C	Any T, Any N, M1

Station 14

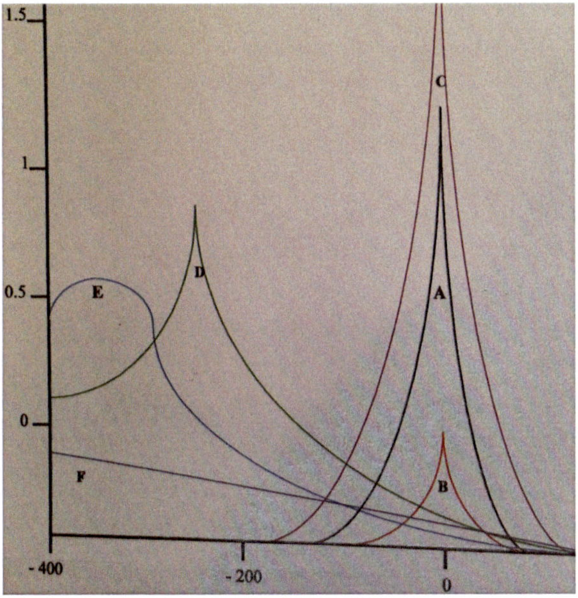

Questions

A. What is the unit of the x-axis?

B. What is (i) the unit of the y-axis and (ii) the normal range?

C. What are the intensities of the sound used in (i) a 3 month old baby and (ii) a 3 year old child?

D. What other useful information is provided on a tympanogram?

E. Give an example of a condition that corresponds with traces A-F.

Answers (Station 14)

Tympanogram traces

A. daPa

B. (i) ml (per equivalent air volume) and (ii) 0.3-1.6ml

C. (i) 1000Hz and (ii) 226Hz

D. Canal volume (nornal adult range 0.6 – 1.5 ml; children 0.4 – 0.9 ml).

E. A normal, B low compliance probably due to fixed ossicles (eg otosclerosis); C flaccid tympanic membrane or dislocated ossicles, D retracted tympanic membrane, E resolving OME, F glue ear.

REVISION NOTES

- The aim of this question is to test your understanding of tympanograms. You may be asked to draw one or more traces in the examination, so it is advisable to learn the units of the x-and y-axis.
- Tympanometry is used to measure tympanic membrane compliance and also to detect middle ear pathology.
- The British Society of Audiology offers the following as a guide to normal values:
  - Middle ear pressure: -50 to +50daPa in adults (-150daPa in children)
  - Middle ear compliance: 0.3 to 1.6cm^3
- The differentiation between OME and a perforation from the tympanogram is based on the canal volume, which will be larger if a perforation is present.
- A healed perforation with monomeric segment of tympanic membrane may give rise to a bifid tympanogram (Figure 14.1).

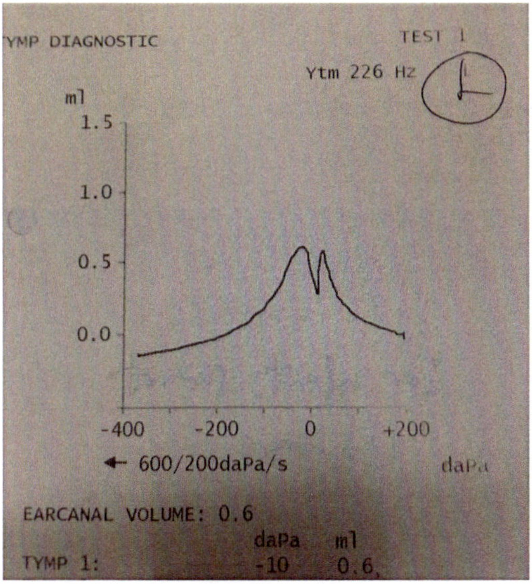

Figure 14.1 Bifid tympanogram due to a large monomeric segment of the tympanic membrane.

- Patients with normal hearing would have a sharp peak type A tympanogram while patients with OME or a perforated tympanic membrane would have a flat type B tympanogram (Figure 14.2).
- **Tympanometry in a nutshell**
  - Tympanometry is an examination used to test the condition of the middle ear and mobility of the TM and the ossicles by creating variations of air pressure in the ear canal.
  - An objective test of middle-ear function
  - A measure of energy transmission through the middle ear.
  - Makes a distinction between sensorineural and conductive hearing loss

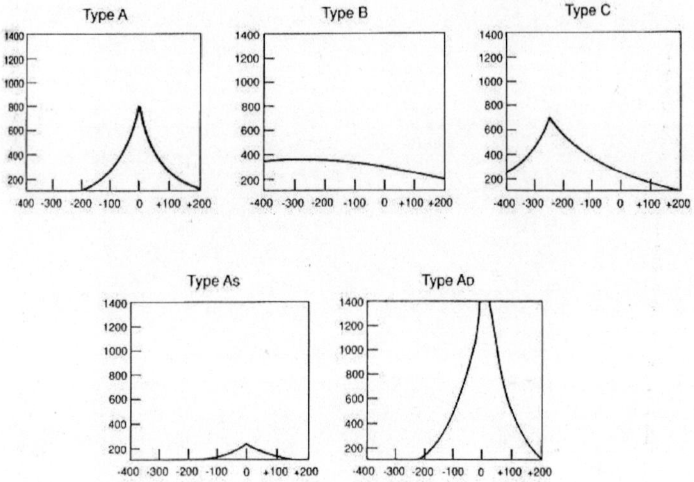

Figure 14.2 Types of tympanograms.

Station 15

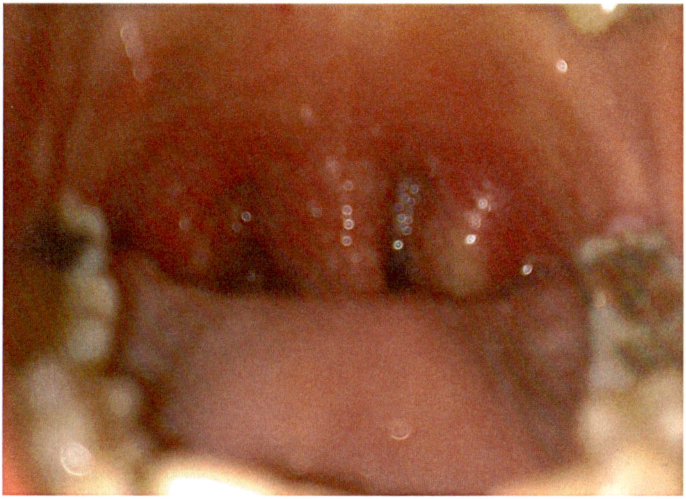

Questions

A. List 2 differential diagnoses.

B. What are the main causative organisms for the diagnoses given above?

C. What would be the patient's presenting symptoms?

D. What are the principles of treatment?

E. What 2 blood tests would be useful to aid diagnosis?

F. List 3 absolute (not relative) indications for tonsillectomy.

G. List 5 complications of this condition.

Answers (Station 15)

Clinical photograph o fa patient with acute tonsillitis.

A. Acute tonsillitis
Glandular fever

B. Group A beta haemolytic streptococcus
Epstein Barr Virus

C. Sore throat
Odynophagia
Otalgia

Halitosis
Dehydration

D. Analgesia, fluid rehydration and antibiotics (to prevent secondary complications in the case of viral tonsillitis).

E. Full blood count and monospot test.

F. Severe obstructive sleep apnoea, suspected malignancy and strep carrier with recurrent endocarditis.

G. Peritonsillar abscess, retropharyngeal abscess with inferior extension to mediastinium, septicaemia, infective endocarditis and glomerulonephritis.

Revision Notes

- The main differential diagnoses in this case are acute tonsillitis and glandular fever.
- Full blood count and liver function test are important investigations as patients with glandular fever may have raised lymphocyte count, low platelets and deranged liver function tests.
- A positive Monospot test is highly suggestive of glandular fever. The test detects heterophile antibodies produced by human in response to EBV infection. It has a **sensitivity** between 70-92 percen and a **specificity** between 96-100 percent.
- The treatment of acute tonsillitis is with Penicillin V, while the treatment for glandular fever is supportive with analgesia and adequate hydration.
- Patients with glandular fever should be advised to avoid contact sports for 6-8 weeks as glandular fever can lead to hepatosplenomegaly.
- Recurrent tonsillitis of more than 7 episodes per year is one of the indications for tonsillectomy according to the Scottish Intercollegiate Guidelines Network (SIGN) guidelines.
- Necrotising tonsillitis can occur in haemolytic streptococci infection (scarlet fever), diphtheria and

Vincent's angina (fusiform bacteria and spirochetes).

- In chronic recurrent tonsillitis the crypts can contain tonsilloliths (stones). Tonsilloliths are made up of food particles, cellular detritus, fibrin, granulocytes, bacteria and fungi.
- Tonsillitis can give rise to life-threatening complications such as mediastinal abscess, which usually requires a thoracotomy to drain (Figures 15a and b) in combination with cervical drainage of a parapharyngeal collection of pus (Figure 15.c).

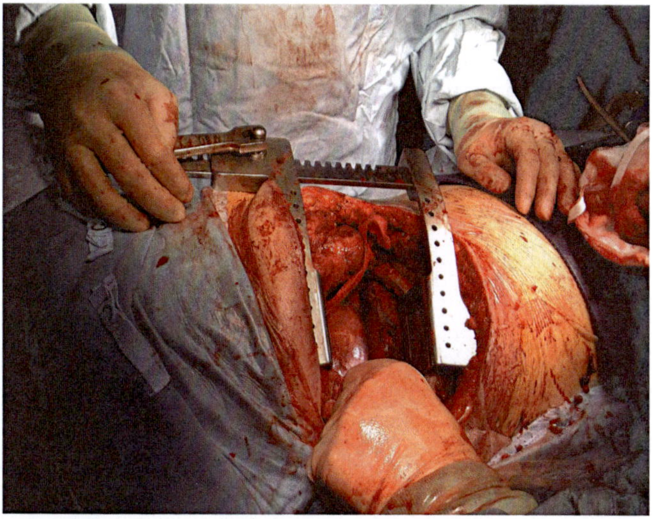

Figure 15a Right-sided thoracotomy to drain a mediastinal abscess secondary to tonsillitis (patient lying on the left side).

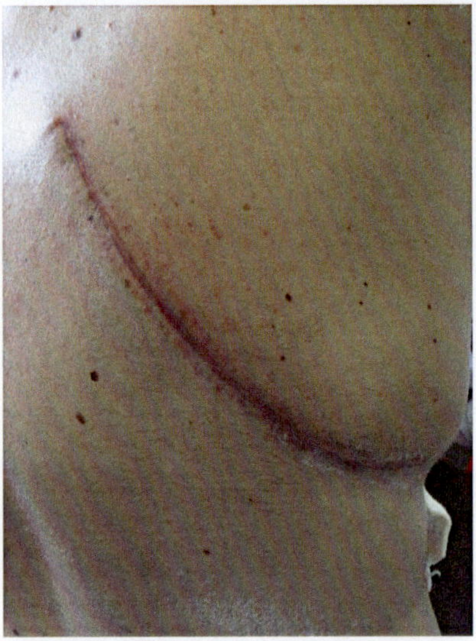

Figure 15b Thoracotomy scar of the patient shown in Figure 15a.

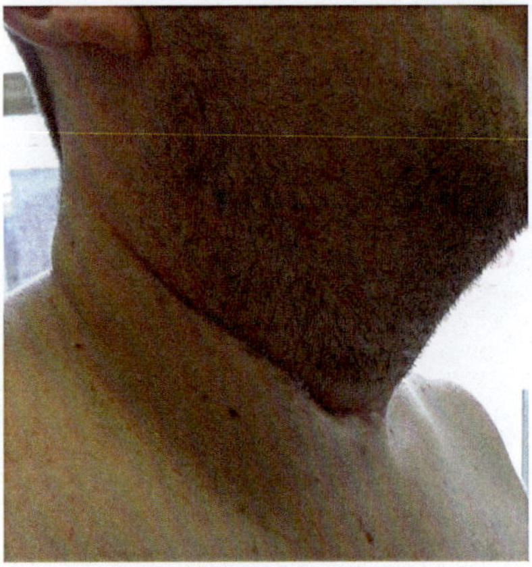

Figure 15c Scar from cervical drainage of a parapharyngeal abscess in the above patient

Station 16

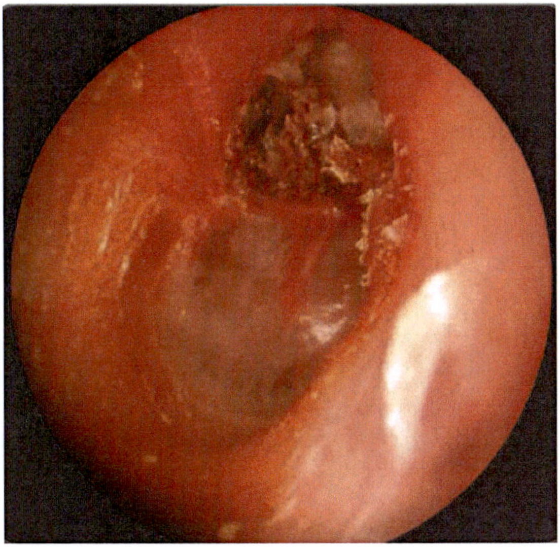

Questions

A. What is the diagnosis?
B. What type(s) of deafness can this cause and why?
C. List 4 symptoms associated with this condition.
D. What are the treatment options if the ear is wet?
E. List 4 complications of surgery.

Answers (Station 16)

Clinical photograph of attic cholesteatoma

A. Attic cholesteatoma.
B. Conductive hearing loss as it may erode and discontinue the ossicular chain. However, it may also cause a mixed hearing loss due to erosion into the labyrinth or inner ear and the ossicles but the cholesteatoma itself is in contact with the inner ear to transmit sound.
C. Chronic otorrhoea
Dizziness
Tinnitus
Hearing loss

Imbalance

D. Regular microsuction and topical antibiotic drops such as ciprofloxacin drops

E. **Intra-temporal**: bleeding infection, facial nerve damage, deafness, tinnitus and perilymph fistula.
Extracranial: cellulitis, neck abscesses (Bezold, Citelle, Luc).
Intracranial: Meningitis, brain abscess, CSF otorrhoea, sigmoid sinus thrombosis.
You will notice that the complications of cholesteatoma are similar to the complications associated with acute otitis media.

Revision Notes

- A cholesteatoma is a non-neoplastic but destructive lesion containing layers of keratin in a cavity lined by squamous epithelial tissue. The lesion may be congenital or acquired.
- Congenital cholesteatoma arises from the growth of embryonic epidermal rests (epidermoid formation) behind an intact tympanic membrane.
- Acquired cholesteatoma results from a posterior superior tympanic membrane insult with altered self-clearing and tympanomastoid erosion.
- The main presenting complaints involve chronic foul smelling otorrhoea, hearing loss and dizziness.
- Dizziness may indicate labyrinthine fistula of the lateral semicircular canal.
- The investigation of choice is initially pure tone audiogram and a tympanogram, plus a CT scan of the temporal bone. The classical sign is a soft tissue mass in the Prussak's space with blunting of the scutum (Figure 16.1).
- In the future non-epi diffusion weighted MRI will play a larger role especially in surveillance for recurrent disease).

- The reasons for a CT scan are as follows:
  - o To plan approach (depends on extent of pneumatisation/contracted mastoid; high jugular bulb; low dura).
  - o To check for anatomical abnormalities, especially if syndromic or presence of abnormality around the outside EAC.
  - o To see if facial nerve is dehiscent.
  - o To look for bony destruction and or fistula.
  - o To see extent of soft tissue abnormality (not necessary the extent of disease) especially in cases of poor otomicroscopy.
  - o revision cases.
  - o medicolegal requirement.
- The treatment of this condition can be divided into:

  Conservative: Regular microsuctioning, if patient cannot tolerate surgery (cholesteatoma is a surgical disease).

  Surgical: Tympanomastoid surgery (either keeping the posterior canal wall up or taking it down).
- The main priority of treatment is to make the ear safe by eradicating the disease. The secondary aim is to address hearing loss by reconstruction of the sound transmission mechanism of the middle ear.
- Anatomically the sinus tympani tends to be the site of common recurrence because its poor accessibility.

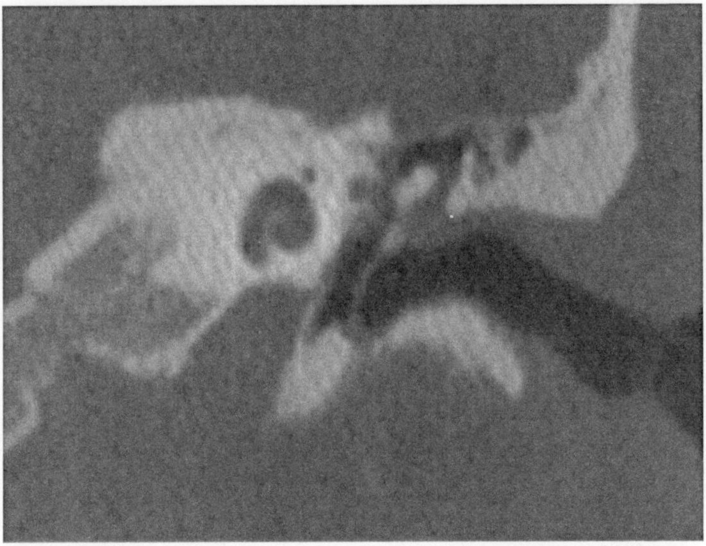

Figure 16.1 CT scan showing a non-dependent soft tissue mass between the ossicle and scutum suggestive of cholesteatoma.

Table 16.1 Summary of the aetiopathogenic theories of congenital and acquired cholesteatoma.

Congenital	Acquired
Epidermoid formation	Basal hyperplasia
Migration	Migration
Amniotic fluid	Retraction pocket
Inclusion	Implantation (iatrogenic, traumatic)
Squamous metaplasia	Squamous metaplasia
Embryonic germ cell proliferation	

Persaud *et al.* An evidence based review of the aetiopathogenic theories of congenital and acquired cholesteatoma. *JLO 2007;121(11): 1013-1019.*

Station 17

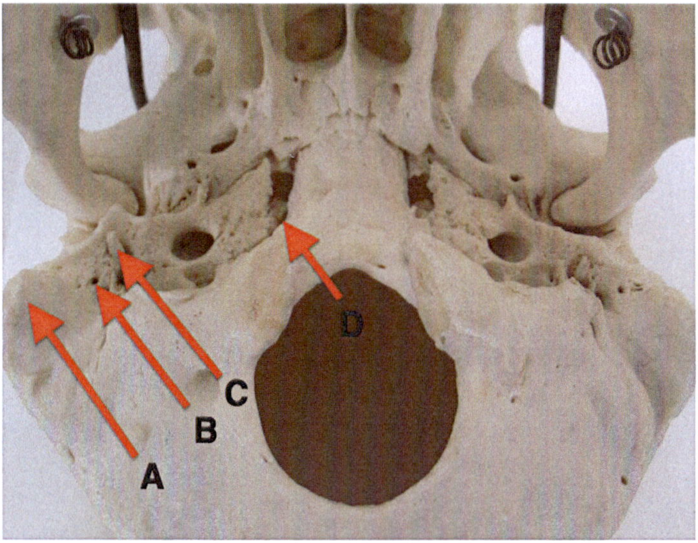

Questions

A. What is structure 'A'?

B. Name 2 muscles that attaches to 'A'

C. What is 'C'?

D. Name 5 structures that attach to 'C'

E. Which nerve runs through the inferior tympanic canal (labelled 'B')?

F. Name one nerve associated with 'D'

G. Which artery accompanies the facial nerve through the stylomastoid foramen?

Answers (Station 17)

Photograph of the inferior view of the skull base

A. Mastoid process

B. Sternocleidomastoid muscle
Posterior belly of diagastric muscle

C. Styloid process

D. Stylohyoid muscle, styloglossus muscle, stylopharyngeus muscle, stylohyoid ligament and stylomandibular ligament.

E. The lesser petrosal nerve.

This nerve is the parasympathetic branch of the glossopharyngeal nerve. It then runs through the middle ear as Jacobson's nerve and eventually enters the infra temporal fossa via foramen ovale to synapse in the otic ganglion. Post ganglionic fibres hitch-hike on the auricular temporal nerve (a branch of the trigeminal nerve) to reach the parotid gland.

F. Greater superficial petrosal nerve.

The greater superficial petrosal nerve is a parasympathetic branch of the facial nerve and together with the deep petrosal nerve, running on the nearby internal carotid artery, forms the vidian nerve which enters the vidian canal to reach the pterygopalatine ganglion (or hayfever ganglion).

G. The stylomastoid artery which is a branch of the posterior auricular artery; this artery is usually encountered before seeing the facial nerve during parotidectomy.

Revision Notes

- It is important to know the anatomy of the skull base (both the superior and the inferior views) especially the structures running through the foramens and also the attachments.

Table 17.1 Important skull base foramen and associated structures.

FORAMEN	ASSOCIATED STRUCTURES
Foramen ovale	Mnemonic 'MALE' **M** – Mandibular division of trigeminal nerve **A** – Accessory Meningeal artery **L** – Lesser petrosal nerve **E** – Emissary veins
Jugular foramen (Figure 17.2)	Glossopharyngeal nerve (CN IX) Vagus (CN X) Accessory nerve (CN XI) Sigmoid sinus
Foramen spinosum	Middle meningeal artery and vein Meningeal branch of mandibular nerve
Stylomastoid foramen (Figure 17.2)	Facial nerve and stylomastoid artery (a branch of the posterior auricular artery).
Foramen lacerum	Greater petrosal nerve (on top of foramen) Internal carotid artery (on top of foramen)

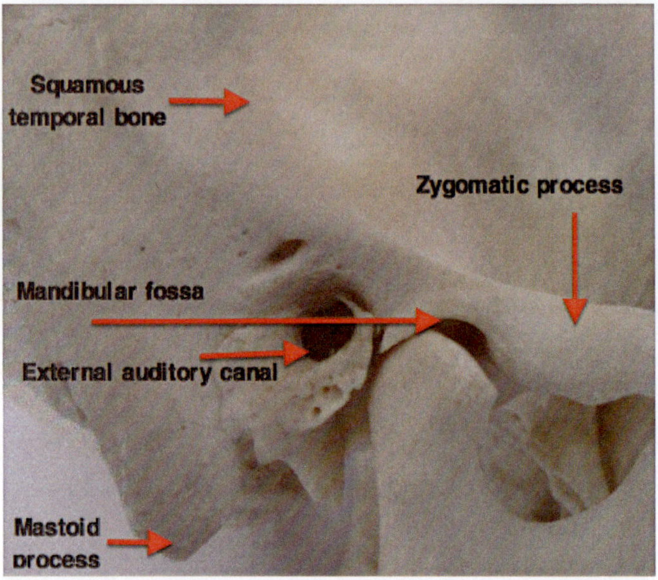

Figure 17.1 Important anatomical structures on the lateral temporal bone.

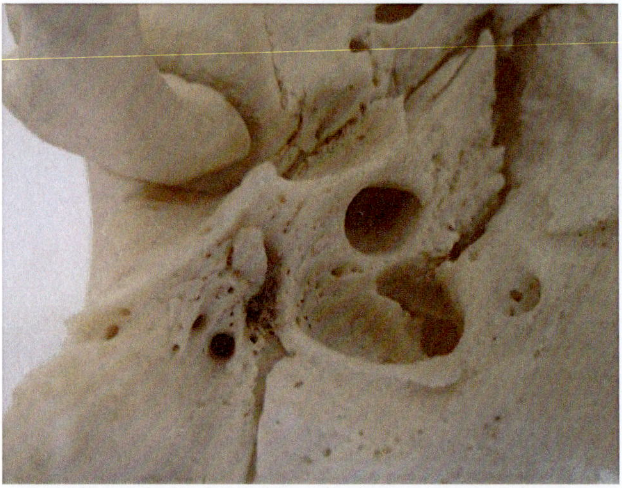

Figure 17.2 Skull base show the relation between the styloid process and the triangle formed by the carotid canal, jugular foramen and stylomastoid foramen.

Station 18

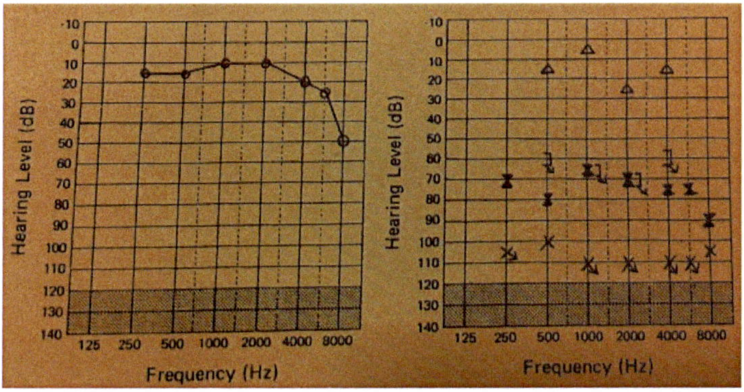

Questions

A. Draw symbol for right unmasked air conduction.

B. Draw symbol for left unmasked air conduction.

C. Draw symbol for unmasked bone conduction.

D. Describe the pure tone audiograms.

E. What are the treatment options for this patient?

Answers (Station 18)

PTA with normal hearing on left and profound SNHL on right

A. O

B. X

C. Δ

D. In the right ear there is normal hearing in the lowfrequencies and mild to moderate hearing loss in 6kHz and 8kHz, respectively. In the left ear there is profound sensorineural hearing loss.

E. Conservative (If it does not affect patient's lifestyle).
Contralateral Routing if Offside Signals (CROS) hearing aid (to reduce the head shadow effect)
Bone conduction hearing aid such as Bone Anchored Hearing Aid (BAHA) (also to reduce the head shadow effect).

Revision Notes

- The differential diagnosis for unilateral sensorineural hearing loss varies based on the patient's age.
- In adults, the differential diagnosis includes:
  Traumatic
  Noise induced hearing loss
  Presbycusis
  Meniere's disease
  Acoustic neuroma
  Infective causes such as meningitis.
- In children, the differential diagnosis can be divided into:
  Congenital: Waardenburg's syndrome, CHARGE syndrome
  Intrauterine infections - TORCHS (Toxoplasmosis, Rubella, CMV, Herpes simplex, Syphillis)
  Neonatal/childhood infection eg meningitis
  Maternal drug/alcohol abuse during pregnancy
  Ototoxic drugs during childhood.

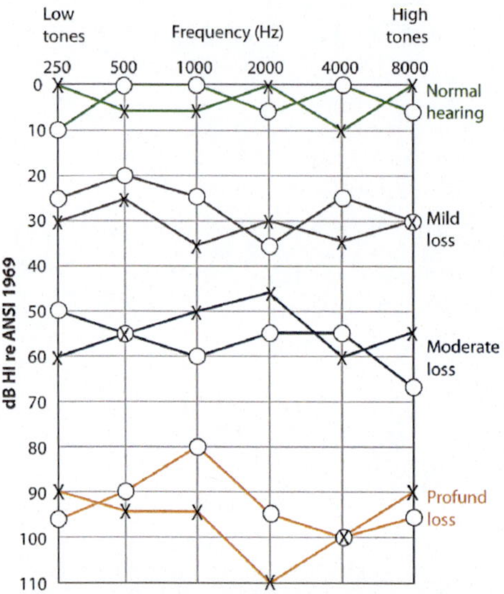

Figure 18.1 Levels of degrees of hearing loss.

Description	Right ear	Left ear
Air conduction (when necessary)	○	X
Air Conduction not masked (shadow point)	●	⧗
Air conduction masked (not changed from previous test)	◒	X▲
Air conduction limit, threshold not found	○↓	X↓
Bone conduction not masked	△	△
Bone conduction masked	[	]
Bone conduction limits, threshold not found	[↓	]↓
Uncomfortable loudness level	└	┘
Uncomfortable loudness level not found	└↓	↓┘
Sound field	~S	~S
Aided	A	A

Table 18.1 Symbols used for audiograms.

Station 19

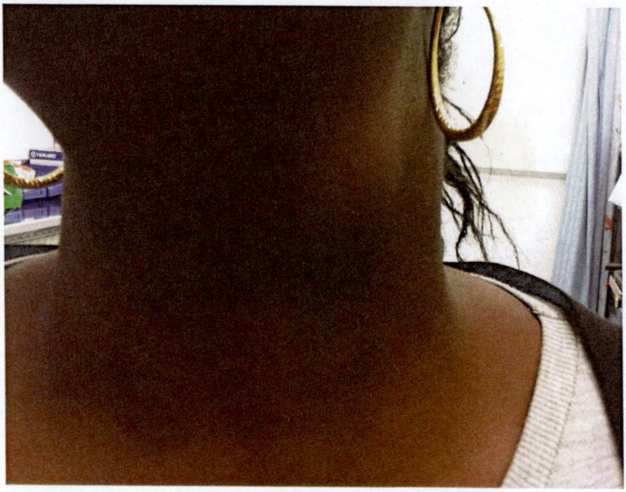

Questions

A. In which neck triangle is the swelling?
B. What is the most likely diagnosis?
C. List three differential diagnoses.
D. What investigation would you perform next?
E. Describe at least 2 management options.

Answers (Station 19)

Clinical photograph of a patient with a left branchial cyst.

A. Anterior triangle.
B. Branchial cyst.
C. Skin – sebaceous cyst, lipoma
Lymphadenopathy
Parotid swelling
Submandibular gland swelling
Carotid body tumour.
D. Ultrasound scan with fine needle aspiration cytology (FNAC).
E. Conservative management by observing for frequency of infections and if the lump is enlarging.

Treat infections with antibiotics.
Surgical excision of branchial cyst.

Revision Notes

- Branchial cysts contain lymphoid tissue and are lined by squamous epithelial tissue.
- There are several theories as to its aetiology but they are mainly thought to arise from squamous epithelium rests within lymph nodes during embryological development.
- They usually present in early adulthood.
- In patients above 40 years old, swelling in this region should be treated as metastatic disease, until proven otherwise.
- Ultrasound and FNAC are the investigations of choice.
- Surgical excision is the treatment of choice.

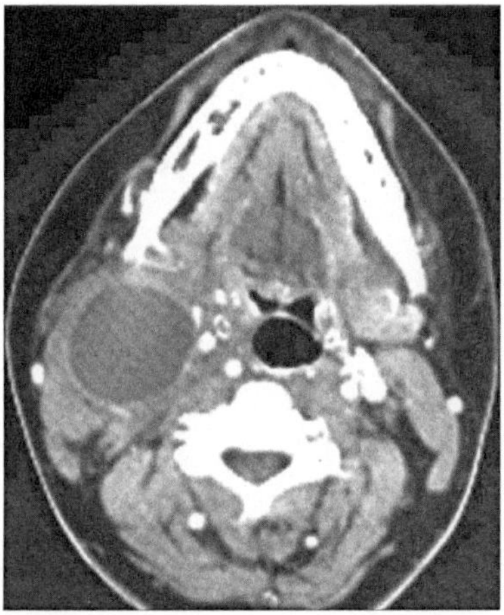

Figure 19.1 Axial CT scan showing a right branchial cyst.

Station 20

Following a hemithyroidectomy, a patient complains of not being able to hit the high notes during her choir practice sessions.

Questions

A. Which nerve has been injured and subsequently which muscle has been affected?

B. Name the other laryngeal muscles and their innervation.

C. Which nerves supply sensation to the larynx?

D. What type of joint articulates the arytenoid to the cricoid cartilage?

E. Name the 4 cartilages of the larynx

Answers (Station 20)

Anatomical question about the larynx.

A. External branch of the superior laryngeal nerve supplies cricothyroid muscle.

B. The other intrinsic laryngeal muscles are:

- i. Thyroarytenoid (vocalis) (paired)
- ii. Lateral cricoarytenoid (paired)
- iii. Posterior cricoarytenoid (paired)
- iv. Transverse arytenoid (unpaired).

These are all supplied by the recurrent laryngeal nerve.

C. The internal branch of the superior laryngeal nerve of the vagus is responsible for sensation above the vocal cord whilst the recurrent laryngeal nerve supplies sensation below the vocal cord.

D. Synovial joint.

E. The 4 laryngeal cartilages are:

- i. Thyroid cartilage
- ii. Cricoid cartilage
- iii. Arytenoid cartilage
- iv. Epiglottis.

Revision Notes

- The external laryngeal nerve may be damaged during cricothyroid, thyroid and lateral pharyngotomy approaches. The nerve is located in Joll's triangle, formed by the midline, strap muscle and superior thyroid pedicle; the floor is formed by cricothyroid muscle (Figure 20.1a).
- The recurrent laryngeal nerve is located in Beahr's triangle, formed by trachea inferior thyroid artery and common carotid artery (Figure 20.1b)
- Cricothyroid muscle is supplied by the external branch of the superior laryngeal nerve of the vagus. This muscle tenses the vocal cords to increase the pitch of voice.
- The other intrinsic muscles of the larynx are the thyroarytenoid (vocalis), lateral cricoarytenoid, posterior cricoarytenoid and transverse arytenoid, these are all supplied by the recurrent laryngeal nerve.
- The internal branch of the superior laryngeal nerve of the vagus supplies sensation above the glottis (Recurrent laryngeal nerve supplies sensation for the glottis and below).
- The arytenoid moves on the cricoid cartilage by means of a synovial joint. It is susceptible to all the disorders that affect the larger synovial joints elsewhere in the body.
- The 4 cartilages of the larynx are the thyroid, cricoid, epiglottis and arytenoid cartilages, these form the framework to which muscles and tendons attach.

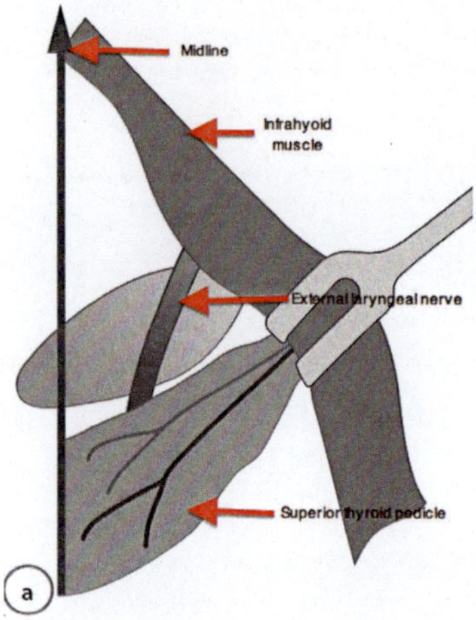

Figure 20.1a Joll's triangle (superior thyroid pedicle, infrahyoid muscle, midline – mnemonic SIM) (Courtesy of Dr Reza Jarral).

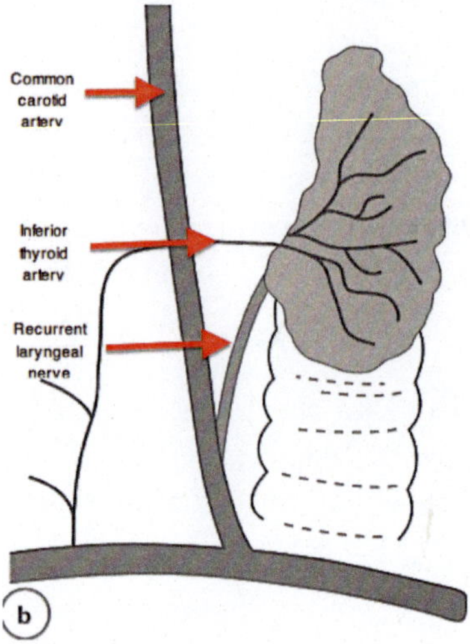

Figure 20.1b Beahr's triangle (trachea, inferior thyroid artery and common carotid artery - mnemonic TIC) (Courtesy of Dr Reza Jarral).

Station 21

A 28 year old patient was noted to cough repeatedly during microsuctioning of her ear canal.

Questions

A. Which nerve is responsible for this problem?

B. List 3 nerves that contribute to the sensory innervation to the pinna?

C. Which 3 nerves which innervates the tympanic membrane?

D. Which nerve innervates the skin over the mastoid bone?

E. Which 2 cervical nerves form the greater auricular nerve?

Answers (Station 21)

A. Arnold's nerve (a branch of the vagus nerve).

B. Facial nerve, vagus nerve and trigeminal nerve and greater auricular nerve.

C. Glossopharyngeal nerve, Trigeminal (auricular temporal) and vagus (auricular branch).

D. Greater auricular nerve.

E. C2 and C3 nerve fibres.

Revision Notes

- Arnold's nerve is a branch of the vagus nerve which innervates the inferior bony canal, the posterior-superior cartilaginous canal and adjacent tympanic membrane and conchal bowl (Figure 21.1). Touching the skin of the ear canal in the areas mentioned triggers this nerve to stimulate.
- The conchal bowl is dually innervated by Arnold's nerve and sensory branch of the facial nerve as illustrated in figure 21.1.
- The pinna is innervated laterally, inferiorly and posteriorly by the greater auricular nerve (derived from the cervical plexus).

- The auriculotemporal branch of the mandibular division of the trigeminal nerve supplies the anterior portion of the pinna.
- The greater auricular nerve runs from Erbs point at the midpoint of the posterior border of sternocleidomastoid muscle to the parotid gland. It divides into anterior branch and posterior branches. The former supplies skin over the angle of the mandible whilst the latter supplies the ear lobe. It is now common practice for ENT surgeons to preserve the posterior branch during to parotidectomies to preserve sensation to the ear lobe.

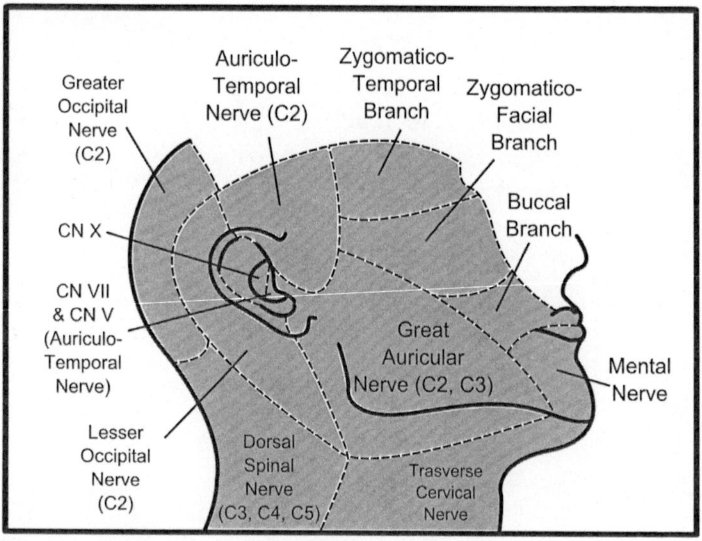

Figure 21.1 Sensory nerve supply around the pinna (Courtesy of Dr Reza Jarral).

Station 22

A 55-year old lady is referred to see you in clinic with a history of vertigo. She has had 4 episodes of vertigo over the last 2 months. Each episode lasts for several hours; she is nauseated and on 2 occasions vomited. Lately, she has been experiencing fullness in her left ear along with some tinnitus.

Questions

A. What is the likely diagnosis?
B. What type of hearing loss would you most likely expect to see on an audiogram?
C. What dietary advice would you give?
D. Name 2 surgical options for treatment?

Answers (Station 22)

A. Meniere's Disease
B. Fluctuating sensorineural hearing loss, initially in the lower frequencies
C. The aim of dietary changes is to regulate the body's fluid shifting. Eating and drinking water at even intervals are specific measures patients can implement to reduce fluid retention. Also limit salt and monosodium glutamate intake and avoid caffeine.
D. Myringotomy tube insertion
Endolymphatic sac surgery.

Revision Notes

- Meniere's disease is characterised by episodic vertigo, fluctuating low frequency sensorinueral hearing loss, tinnitus and aural fullness. It is thought to be associated with endolymphatic hydrops, or dilation of scala media.
- It is a clinical diagnosis and therefore requires exclusion of other possible causes.
- Between episodes, the hearing loss experienced may recover partially, fully or not at all.

- The investigation of choice is a pure tone audiogram (PTA). If it is repeated over a period of time, it will show a stepwise deterioration of hearing. In early attacks, the PTA will show a low frequency sensorineural hearing loss.
- The management of Meniere's Disease can be divided into:

  Dietary changes – as mentioned above

  Lifestyle changes – stopping smoking, managing stress

  Medical – Thiazide diuretics, Vestibular sedatives during acute attacks such as Stemetil, vestibular rehabilitation, hearing aids

  Surgical – Grommet insertion, intratympanic steroid injection, intratympanic gentamicin, endolymphatic sac surgery, vestibular nerve section.
- Bilateral profound hearing losses secondary to Meniere's disease may be rehabilitated with cochlear implants, if air conduction hearing aids are inadequate.

Station 23

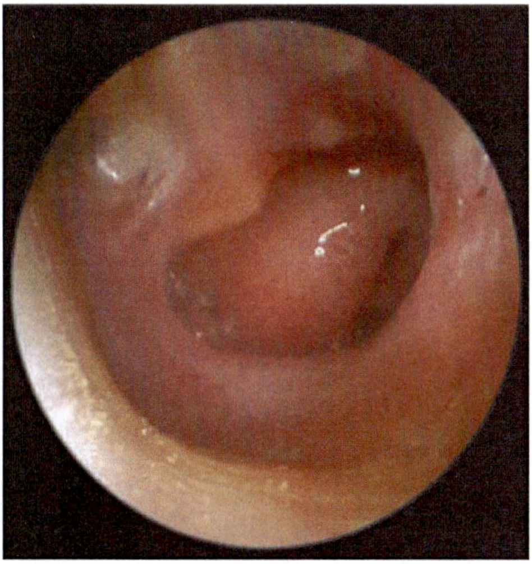

A 34 year old male attends clinic with the complaint of ear discharge. It is intermittent, usually triggered by an upper respiratory tract infection. It is now becoming a nuisance and he would like something done.

Questions

A. Describe the type of perforation shown in the picture.
B. What is the diagnosis?
C. What 3 steps form part of the acute management plan?
D. What are the options for longer-term management?
E. List 3 possible complications associated with surgical closure of tympanic membrane perforations.

Answers (Station 23)

Clinical photograph of active mucosal chronic otitis media (COM).

A. Wet central tympanic membrane perforation.
B. Chronic suppurative otitis media (CSOM) or active mucosal chronic otitis media (inactive mucosal chronic otitis media is also known as a dry perforation).

C. Microbiological swab, microsuctioning and topical antibiotic ear drops, such as Ciprofloxacin

D. **Conservative**: Keep ear dry, bone conduction hearing aid if patient has hearing loss.
Medical: Topical antibiotic drops for infective episodes.
Surgical: Myringoplasty to close the perforation and make ear water-tight.

E. Bleeding, infection, hearing loss, dizziness, taste disturbance, complications of scarring, failure to close perforation.

Revision Notes

- Tympanic membrane perforations can either be central or marginal, wet or dry.
- The aim of the acute management is to render the ear dry.
- Associated nasal symptoms should be treated, eg with a nasal steroid and maybe a short course of anti-inflamatory antibiotics such as clarithromycin (500mg bc for 7days).
- Ciprofloxacin drops are the mainstay, however ENT-UK guidelines approve the use of potentially ototoxic topical antibiotic-steroid preparations as the presence of infection is ototoxic *per se* and reduces permeability across the round window.
- Pre-treatment audiometry must be undertaken.
- Once the ear is dry, the clinical assessment is repeated. At this stage the treatment plan may include the following steps:

  Treatment of underlying nasal disease
  Treatment of intermittent episodes of otorrhoea
  Conservative management
  Hearing aid provision
  Surgical closure – myringoplasty.

Station 24

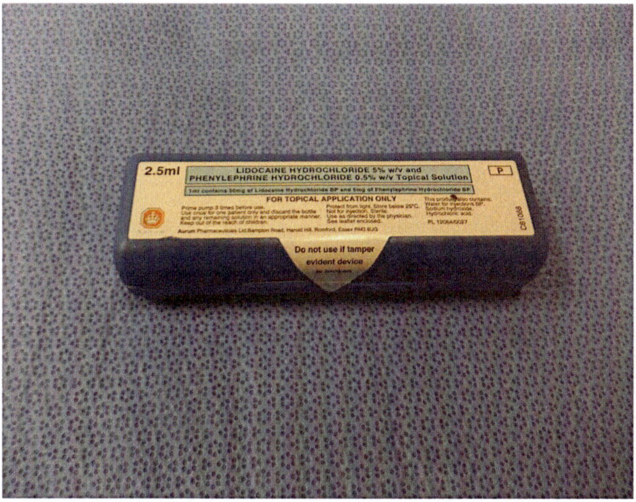

Questions

A. List 2 instances when this Local anaesthetic spray may be used.

B. What is the total dose (mg) of lidocaine present in 2.5mls of 5 % lidocaine?

C. What is the recommended maximum safe dose for plain lidocaine (lignocaine)?

D. What is the recommended maximum safe dose for lidocaine and adrenaline?

E. What are the ingredients of Moffett's solution?

F. What are the side effects of Moffett's solution?

Answers (Station 24)

Picture of co-phenylcaine

A. (1) to decongest the nose prior to nasal surgery and (2) to anaesthetise and decongest the nose prior to flexible nasendoscopy.

B. 125 mg (5% Lidocaine) .

C. 3mg/kg.

D. 7mg/kg.

E. Cocaine, adrenaline and sodium bicarbonate (to free base the cocaine and make it more lipophilic, pKa 8.6).

F. Tachycardia and arrhythmias, hypertension, hyperthermia, sweating and anxiety.

Revision Notes

- Lidocaine is an amide local anaesthetic by acting on the sodium channels to cause a reversible conduction block along nerves.
- The addition of a vasoconstrictor prolongs the action of the local anaesthesia because it delays the local clearance.
- A 1% solution of any drug contains 10miligrams/ml gram. Therefore, a 1% lidocaine solution contains 1000 mg of lidocaine per 100 ml (which is the same as 10 mg/ml).
- A summary of the main characteristics of commonly used local anaesthetics is provided in Table 24.1

Table 24.1 Fundamental characteristics of commonly used local anaesthetics (LA).

LA	Type	Onset of action (mins)	Duration of action (mins)	Preparation	Recommended dose
Lignocaine	Amide	2-4	30-60	Solution 0.5-2% Gel 2% Ointment 5% Spray1-4%	3mg/kg 7mg/kg with adrenaline
Prilocaine	Amide	2-4	30-90	Solution 0.5-2%	6mg/kg
Lignocaine & prilocaine (EMLA)	Amide	60	60	EMLA in a tube containing 5g or 30mg (lignocaine2.5% and prilocaine 2.5%)	Cream 25mg/ml prilocaine and 25mg/ml lignocaine 0.8ml/10kg.
Bupivacaine	Amide	10-20	120-240	Solution 0.25% and 0.5% (with/without) 1;80,000-200,000 adrenaline solution.	2mg/kg
Cocaine	Ester	15-30	60	Moffett solution 1ml of 10% cocaine, 1ml of 8.4% sodium bicarbonate, 1ml of 1;1000 adrenaline and 3 mls of normal saline.	1.5-3mg/kg

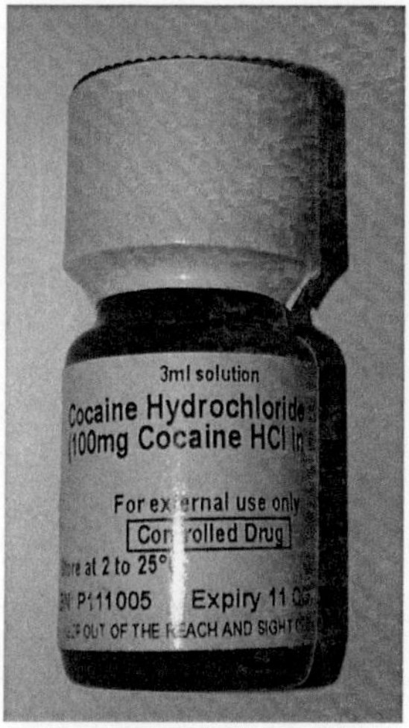

Figure 24.1 Cocaine solution is stored in a dark bottle because it is light sensitive.

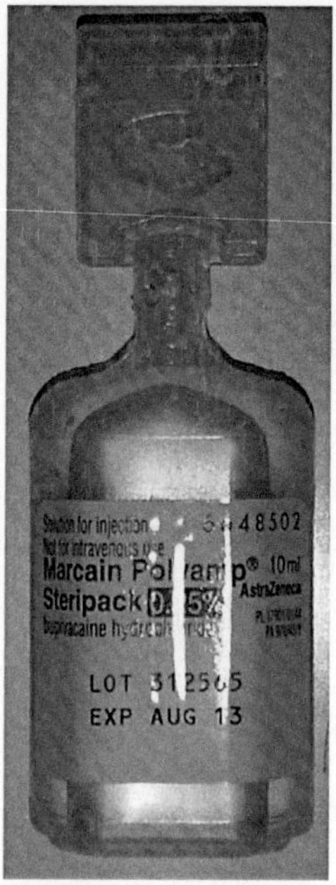

Figure 24.2 Marcaine (bupivacaine) comes in a clear plastic container as it is not light sensitive.

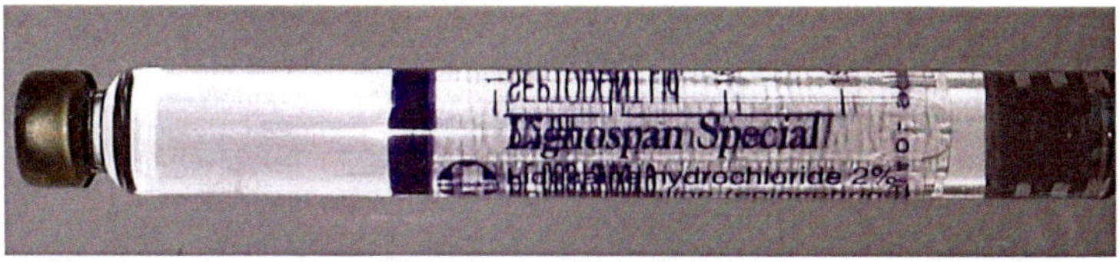

Figure 24.3 Cartridge of Lignospan (lignocaine hydrochloride 2% and adrenaline 1:80, 000) used commonly in nasal surgery.

Station 25

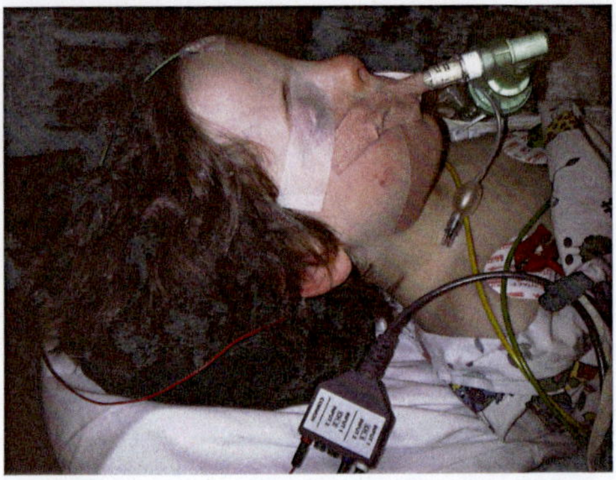

Questions

A. What is the incidence of deafness in newborns?

B. Name 3 causes of hearing impairment in children.

C. What 2 tests are used in the national newborn hearing screening programme.

D. What happens when a baby fails the screening tests?

E. What test is the child undergoing in the picture above?

Answers (Station 25)

A child having a diagnostic ABR.

A. 1:1000.

B. Genetic factors
Congenital infections (TORCH: toxoplasmosis, rubella, CMV, herpes simplex)
Meningitis
Intensive care unit for more than 48 hours
Craniofacial abnormalities.

C. Automated oto-acoustic emission (AOAE).
Automated auditory brainstem response (AABR).

D. The maximum **screening** tests for a normal baby are (i) **automated** OAE (ii) repeat automated OAE - if no clear response is detected in the first test and (iii) **automated** ABR. If the baby fails the screen process he/she is referred to the local centre or hospital for further investigations, including tympanometry, a **diagnostic** OAE and a **diagnostic** ABR.

E. Diagnostic ABR (tone pips ABR is the gold standard diagnostic test).

Revision Notes

- The national newborn hearing screening programme was introduced in March 2006.
- The target condition for the screen is bilateral, permanent hearing impairment (sensorineural or permanent conductive) averaging 40dB or more.
- The two screening tests used are automated OAE and automated ABR; these are basic tests and the results are either pass or fail.
- Diagnostic OAEs and ABRs offer thresholds and are more frequency specific.
- There are 2 protocols in use, one for healthy babies and another for special care baby unit and neonatal intensive care unit SCBU and NICU) babies who have a higher risk of hearing impairment.
- High risk babies are screened with both automated OAE and automated ABR.
- If deafness is detected after a battery of tests, the new born is aided accordingly.
- Facts about otoacoustic emissions (OAEs):
  - Small sounds generated by healthy outer hair cells in response to a click stimulus
  - Impaired cochleae do not produce OAEs
  - High correlation between OAEs and normal audiometric thresholds (better than 30dBHL)
  - No correlations between size of OAEs and threshold level
  - Retrocochlear disorders are not identified by OAEs.

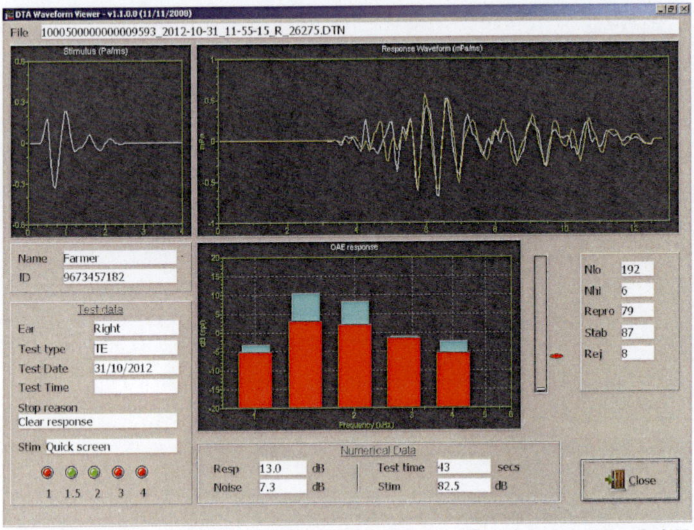

Figure 25.1 New simplified format of a diagnostic OAEs with clear responses (clear responses of at least 6dB in 2 of the 5 frequency bars are needed to pass).

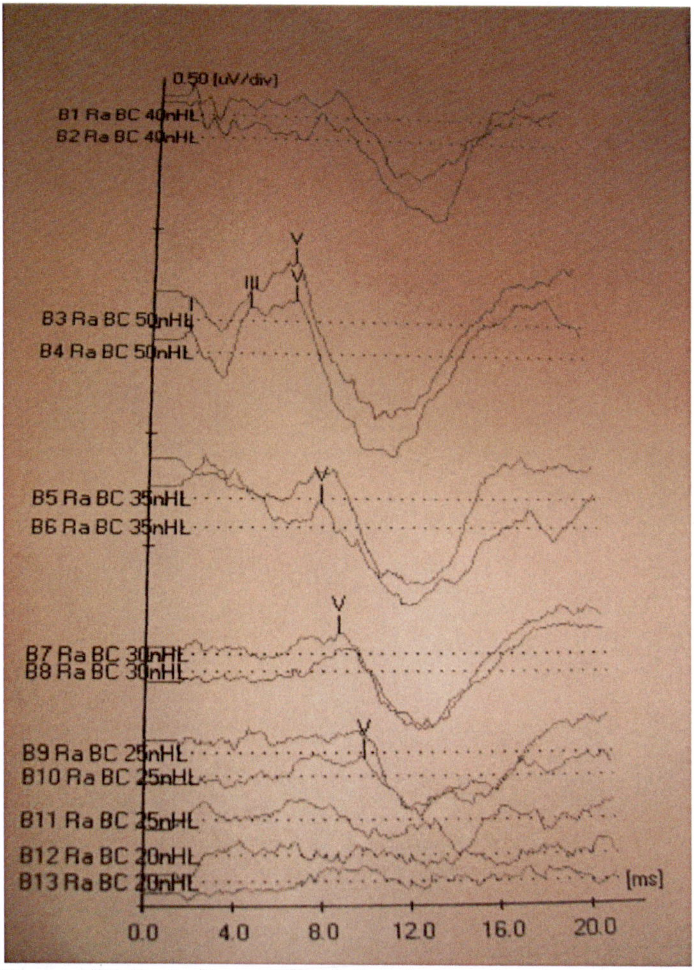

Figure 25.2 A diagnostic ABR printout (hearing threshold is less than or equal to 30dB HL – a subjective interpretation).

- Stimuli in clinical audiology
    - A click stimulus is not frequency specific:
        - A narrow band click stimuli is 2-4kHz.
        - A broad or wide band click stimuli is 1-4kHz.
    - A tone is frequency specific:
        - A tone burst has an overall length >20ms.
        - A tone pip has an overall length <20ms.
    - Additional information
        - Tone burst has a defined start (rise time), duration (plateau) and end (fall time); the plateau is longer than the rise/fall time.
        - Tone pips usually has a plateau which is the same or shorter than the rise/fall time.

Station 26

Scenario:

A 43-year-old woman presents to her GP with a swelling in her neck. On direct questioning she admits to being rather tired recently, but she is otherwise well. She has a family history of thyroid disease. Examination is normal apart from a diffuse goitre. The GP requests thyroid function tests and the results are as follows: TSH 6.5 (0.3-5.5), FT4 10 (10-22), TPO antibodies >1000 (<50).

Questions

A. What is the most likely diagnosis?
B. What investigations would be helpful to confirm the diagnosis?
C. What symptoms are likely to be present?
D. What treatment may be helpful in the long term
E. List 4 indications for surgery.

Answers (Station 26)

A. Hashimoto's thyroiditis.
B. ESR
Anti-thyroglobulin Antibodies
TSH receptor antibodies to rule out Grave's disease.
C. Depression
Weight gain
Hair loss
Fatigue
D. Thyroxine
E. Suspicion of lymphoma
Difficulty breathing or swallowing
Cosmesis
Pressure symptoms.

Revision Notes

- Hashimoto's thyroiditis an autoimmune disease in which the thyroid gland is infiltrated by a variety of cell- and antibody-mediated immune processes.
- The symptoms of Hashimoto's thyroiditis include psychosis, weight gain, depression, mania, sensitivity to heat and cold, paresthesia, fatigue, panic attacks, hypoglycaemia, high cholesterol, constipation, migraines, muscle weakness, cramps, memory loss, infertility and hair loss.
- Diagnosis is made by detecting elevated levels of anti-TPO antibodies in the serum.
- On gross examination, there is often presentation of a firm goitre that is not painful to the touch. Other symptoms seen with hypothyroidism depends on the current state of progression of the response, especially given the usually gradual development of clinical hypothyroidism.
- Testing for TSH, Free T3, Free T4, and the anti-thyroglobulin antibodies (anti-Tg), anti-thyroid peroxidase antibodies (anti-TPO) and anti-microsomal antibodies can help obtain an accurate diagnosis.
- Earlier assessment of the patient may present with elevated levels of thyroglobulin.
- Hypothyroidism is the end product and this requires thyroxine replacement therapy.

Table 26.1 Thyroid conditions and levels of TSH, FT4 and antibodies in the blood.

THYROID DISEASE	TSH	FT4	ANTIBODIES
Post partum thyroiditis	low	high	normal
Sick euthryoid (eg elderly patient with normal TFT)	normal	normal	normal
Grave's disease(type 5 hypersensitivity reaction)	very low	high	TPO mildly elevated TSH Receptor-antibodies elevated
Hashimoto's disease (thyroid gland eventually replaced by lymphoid tissue, at risk of developing lymphoma)	high	normal/low in early stages, very low in late stages	TPO very high (>1000)
Toxic Multinodular goitre	low	high	normal

Station 27

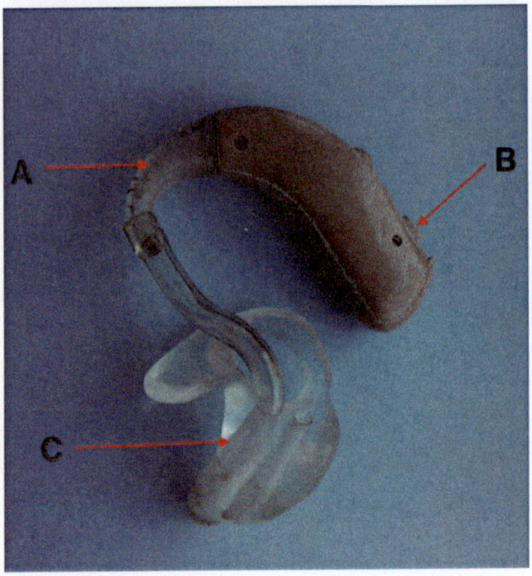

Questions

A. This hearing aid is for which ear?
B. Label A, B, C
C. What material is the hearing aid made of?
D. List 2 reasons why the hearing aid whistles.

Answers (Station 27)

Picture of behind the ear (BTE) hearing aid.

A. Left ear
B. A – ear hook
B – switch
C – ear mould
C. Acrylic
D. The hearing aid whistles when the microphone is too close to the speaker or when the ear canal is impacted with wax.

Revision Notes

- Behind the ear hearing aid is one of the most commonly used hearing aids for mild to severe hearing loss.
- It is useful to pay a visit to the audiology department and familiarise yourself with the different types of BTE hearing aids available and the location of the microphone, battery, tubing and T, M, O switch.
- The T, M, O switch stands for Telecoil, Microphone, Off.
- Hearing aids are getting smaller and smaller with patients now also using in the ear hearing aids although these devices are not as useful for severe hearing loss.
- BTE hearing aids are reliant on the patient having good air conduction.

Station 28

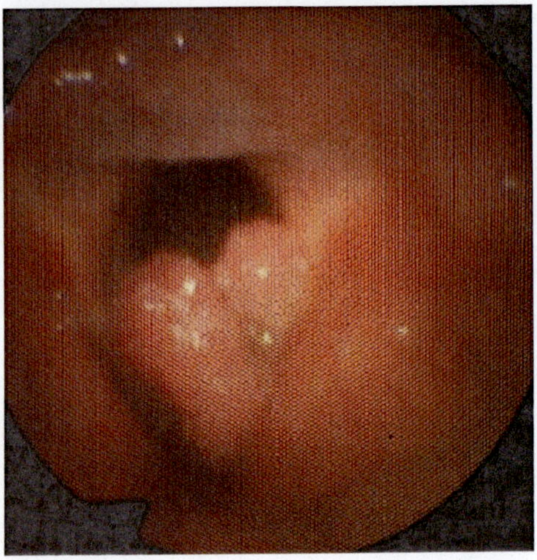

Questions

- **A.** What is the most likely diagnosis seen in this larynx?
- **B.** What is the aetiology of this condition?
- **C.** What symptoms would the patient present with?
- **D.** What is the surgical management of this condition?
- **E.** List 2 adjuvant treatment.
- **F.** What surgical procedure is avoided if possible and why?
- **G.** Why might this condition decrease in incidence in the future?

Answers (Station 28)

Clinical photograph of vocal cord papillomatosis.

- **A.** Laryngeal papillomatosis
  Squamous cell carcinoma
- **B.** Human Papillomatosis Virus (HPV) types 6 and 11; the latter is more aggressive.
- **C.** Hoarse voice
  Stridor
  Shortness of breath

In children they may have a weak cry, chronic cough and noisy breathing.

D. Surgical debridement ideally using a microdebrider; some units still use laser but this may cause an airway fire, spread the virus further into the airway or onto the operator!

E. **Adjuvant treatments**: Alpha interferon and antivirals such as intralesional Cidofivir.

F. Tracheostomy is avoided as the papillomatous lesions may spread and implant around the tracheostomy and also spread lower down into the lungs.

G. HPV vaccination using Gardasil.

Revision Notes

- The cluster of grape like lesions on the vocal cords in the picture above is characteristic of laryngeal papillomatosis.
- The papillomas appear to proliferate on squamous epithelium mainly so seedlings of papillomas lower down the respiratory tree suggests metaplasia.
- Frequent recurrence of the disease may require adjuvant treatment in addition to surgery.
- Medical treatment may also include indole-3-carbinol (cabbage juice derivative) and immunostimulants.
- During surgical treatment, care must be taken to avoid webbing of the anterior commissure.
- Tracheostomy is avoided to prevent seeding of the lesion further down in the airway.

Station 29

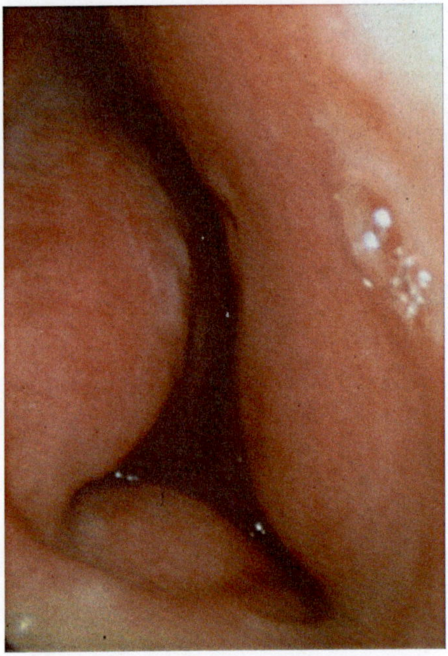

Questions

A. What is the diagnosis?

B. What symptoms would patients present with?

C. List 4 non-allergic causes of this condition.

D. What are the 3 groups of medication used to treat this condition?

E. List 3 surgical techniques to treat this condition.

Answers (Station 29)

Clinical photograph of an enlarged inferior turbinate and rhinorrhoea.

A. Inferior turbinate hypertrophy associated with rhinorhoea.

B. Nasal obstruction
Discharge

Post nasal drip
Symptoms of sinusitis such as facial pain.

C. Infection
Neoplasia
Congenital
Rhinitis medicamentosa.

D. Steroids
Antihistamines
Leukotriene antagonists.

E. Out fracture of turbinates
Submucous diathermy
Turbinate trimming.

Revision Notes

- Another cause for enlarged turbinates is allergic rhinitis.
- Computerised tomography (CT) scan of the paranasal sinuses would be a useful investigation as patients may also have underlying sinusitis.
- Rhinitis medicametosa arises from the prolonged use of nasal vasoconstrictors such as Oxymetazoline. The treatment of this condition includes stopping the nasal vasoconstrictors and commencing on a prolonged course of topical nasal steroids such as Mometazone (Nasonex).
- Because of the risk of rhinitis medicamentosa, patients are usually advised to use nasal vasoconstrictors for only one week.
- Following surgical intervention, such as FESS< patients must be warned that their symptoms may return, especially if there is an allergic cause.

Station 30

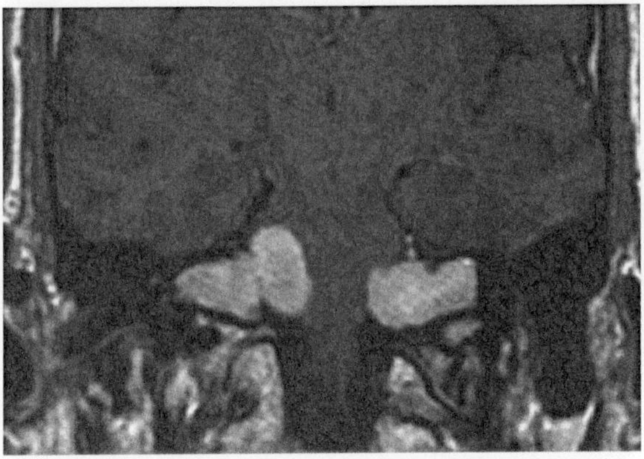

Questions

A. What is the plane of this image?

B. What is this investigation?

C. What is the differential diagnosis for lesions occurring in the cerebellar pontine angle?

D. What is the most likely diagnosis?

E. What condition is most likely associated with the above finding?

F. Name 2 other central nervous system lesions which may be associated with this condition.

Answers (Station 30)

Coronal MRI scan of brain with contrast showing bilateral acoustic neuromas in a patient who is complaining of bilateral tinnitus.

A. Coronal plane.

B. T1-weighted contrast Magnetic Resonance Imaging (MRI).

C. Acoustic neuroma
Meningioma
Epidermoid cyst
Cholesteatoma.

D. Bilateral acoustic neuromas.
E. Neurofibromatosis Type II.
F. Ependymomas and meningiomas (see Figures 30.2 and 30.3).

Revision Notes

- Patients with acoustic neuroma usually presents with tinnitus and hearing loss.
- Patients may also present late with symptoms of raised intracranial pressure and cerebellar dysfunction.
- Bilateral acoustic neuromas are associated with Neurofibromatosis type 2, an autosomal dominant condition associated with a mutation on chromosome 22.
- Schwanomas may also exist in a cystic form (Figure 30.1).
- A pathonomonic sign of inheritance is juvenile sub-capsular cataract.
- The gold standard investigation for acoustic neuroma is Magnetic Resonance Imaging (MRI).
- Audiometry would show a sensorineural hearing loss.
- The management of acoustic neuroma could be divided into:
    - Watchful waiting if patient asymptomatic with serial Magnetic Resonance Imaging
    - Stereotactic radiosurgery such as gamma knife
    - Surgical excision which could be translabyrinthine, middle fossa or retrosigmoid approach.
- Retrocochlear pathology, such as a vestibular schwannoma is associated with poor speech discrimination. Therefore residual hearing may not be useful and can be sacrificed during surgery.
- If surgery is performed to remove the lesion, the hearing loss is rehabilitated with an auditory brainstem implant

(ABI) at the time of primary surgery. The implant is placed onto the brainstem via the lateral opening of the 4th ventricle (Foramen of Luschka).

- **Basic key information pertaining to MRI and CT:**
  - Terms: low or high **signals/intensity** (with CT use the term hypo- or hyper- **dense**)
  - Low signal is black, High signal is white
  - T2 Water White (WW) i.e high signal
  - T1 Water Black, i.e. Low signal
  - Fat is high signal on both T1 and T2
  - Contrast (gad) is only given in T1; contrast may be seen in blood vessels or in choroid plexus.
  - Normally: T2 then T1 then T1 with contrast
  - Very black areas: Bone, Air, Flowing blood (flow voids)
  - When looking at a MRI consider the following plan: 'PCAP' – **P**lane, **C**ontrast given, **A**natomical location and **P**athology demonstrated [similarly when looking at a CT scan consider PwCAP – Plane, **w**indow (soft tissue or bone), Contrast given, Anatomical location and Pathology demonstrated].

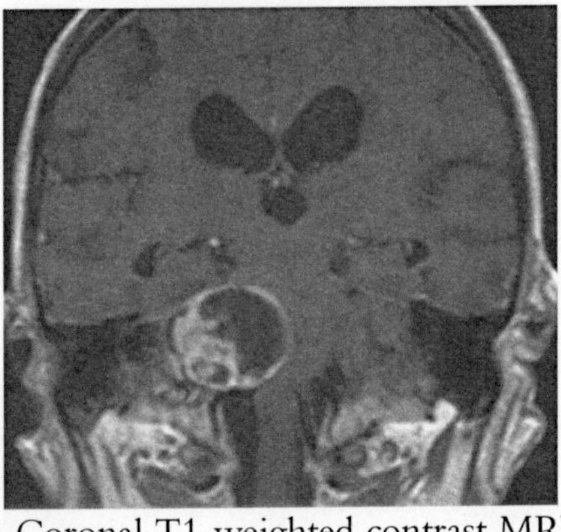

Figure 30.1 Coronal T1-weighted contrast MRI showing a cystic schwannoma.

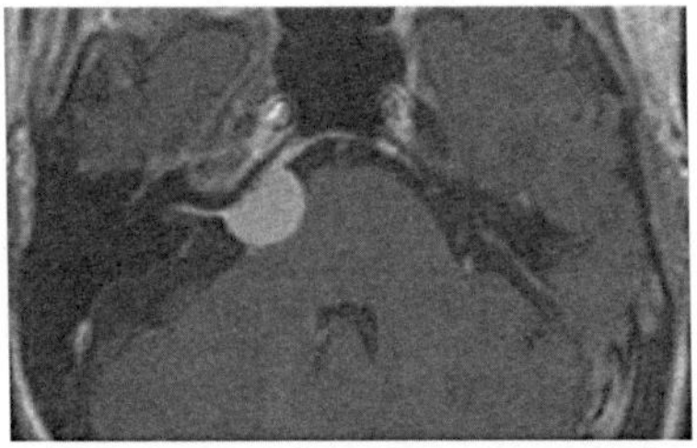

Figure 30.2 MRI scan showing a meningioma in the cerebellar pontine region (notice the characteric bilateral dural tails and broad base).

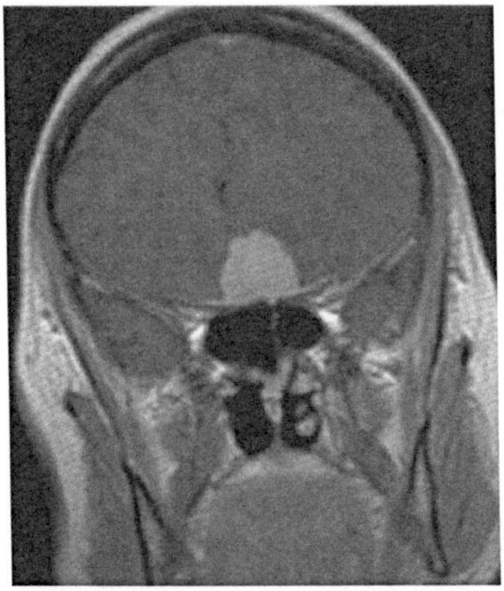

Figure 30.3 Olfactory groove meningioma (this patient presenting complaint was anosmia).

Station 31

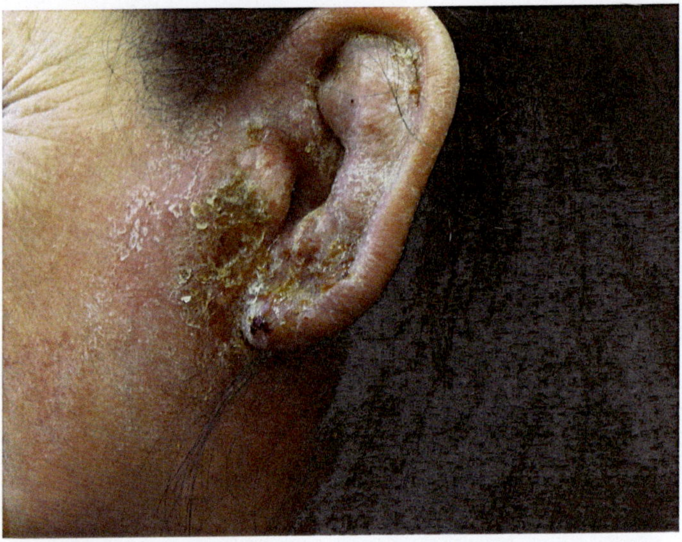

Questions

A. What is the diagnosis?

B. Name 2 groups of patients in which this condition is commonly seen.

C. What is the treatment?

D. What is this condition called if the aetiology is fungal?

E. Name 2 bacterial and 2 fungal organisms commonly associated with this condition.

Answers (Station 31)

Clinical photograph of a patient with severe otitis externa.

A. Otitis externa.

B. Swimmers/surfers
Immunocompromised patients such as diabetics or transplant patients.

C. Microbiological specimen
Regular microsuction
Topical antibiotic drops with steroids

Insertion of a pope wick if there is extensive oedema of the external auditory canal to facilitate the antibiotic drops to reach the deep ear canal by capillary action.

D. Otomycosis.

E. Staphylococcus aureus
Pseudomonas aeruginosa
Aspergillus niger
Aspergillus albicans.

Revision Notes

- Otitis externa is the inflammation of the skin lining the external auditory canal.
- Other conditions predisposing to otitis externa include humidity, heat, trauma and chronic skin diseases such as psoriasis and eczema.
- The aetiology of this condition is usually bacterial (90%).
- The complications of untreated disease include spread to temporal bone (malignant otitis externa), especially if the patient is immunocompromised. Spread of the infection to the petrous apex may lead to retro-orbital pain and 6th cranial nerve palsy (Gradenigo's syndrome).
- Otitis externa is an immunocompromised patient should raise suspicion of malignant otitis externa or necrotizing otitis externa. This condition is associated with considerable morbidity and mortality and requires long term intravenous antibiotics and sometimes surgical debridement.

Station 32

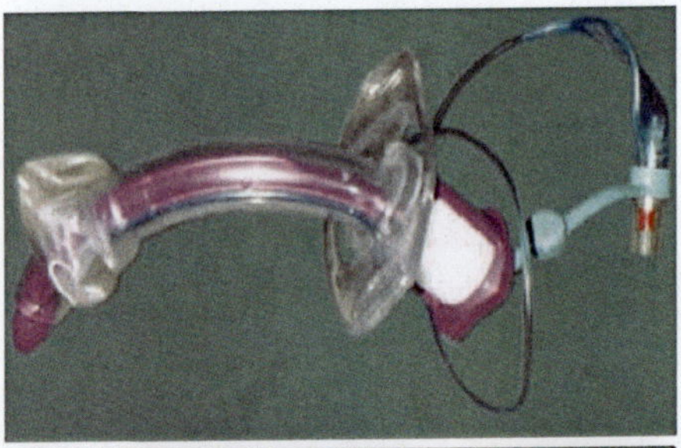
1.

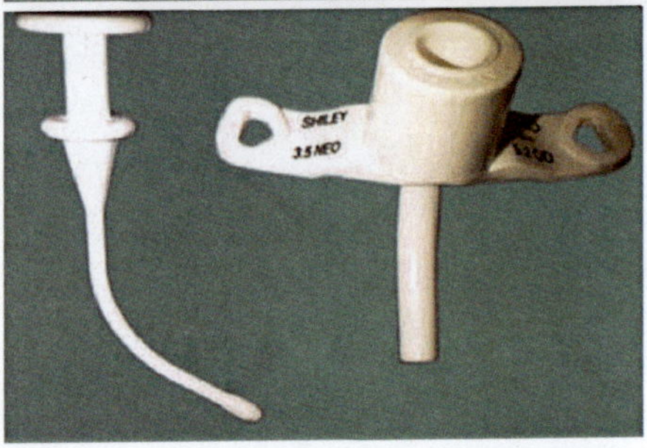

2.

Questions

A. What is picture 1?
B. What is picture 2?
C. Why are paediatric tracheostomy tubes uncuffed?
D. List 3 indications for an uncuffed tracheostomy tube.
E. What are the complications of tracheostomy?

Answers (Station 32)

Pictures of tracheostomy tubes.

A. Cuffed adult tracheostomy tube.
B. Neonatal tracheostomy tube.
C. To reduce the risk of subglottic stenosis.
D. Children
Vocalisation
Upper airway obstruction.

E. **Early** – bleeding, infection, recurrent laryngeal nerve injury, surgical emphysema, pneumothorax, tube displacement and tube obstruction.
Late – tracheocutaneous fistula, tracheoesophageal fistula, tracheal stenosis, tracheoinnominate artery fistula.

Revision Notes

- There is a range of different tracheostomy tubes and it is important to be able to differentiate between a cuffed and an uncuffed tracheostomy tube, if it has an adjustable flange, fenestrations or inner tube.
- The inner tube is longer than the tracheostomy tube so it collects secretions and allows removal and cleaning of the tube without the need to remove the tracheostomy tube.
- An adjustable flange tube (Figures 32.1 and 32.2) is used for patients with larger necks or increased pretracheal space.
- Some tracheostomy tubes have fenestrations to allow speech in patients. These patients will need to be able to protect their own airway. Thus these tubes are useful to aid weaning in patients.

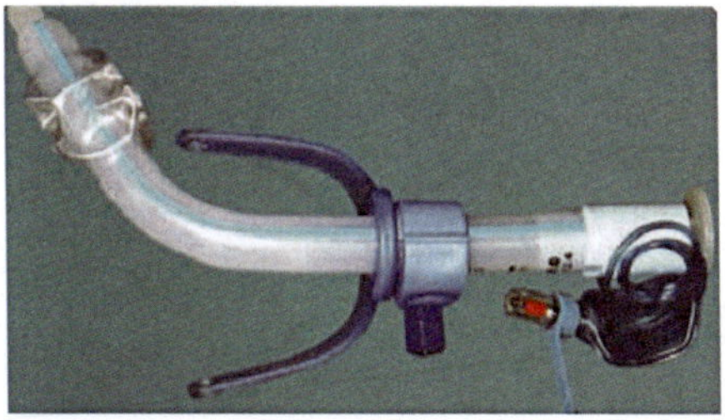

Figure 32.1 Adjustable flange tracheostomy tube (requires air to fill cuff).

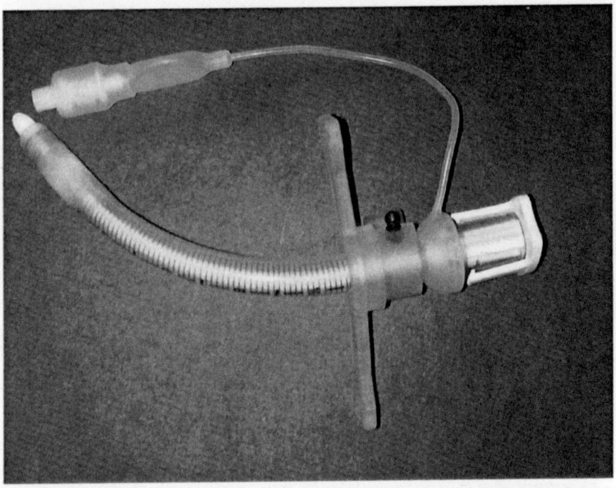

Figure 32.2 Bivona adjustable flange tracheostomy tube (requires water to fill cuff).

Station 33

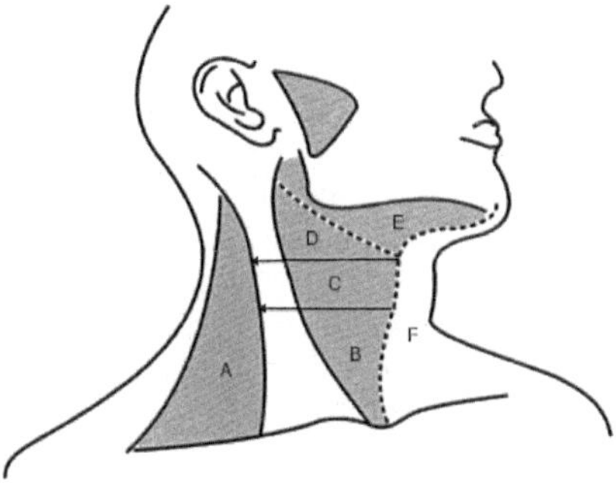

Questions

A. Name neck levels A, B, E.

B. What structures could be damaged during neck dissection of area B?

C. What are the 3 structures that may be preserved in modified radical neck dissection?

D. If doing lymph node excision in area A, which nerve is at risk?

E. To which area does the lymphatic drainage of the tongue tip go to?

F. Following a neck dissection, a patient complains of numbness over the lateral aspect of the forearm. Which dermatome is affected?

Answers (Station 33)

Picture of neck levels.

A. A – Level V
B – level IV
E – level I

B. Corotid sheath and it's structures such as internal jugular vein, carotid artery and vagus nerve, Spinal accessory nerve
Brachial plexus
Pleura.

C. Accessory nerve
Sternocleidomastoid muscle
Internal jugular vein.

D. Accessory nerve.

E. Level I (Area E).

F. C6 (see Figure 33.6).

Revision Notes

- Lymph nodes in the neck (Figure 33.1) are divided into 6 different levels (Figure 33.2, Table 33.1); this should not be confused with neck triangles (Figure 33.3) or the three trauma zones in the neck (Figure 33.4, Table 33.2).
- Level I contain the submental and submandibular lymph nodes.
- Level II contains lymph nodes around the upper third of the internal jugular vein while levels III and IV are lymph nodes around middle and lower third of the internal jugular vein respectively.
- Level V consists of lymph nodes in the posterior triangle while level VI is the anterior lymph nodes containing paratracheal and perithyroidal lymph nodes.
- Oral cavity tumours commonly spread to levels I, II and III while laryngeal tumours would spread to levels II, III and IV.
- In vary rare cases, patients may require bilateral radical neck dissection. The main complication from this procedure is increased intracranial pressure due to removal of both internal jugular veins. This surgery is possible because of the emmissory veins which connect the intracranial venous system with the extracranial system. These patients will need to be nursed sitting up in the bed and may also require mannitol to reduce the intracranial pressure.

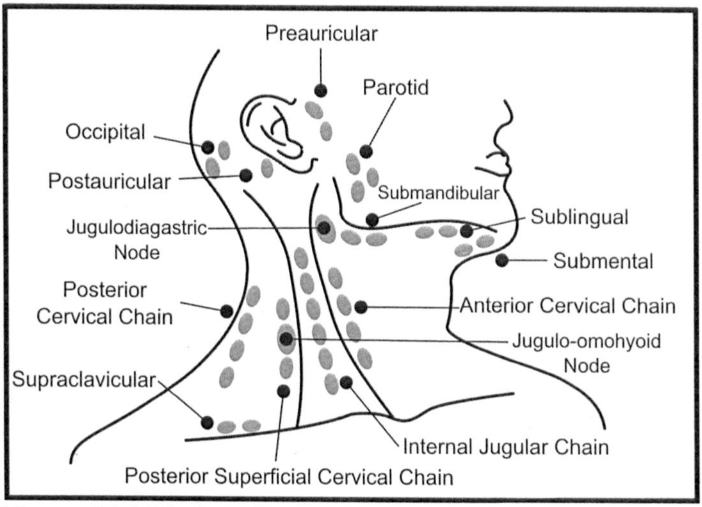

Figure 33.1 Neck nodes.

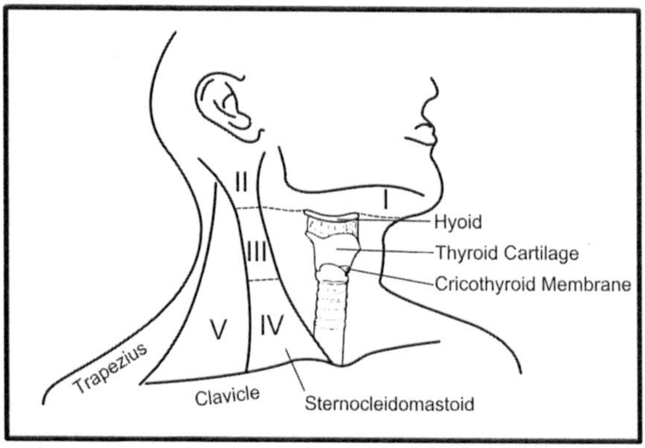

Figure 33.2 Neck levels.

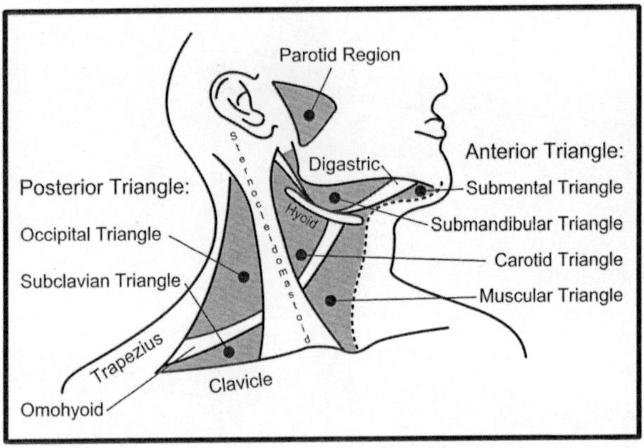

Figure 33.3 Neck triangles with sub-divisions

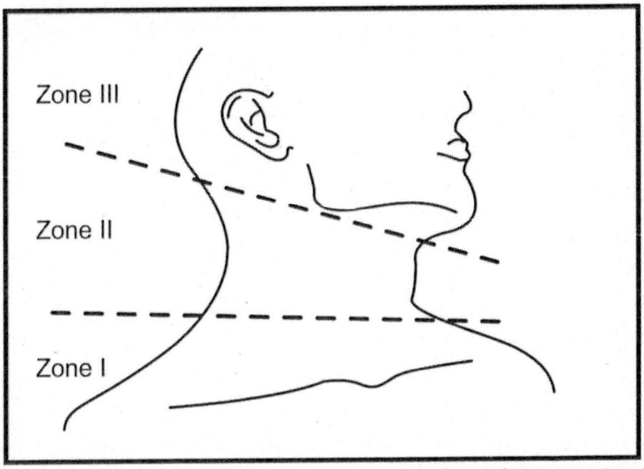

Figure 33.4 Neck trauma zones (I clavicle to cricoid, II cricoid to angle of mandible, III angle of mandible to skull base).

Table 33.1 Levels in the neck according to Head and Neck surgeons.

Levels	Boundaries
I	Hyoid bone and body of mandible; anterior and posterior bellies of digastric
II	Skull base to hyoid and across to posterior margin of sternocleidomastoid muscle
III	Hyoid to lower border of cricoid and across to posterior margin of sternocleidomastoid muscle
IV	Clavicle to lower border of cricoid and across to posterior margin of sternocleidomastoid muscle
V	Clavicle to skull base and between posterior border of sternocleidomastoid muscle to anterior border of trapezius muscleclavicle to

Table 33.2 Zones in the neck according to trauma surgeons.

Zones	Limits	Vulnerable structures	Comments
III	Area between the angle of the mandible and skull base	Internal jugular vein, internal internal carotid artery, parotid and submandibular gland, pharynx oral cavity and vertebrobasilar complex.	Rapid surgical access is hampered and may require mandibular disarticulation or mandibulotomy for access to the great vesssels.
II	Area between the lower border of the cricoid	Internal jugular vein, common carotid artery, external carotid artery and	Easy to access and associated with good prognosis.

	cartilage and the angle of the mandible	branches, internal carotid artery, vertebral artery and spinal cord.	
I	Area between the upper border of the clavicle and the lower border of the cricoid	Apex of lungs, trachea, oesophagus, aortic arch, branchiocephalic veins, contents of carotid sheath.	Poor access and rapid blood loss means that the mortality rate is high from injuries in this area, especially in non-trauma units.

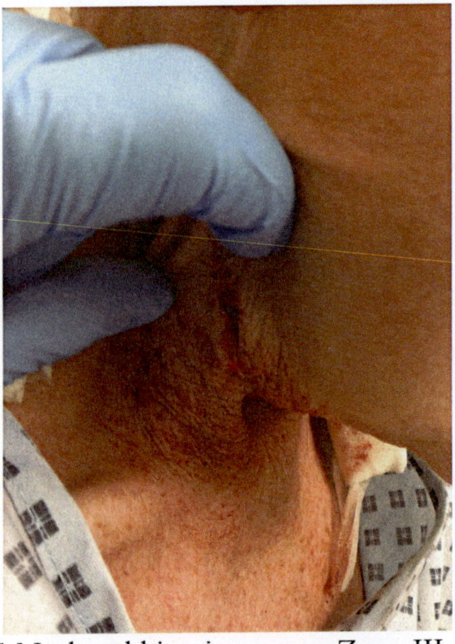

Figure 33.5 Neck stabbing in trauma Zone III caused by a scissors (fortunately did not reach the internal jugular vein).

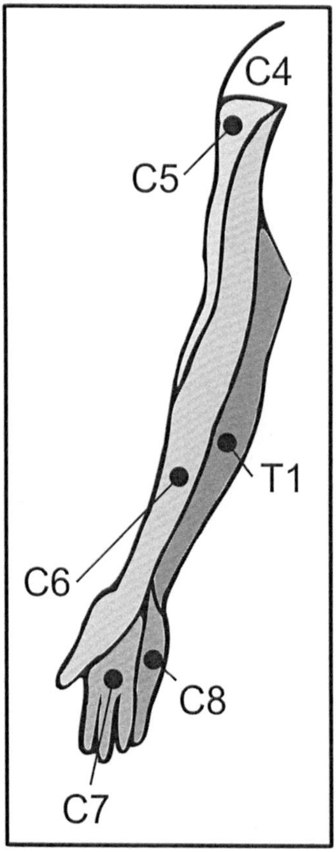

Figure 33.6 Dermotome distributions of the upper limb (note T1 nerve supplies medial forearm).

Station 34

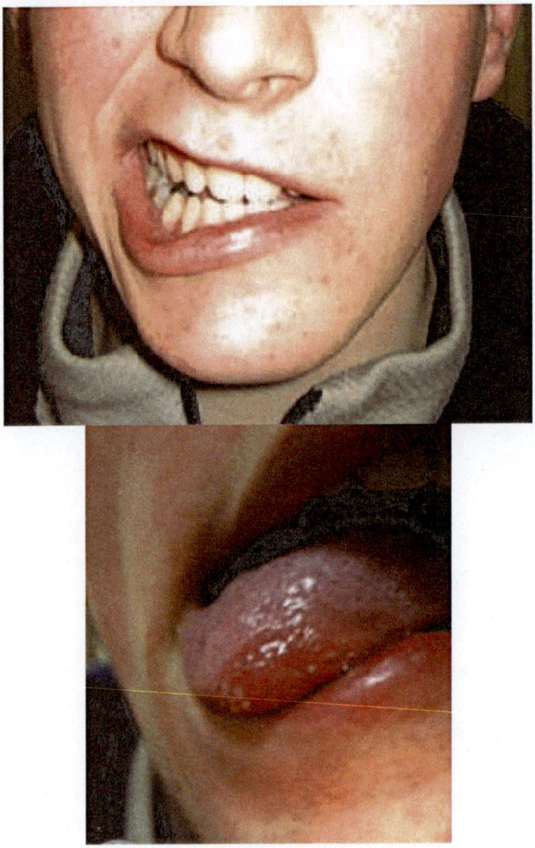

Questions

A. What is the diagnosis?

B. What is the causative organism?

C. Where does the organism remain dormant?

D. What would the stapedial reflex be in this patient?

E. What sound intensity level is required to elicit stapedial reflexes?

F. What are the systemic manifestations of this condition in immunocompromised individuals?

G. Name one grading system for the above condition.

Answers (Station 34)

Clinical photographs of patient with unilateral LMN CN VII palsy and vesicles on the tongue in the distribution of chorda tymapani.

A. Ramsay Hunt syndrome (left lower motor neuron facial nerve palsy with vesicles in the distribution of chorda tympani).

B. Herpes zoster virus.

C. Geniculate ganglion of the facial nerve.

D. High compliance due to lack of stapedial muscle action.

E. 85dB

F. Meningitis
Encephalitis
Disseminated spread of infection across multiple dermatomes
Atypical pneumonia.

G. House-Brackmann Grading system.

Revision Notes

- Painful vesicular lesions due to Herpes Zoster virus and a lower motor neuron Facial Nerve palsy is also known as Ramsay Hunt Syndrome.
- Following initial infection with the chicken pox virus (Varicella Zoster virus), the virus lies dormant in the geniculate ganglion, which has the cell bodies of chorda tympani nerve.
- The virus is re-activated in times of stress, aging or immunosuppresion.
- Vesicular lesions could be seen in the pinna (Figure 34.1), palate or on the tongue.
- Rarely, there is involvement of the eighth cranial nerve causing vertigo, tinnitus and hearing loss.
- Prompt treatment with neuropathic analgesia, steroids and antiviral agent is recommended to reduce the risk of

complications such as permanent facial muscle weakness and deafness.

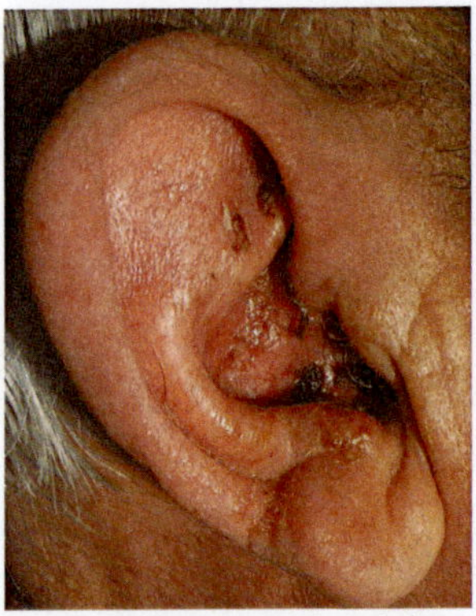

Figure 34.1 Clinical photograph of herpes zoster oticus affecting the sensory branch of the facial nerve to ear (this patient had Ramsey Hunt syndrome).

Table 34.1 House-Brackmann grading system for facial nerve palsy.

Grade	Definition
I	Normal symmetrical function in all areas
II	Slight weakness noticeable only on close inspection Complete eye closure with minimal effort Slight asymmetry of smile with maximal effort Synkinesis barely noticeable, contracture, or spasm absent
III	Obvious weakness, but not disfiguring May not be able to lift eyebrow **Complete eye closure** and strong but asymmetrical mouth movement with maximal effort

	Obvious, but not disfiguring synkinesis, mass movement or spasm
IV	Obvious disfiguring weakness Inability to lift brow **Incomplete eye closure** and asymmetry of mouth with maximal effort Severe synkinesis, mass movement, spasm
V	Motion barely perceptible Incomplete eye closure, slight movement corner mouth Synkinesis, contracture, and spasm usually absent
VI	No movement, loss of tone, no synkinesis, contracture, or spasm

Adapted from: House JW, Brackmann DE. Facial nerve grading system. *Otolaryngology Head and Neck surg 1985; 93(2):146-147.*

Station 35

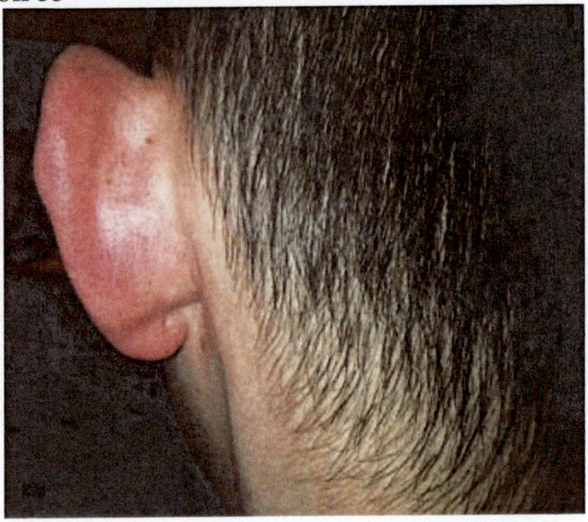

Questions

A. What is the diagnosis?
B. What is the cause for this?
C. What is the management for this condition?
D. When is the advisable time to offer treatment for this condition?
E. Would the management be different if this condition presented in a neonate?

Answers (Station 35)

Clinical photograph of a left prominent ear.

A. Prominent ears (Bat ears).
B. Lack of antihelical fold, deep conchal bowl and protruding lobule.
C. Conservative or surgical with surgical treatment being offered is pinnaplasty.
D. Pre-school years to avoid patient getting teased in school.
E. Yes, the use of an ear splint would be an effective treatment.

Revision Notes

- Prominent ears can cause teasing and bullying that can carry on into adult life.
- Treatment options include camouflaging technique and otoplasty surgery.
- The main surgical techniques to address the anti helix are anterior scoring of the cartilage, posterior cartilaginous trenches made with a diamond burr and the Mustarde suturing method.
- Complications of surgical treatment are bleeding, infection, pinna haematoma, cartilage necrosis, asymmetry, telephone ear deformity and patient dissatisfaction.

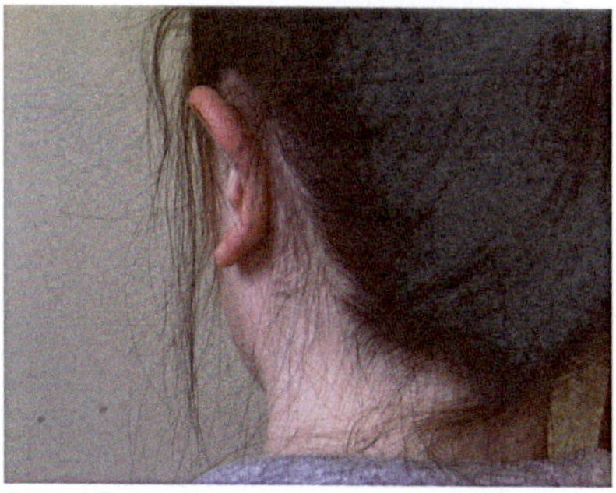

Figure 35.1 Telephone ear deformity following pinnaplasty.

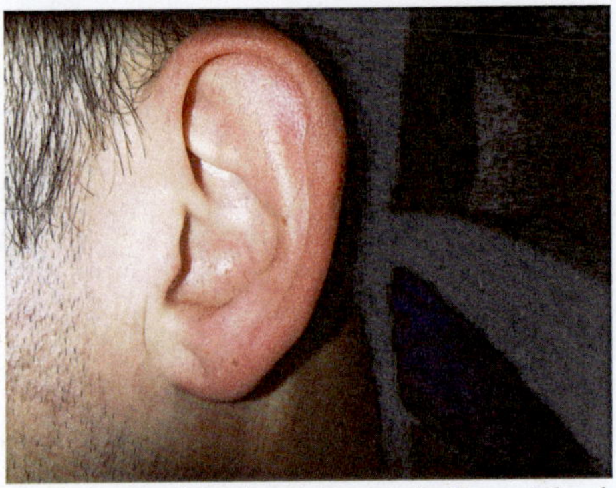

Figure 35.2a Underdeveloped anti-helix with the concha-scaphoid angle greater than 90 degrees.

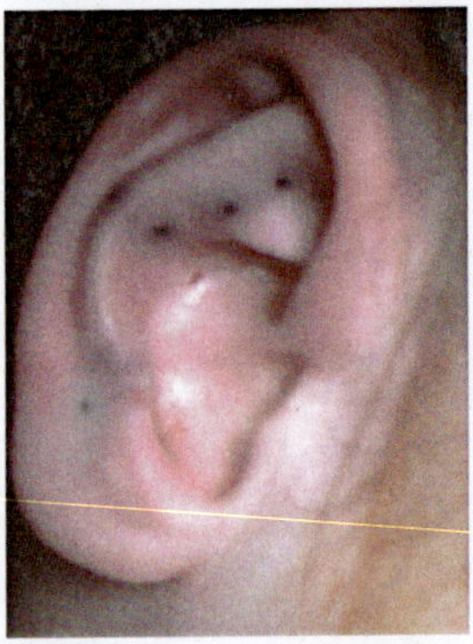

Figure 35.2b Clinical photograph showing correction of prominent ear with clearly defined antihelix and the concha-scaphoid angle less than 90 degrees.

Station 36

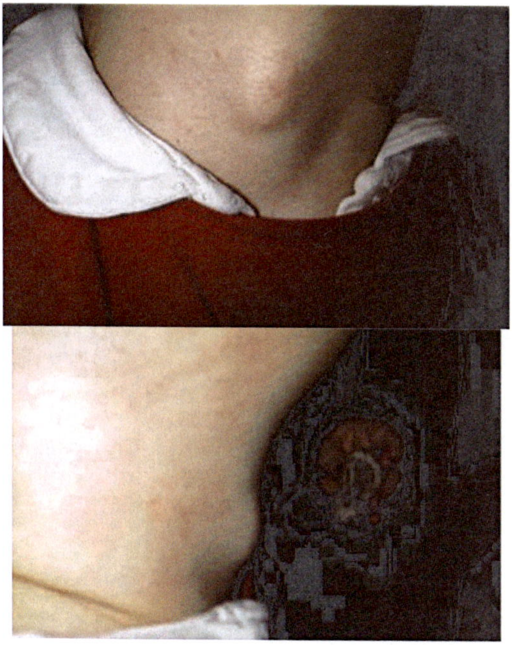

Questions

A. What is the diagnosis if the patient is 4 years old?
B. What is the embryological origin of this swelling?
C. What symptoms and signs would the patient present with?
D. How would you further investigate this condition?

Answers (Station 36)

Clinical photograph of a thyroglossal duct cyst.

A. Thyroglossal duct cyst.
B. The cyst is present due to a persistent duct following the migration of the thyroid gland from the tongue base to anterior of the trachea in the neck.
C. Midline swelling in neck with intermittent increase in swelling and pain due to infections. Patient may have

dysphagia and dyspnoea if lump is large. The lump would move with tongue protrusion.

D. Ultrasound scan
Radio-iodine uptake scan (Prior to excision as there may be active thyroid tissue in the cyst)
MRI.

Revision Notes

- A thyroglossal duct cyst can occur anywhere along the developmental path of the thyroid gland.
- The majority of thyroglossal cysts occur in the midline while 10% occur on the left side and only 1% on the right.
- They should not be incised and drained because this would result a persistent discharging sinus.
- Failure to remove the body of the hyoid bone during surgery for a thyroglossal duct cyst leads to a recurrence rate of 80–85%.
- Sistrunk's procedure is the technique of choice as it involves the removal of the body of the hyoid bone and reduces the risk of recurrence.
- Postoperative accumulation of infection or haematoma may push the tongue base up into the airway and give rise to a 'Ludwig's' angina type of airway emergency.

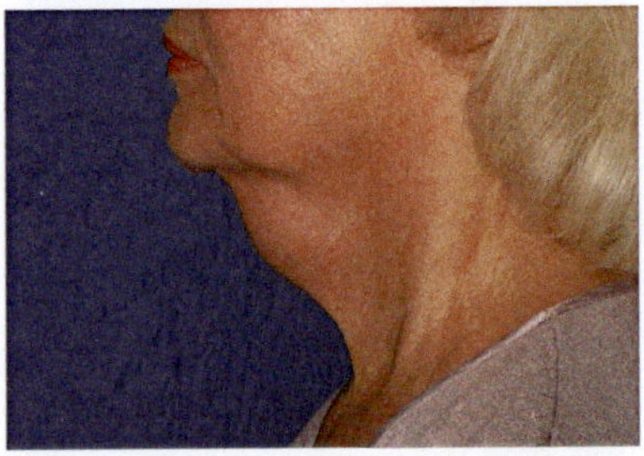

Figure 36.1a Thyroglossal duct cyst may also be present in late adulthood.

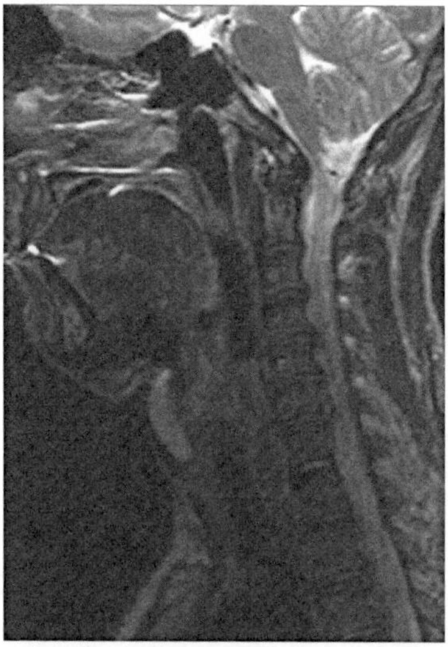

Figure 36.1b Sagittal MRI showing a thyroglossal duct cyst.

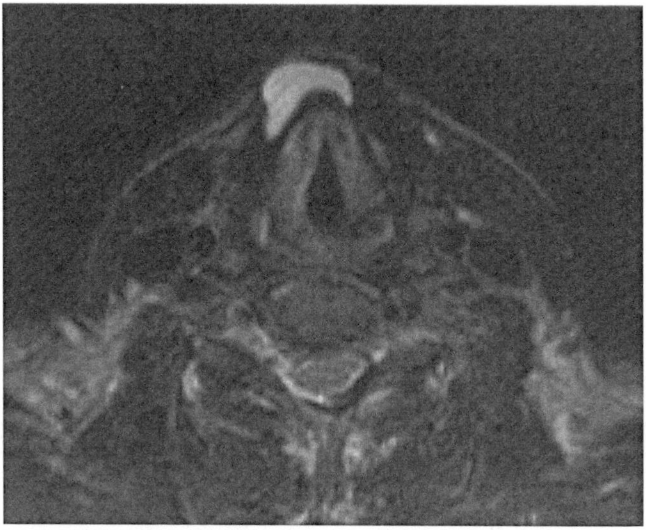

Figure 36.1c Axial MRI showing a thyglossal duct cyst.

Station 37

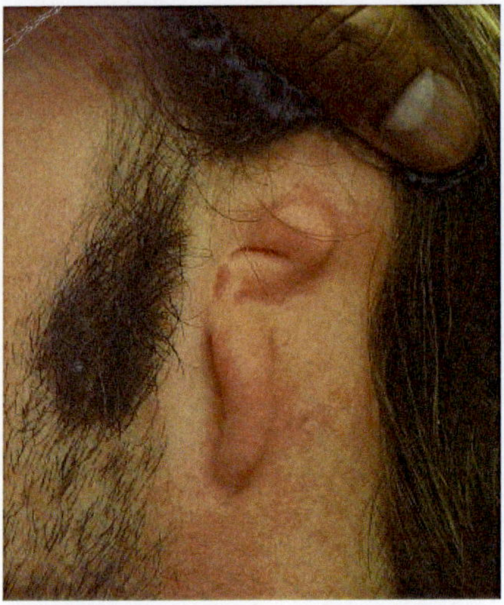

Questions

A. What do we call this condition and what is the medical name for total absence of the pinna?

B. What type of hearing loss is associated with this condition?

C. List 2 associated syndromes.

D. What type of hearing aid is suitable for this condition?

Answers (Station 37)

Clinical photograph of a patient with microtia.

A. Microtia and Anotia.

B. Conductive hearing loss (30-60 dB CHL).

C. Goldenhar syndrome and Treacher-Collins (also Pierre-Robin and CHARGE syndrome).

D. Bone conduction hearing aid (BCHA), eg BCHA on a soft band trial and then a BAHA.

Revision Notes

- Microtia results in functional and cosmetic issues.
- Canal atresia is usually present with microtia.
- For management of a patient with microtia, it is important to know if the condition is unilateral or bilateral and if the patient is syndromic.
- A multidisciplinary team is required for proper management, especially if the patient is syndromic.
- Surgical reconstruction is challenging because of abnormal middle ear anatomy or disease, eg facial nerve anomalies and cholesteatoma.
- Reconstruction of the pinna is usually done after the age 6-8 when the ribs are of adequate size for rib cartilage graft reconstruction and, in the case of unilateral microtia, when the other pinna reaches normal adult size (for comparison).
- A prosthetic ear is the alternative for cosmetic reconstruction.
- A bone anchored hearing aid is commonly used for the rehabilitation of hearing loss because of canal atresia. This involves the osteointegration of a titanium screw into the skull (figure 37.1) onto which the processor is attached (Figure 37.2).

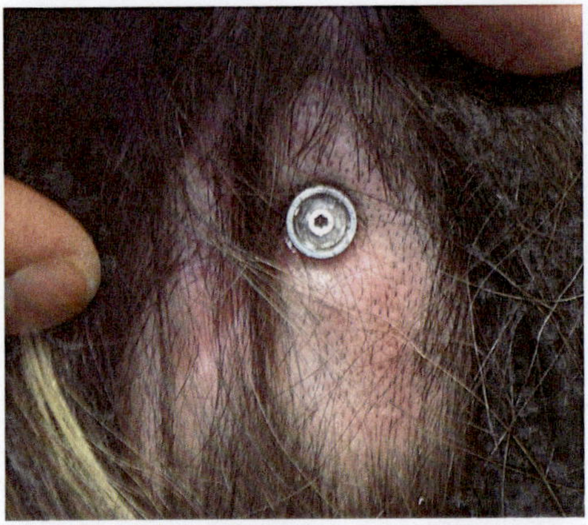

Figure 37.1 BAHA Titanium screw implanted into the skull.

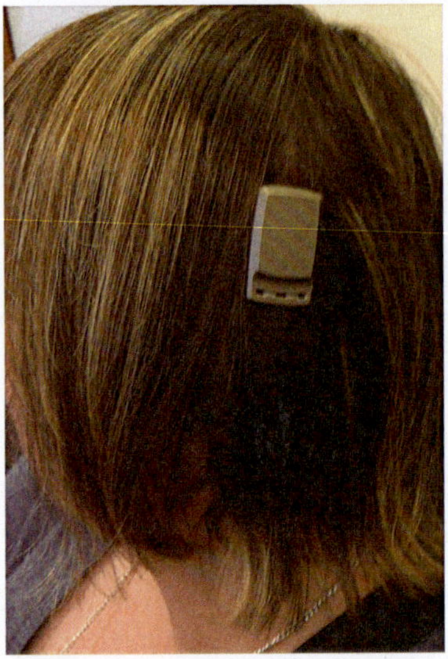

Figure 37.1 BAHA processor attached to titanium screw.

Station 38

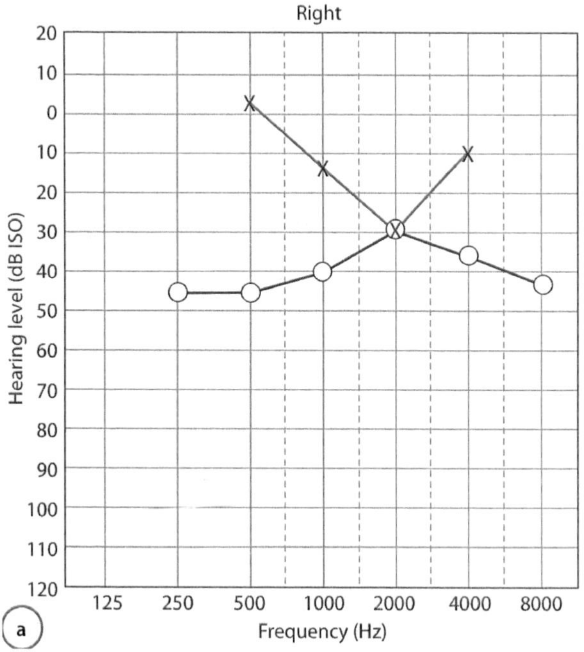

Questions

A. What is this investigation?

B. What is the dip at 2kHz called?

C. What is the most likely diagnosis?

D. What are the treatment options?

E. What further audiometric test would you do to confirm your diagnosis?

Answers (Station 38)

PTA with Conductive hearing loss – Cahart's notch.

A. Pure tone audiometry.

B. Cahart's notch.

C. Otosclerosis.

D. Conservative with hearing aids or surgical by stapedectomy.

E. Tympanometry to rule out fluid in the middle ear and stapedial reflexes; a speech audiogram is also important to invistigate if the cochlea is involved.

Revision Notes

- Often patients will present with family history of hearing loss as otosclerosis is an autosomal dominant metabolic bone disease with incomplete penetrence; nearly 85% of patients will have bilateral disease.
- Otosclerosis affects the otic capsule endochondral layer where mature lamellar bone is replaced by soft woven bone of greater cellularity and vascularity.
- Anterior of the oval window (fissula ante fenestrum) is the commonest site affected; other sites affected include posterior to the oval window (fissula post fenestrum), semicircular canals, the round window and the cochlea.
- Otosclerosis manifests as a conductive hearing loss with a normal tympanic membrane and absent stapedial reflex.
- On examination, the patient may have a faint pink tinge on the cochlear promontory known as the Schwartz's sign (Figure 38.1).
- The conductive hearing loss is due to the reduced mobility of the stapes footplate and hence reduced conduction of sound.
- Aetiopathogenic theories are:
    - (a) it is an expression of persistent measles virus infection of otic capsule-derived bone,
    - (b) it is an expression of a genetic mutation in collagen metabolism which is only expressed in bone derived from the otic capsule.
    - (c) it is an expression of autoimmunity to type II collagen.

- Late stages of otosclerosis may show a high frequency sensorineural hearing loss when the cochlear becomes damaged.
- Surgical treatment involves replacing the stapes (stapedectomy) with prosthesis (eg Teflon piston, Figures 38.2a and b).
- The minimum requirements for stapedectomy are at least a 15 dB conductive hearing loss with at least 60% speech discrimination; hence the importance of performing speech audiogram in affected patients (poor speech discrimination reflects cochlear otosclerosis, Figure 38.3).
- Complications of surgical treatment:

  Early: Bleeding
  Dead ear
  Facial nerve palsy
  Perilymph fistula
  Vertigo
  Tinnitus
  Displacement of prosthesis from incus

  Late: Secondary perilymph fistula
  Necrosis of long process of incus

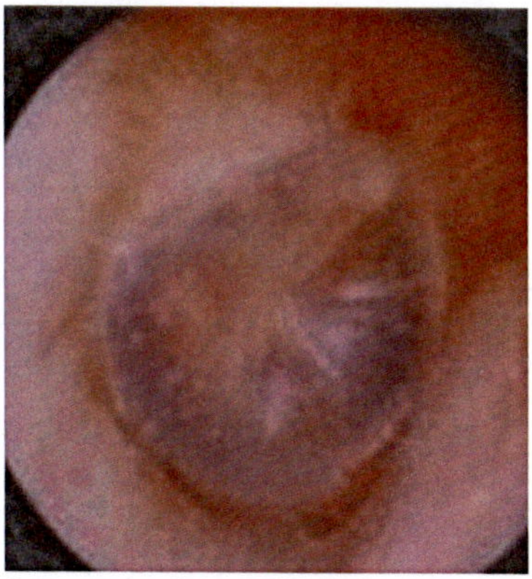

Figure 38.1 Schwartz's sign of active otospongiosis.

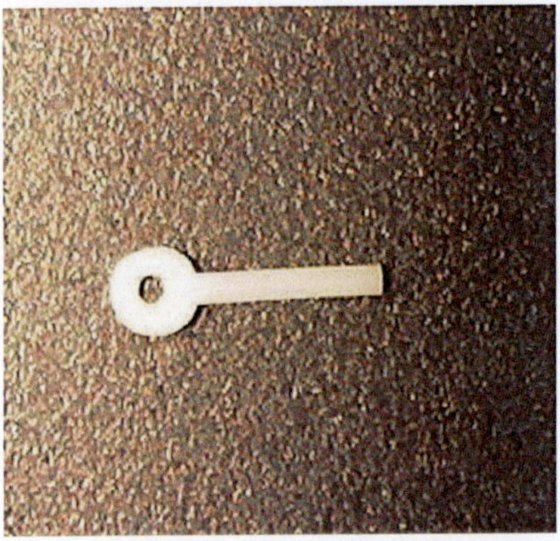

Figure 38.2a A Teflon piston before expansion to fit around the long process of Incus

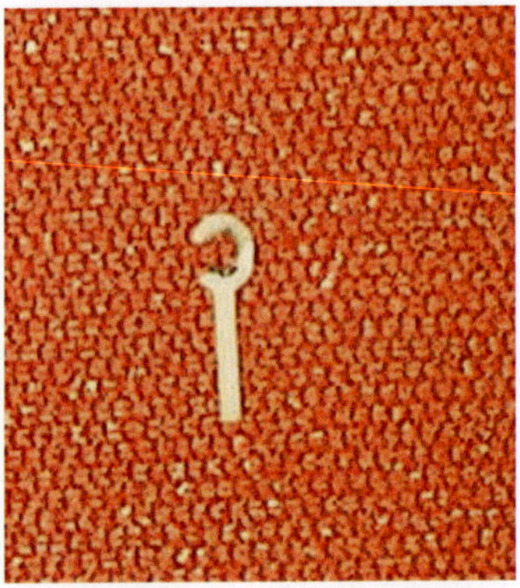

Figure 38.2b A Teflon piston after expansion to fit around the long process of Incus

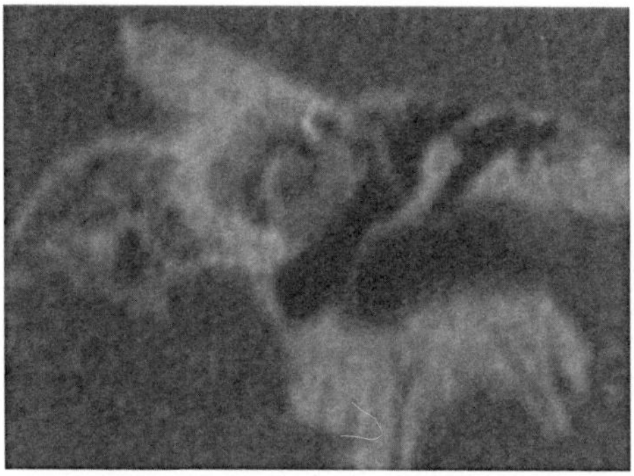

Figure 38.3 A CT scan showing cochlear otosclerosis (note the double density around the snail-like structure).

Station 39

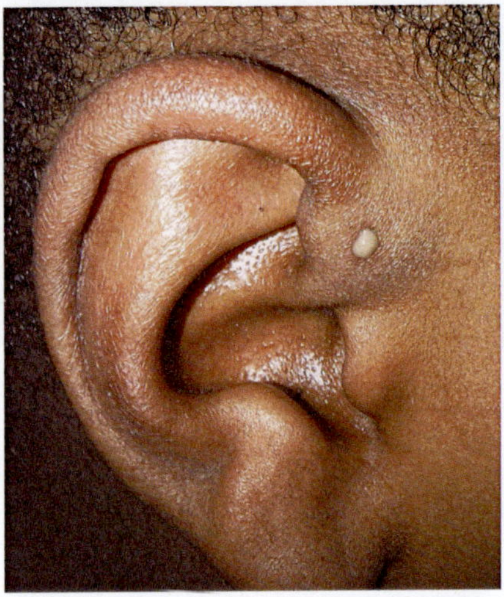

Questions

A. What is the pathology shown in the clinical photograph?

B. What is the embryological orgin of this abnormality?

C. Which syndrome might this abnormality be associated with?

D. Briefly explain how this lesion is treated surgically (assuming the patient is fully consented, appropriately draped, supine and anaesthetised).

E. List 4 complications of surgery.

Answers (Station 39)

Clinical photograph of a discharging preauricular sinus or pit.

A. Preauricular sinus or pit.

B. Incomplete fusion of the Hillock of His.

C. Brachio-oto-renal syndrome consisting of an additional discharging pit in the neck, hearing loss and kidney dysfunction.

D. Elliptical incision followed by dissection down to temporalis fascia and cartilage of the root of helix, which may be resected. Methylene blue may be helpful.

E. Bleeding, infection, scar, re-occurrence if inadequately excised.

Revision Notes

- The pinna is formed from 6 hillocks of His derived from branchial arches 1 and 2.
- A preauricular sinus is not a first branchial arch abnormality.
- Asymptomatic preauricular sinuses are usually left alone.
- An infected preauricular sinus (Figure 39.1) is initially treated with antibiotics and then booked for interval surgery (Figure 39.2a and 39.2b). The facial nerve is not an issue during surgical resection as it deep to the abnormality.

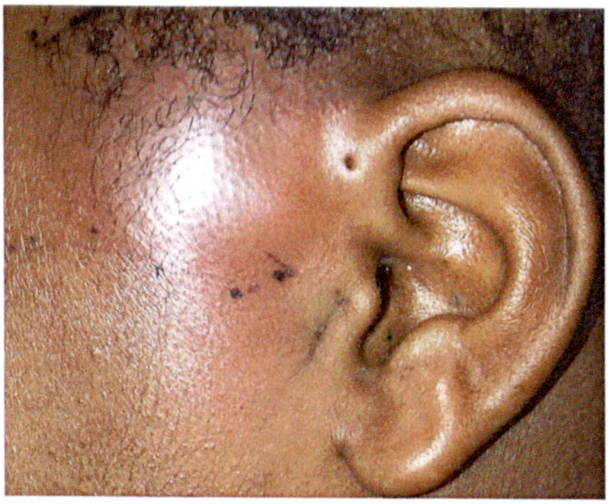

Figure 39.1 Infected preauricular sinus.

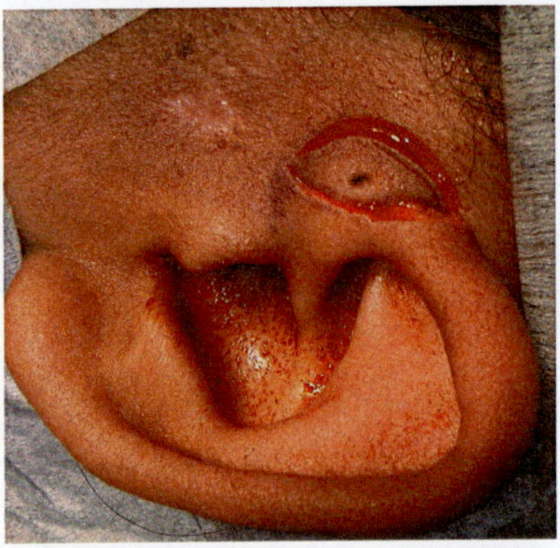

Figure 39.2a Incision to remove a preauricular sinus.

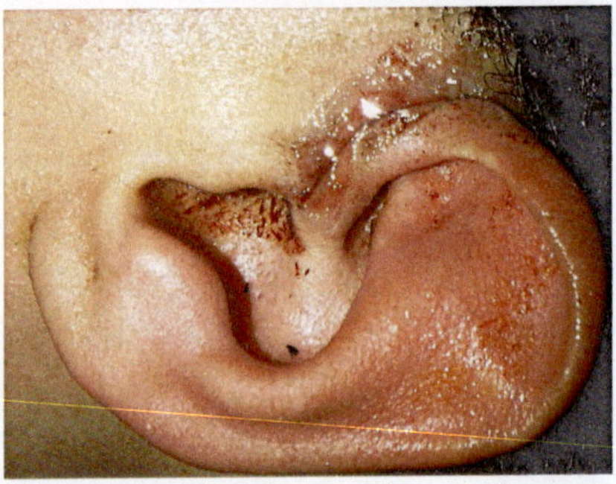

Figure 39.2b Tissue glue used to close incision after removal of a preauricular sinus (this avoids the need to remove stitches. Dissolvable stitches may also be used).

Station 40

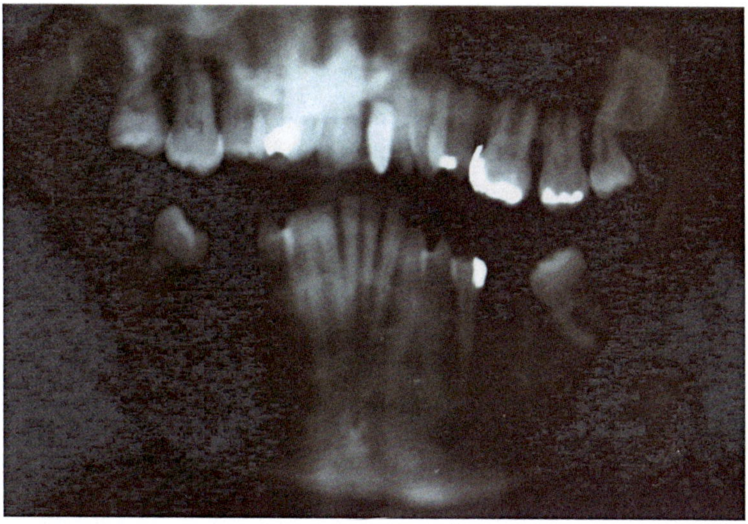

Questions

A. What does the X-ray show?
B. What other investigations could be used to assist in diagnosis?
C. What symptoms may this patient present with?
D. List 4 treatment options for this condition.
E. What determines which surgical approach is used?
F. If hypertension, palpitation, hypercalcaemia and renal calculi (urolithiasis) were also present, which syndrome might this be associated with?

Answers (Station 40)

X- ray showing submandibular gland stone.

A. Submandibular gland stone.
B. Sialogram or ultrasound.
C. Pain worse on eating
Submandibular swelling
Abscess formation
Pyrexia.

D. Conservative treatment initially by hydration, analgesia and sialogogues.
If symptoms are persistent, lithotripsy is a non invasive technique of removing the stone. Therapeutic sialoendoscopy to remove the stone is possible as well.
Surgical treatment includes excision of stone by widening the duct or submandibular gland excision.

E. Site and size of the stone.

F. Multiple Endocrine Neoplasia Type IIA (MEN2A) (Table 40.1).

Revision Notes

- Formation of stones in the salivary glands and their ducts is also known as sialolithiasis.
- The stones are commonly composed of calcium and hydroxyapatite.
- 8 in 10 occur in the submandibular duct, whilst 1 in 20 occur in the parotid and only 1 in 50 occur in the sublingual glands.
- Around 90% of submandibular stones are radio-opaque, but only 10% of parotid stones are radio-opaque.
- Sialography, involves injecting dye into the salivary duct openings to enable visualisation of stones and strictures in the ducts, is 100% reliable in making the diagnosis if duct cannulation occurs.
- Lithotripsy has been shown to be effective in the management of small stones (<7 mm) only while larger stones will require surgical removal.

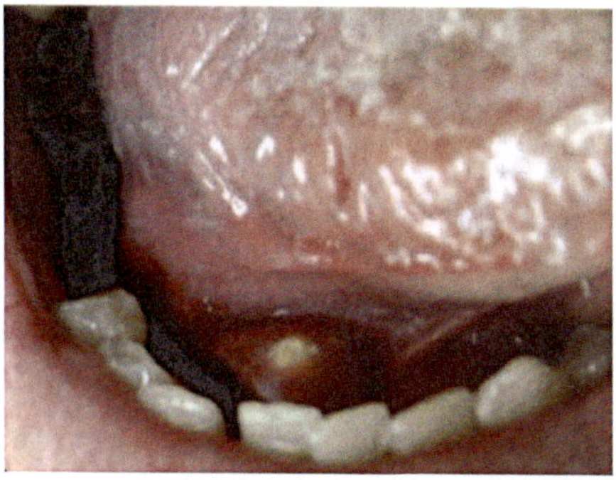

Figure 40.1 Clinical photograph showing a calculus in right Wharton's duct of the submandibular gland.

Table 40.1 Summary of multiple endocrine neoplasias (MEN).

Syndrome	Neoplasias	Features
MEN1	Parathyroid Pancreas Pituitary	Hypercalcaemia, renal stones, hypoglycaemia, galactorrhoea, acromegaly
MEN2A	Medullary cell Phaeochromocytoma Parathyroid	Hypertension, palpitations, hypercalcaemia, urolithiasis
MEN2B	Medullary cell Phaeochromocytoma Multiple neuromas	Marfanoid appearance

Station 41

A 66 year old man presents with severe epistaxis. He is taking warfarin because of a metallic heart valve.

Questions

A. Following anterior nasal packing, what tests would you perform?

B. What other treatment would you institute? List 5.

C. What would you inform the nurses in the ward to monitor?

D. If patient continues to bleed what are the other treatment options?

E. Name the 4 arteries that make up Kisselbach plexus in Little's area?

Answers (Station 41)

A. Full Blood Count
Urea and Electrolytes
Liver Function Test
Coagulation Screen including International Normalised Ratio (INR)
Cross match blood.

B. Oral antibiotics
Analgesia
Intraveneous fluids
Stop warfarin
Commence heparin infusion
If there is active profuse bleeding, reversal of warfarin with vitamin K may be needed.

C. Monitor for any further bleeding and patient's observations such as respiratory rate, blood pressure and heart rate.

D. Posterior nasal packing with Foley catheter and Bismuth Iodoform Paraffin Paste packing or surgical treatment by sphenopalatine artery ligation.

E. **L**abial artery (superior)

Ethmoidal artery (anterior)
Greater palatine artery
Sphenopalatine artery
(mnemonic: **LEGS**).

NB: The sphenopalatine artery also contributes to a posterior plexus of arteries (**Woodruff's plexus**) located on the lateral nasal wall behind the inferior turbinate.

Revision Notes

- There are many causes for epistaxis which could be divided into local or systemic causes.
  Local causes: Idiopathic
  Trauma
  Neoplasia
  Iatrogenic
  Systemic causes: Anticoagulation
  Hypertension
  Hereditary Haemorrhagic Telangiectasia
- The mainstay of treatment is to identify the cause and reverse it. Generally the majority of epistaxis is from Littles area (Figure 41.1) which can be easily cauterised (Figure 41.2).
- The ladder of epistaxis management involves:
  1. External pressure to anterior aspect of nose and ice
  2. Nasal cauterisation (works in the majority of cases of anterior epistaxis, if done properly)
  3. Anterior nasal packing (Merocel, Rapid Rhino)
  4. Posterior nasal packing (Foley's catheter and Bismuth Iodoform Paraffin Paste or Rapid Rhino)
  5. Surgical intervention

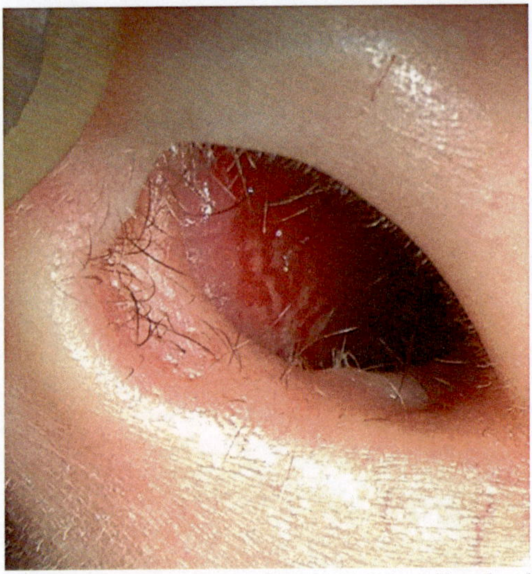

Figure 41.2 Left Little's area showing Kisselback plexus.

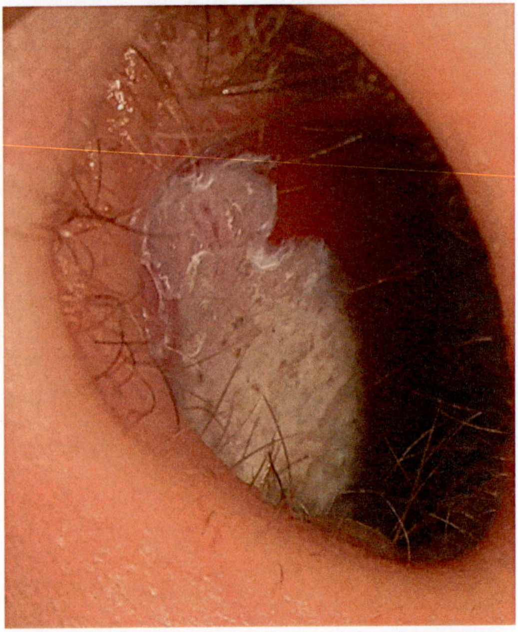

Figure 41.2 Little's area cauterised with silver nitrate.

Station 42

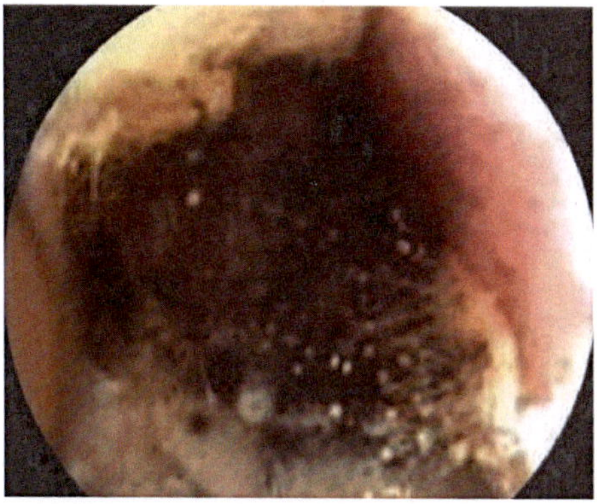

Questions

A. What is the diagnosis?
B. What symptoms is the patient most likely to complain of?
C. Name 2 likely causative organisms?
D. List 4 predisposing factors for this condition.
E. What is the management of this condition?

Answers (Station 42)

Picture otomycosis of external ear canal.

A. Otomycosis
B. Itching
Otorrhoea
Otalgia.
C. Aspergillus Niger
Candida Albicans.
D. Diabetes
Immunosuppresion
Poor hygiene
Increased ear moisture.
E. Regular microsuction
Topical antifungals such as Canestan ®
Keep ears dry.

Revision Notes

- Otomycosis is fungal otitis externa.
- The cause of this condition may be due to immunosuppression, diabetes as mentioned above or also prolonged topical antibiotic use.
- On examination, Aspergillus Niger will usually have multiple black conidiophores as evidenced in the picture above.
- Patients with this condition will need prolonged use of topical antifungals for at least 2 weeks after the fungal infection has cleared as the spores may persist after.

Station 43

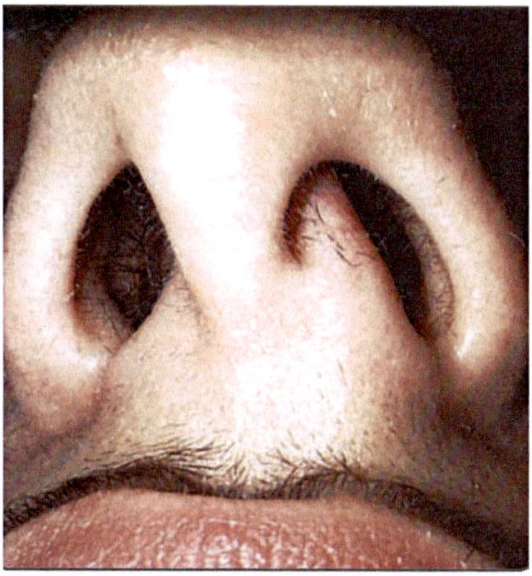

Questions

A. What is the diagnosis?
B. What are the possible causes?
C. Why is timing important in the treatment of this condition if it is due to trauma?
D. What are the indications for surgery? List 2..
E. If a child presents with a nasal fracture, when is the best time to perform operative intervention?
F. What are the complications of surgical treatment?

Answers (Station 43)

Picture of nasal septal deviation.

A. Deviated nasal septum with dislocation of the caudal end of the septum to the left
B. Trauma or congenital.
C. Bones heal within 2-3 weeks, timing is important as once the bones are healed, it will be very difficult to perform manipulation under anaesthesia.
D. Symptomatic nasal obstruction
Cosmetic deformity.

E. Late teenage years to allow full growth of facial bones.

F. Pain
Bleeding
Infection
Septal haematoma
Saddle nose deformity
Epistaxis.

Revision Notes

- Nasal trauma does not necessarily mean nasal bone fracture; it may also involve the septum (fracture/dislocation).
- When patients present with nasal fractures, it is important to also rule out other injuries such as head injury, facial bone fractures or even skull base fractures.
- Septal haematoma will need to be excluded as well. If present, it will need to be drained either by needle aspiration or incision and drainage to prevent cartilage necrosis which may lead to septal perforation or saddle nose deformity.
- During a patient's first presentation with suspected nasal fracture, soft tissue swelling and haematoma makes assessments difficult. These patients should be re-assessed in about 7 days once the soft tissue swelling has settled.
- It is possible to manipulate fractured nasal bones under anaesthesia if the patient presents within up to 21 weeks using Walsham's forceps.
- If the patient presents late, surgical correction will be required by septorhinoplasty.

Station 44

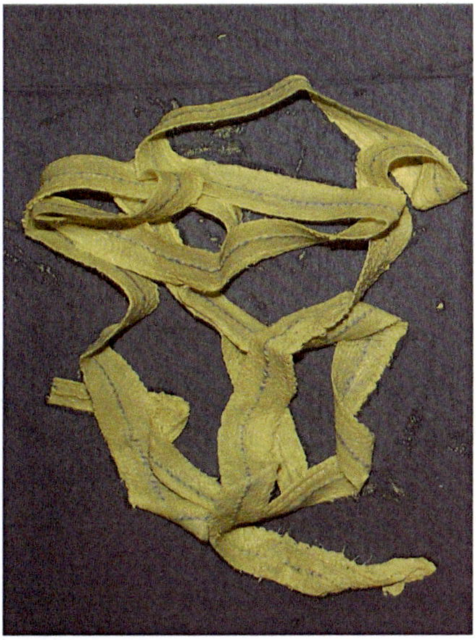

Questions

A. What is the item shown?
B. What is the main ingredient?
C. Name 2 ENT uses of this item.
D. What ingredient is the common cause for an allergic reaction?
E. What type of hypersensitivity reaction may be associated with its use?
F. Why is it necessary to remove this packing prior to embolisation?

Answers (Station 44)

Picture of BIPP.

A. Bismuth iodoform paraffin paste (BIPP).
B. Iodine.
C. BIPP is used following ear surgery, particularly myringoplasty and mastoid surgery. It is also used to

pack the nasal cavity, especially in cases of posterior epistaxis.

D. Iodine (Iodoform).

E. Type IV hypersensitivity reaction.

F. Because the radio-opaque magnetic string is indistinguishable from the blood vessels.

Revision Notes

- Bismuth iodoform paraffin paste (BIPP) and ribbon gauze. BIPP is an astringent and antiseptic dressing which slowly releases iodine over time.
- Allergic reactions are usually a type IV hypersensitivity reaction, also known as a delayed hypersensitivity reaction.
- An inflammatory reaction occurs typically 48-72 hours after exposure to the antigen, it is mediated by T-cells.
- Patients who are previously exposed to BIPP are at an increased risk of developing an allergic reaction.
- If a patient starts to bleed after removal of BIPP packing at the time of embolisation, one can re-pack the nose with plain ribbon gauze.

Station 45

A patient presents to clinic two weeks post right submandibular gland excision. She complains that the right side of her tongue feels numb.

Questions

A. What are the indications for submandibular gland excision?
B. Which nerve is most likely to have been damaged?
C. What other nerves are at risk during submandibular excision?
D. Name the 4 extrinsic muscles of the tongue
E. Name 2 complications of submandibular excision

Answers (Station 45)

A. Chronic sialadenitis
Pain
Malignancy
Management of drooling.
B. Lingual nerve.
C. Marginal mandibular nerve
Hypoglossal nerve.
D. Genioglossus
Hyoglossus
Styloglossus
Palatoglossus.
E. Pain
Bleeding
Infection
Nerve injury.

Revision Notes

- The marginal mandibular branch of the facial nerve is most at risk during the incision. However a carefully placed incision, approximately two patient finger breadths below the angle of the mandible will usually avoid injury to this nerve.

- The lingual nerve supplies sensation to the mucosa of the anterior two-thirds of the tongue.
- The hypoglossal nerve (lies on the hyoglossus muscle) provides motor innervation to the tongue muscles. Damage to the nerve causes wasting of the muscle on the same side (Figure 45.1)
- Failure to ligate the submandibular duct may also lead to extravasation retention cyst formation as the sublingual duct of Rivinius drains into the distal part of submandibular duct.
- A common reason for submandibular gland excision is the presence of a stone in the hilum of the duct (Figures 45.2 and 45.3)

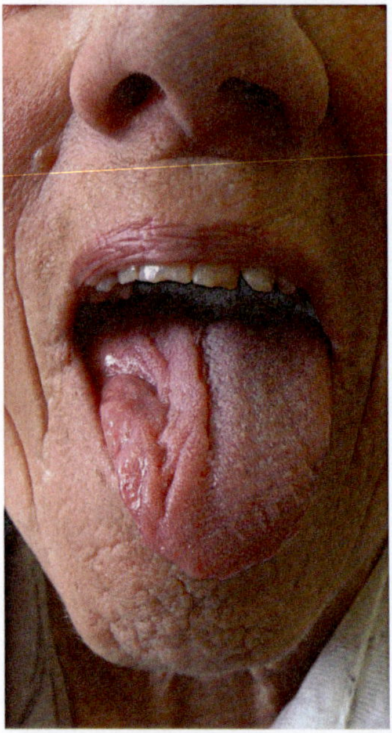

Figure 45.1 Right hypoglossal nerve palsy (notice the wasting of the tongue muscles on the right side).

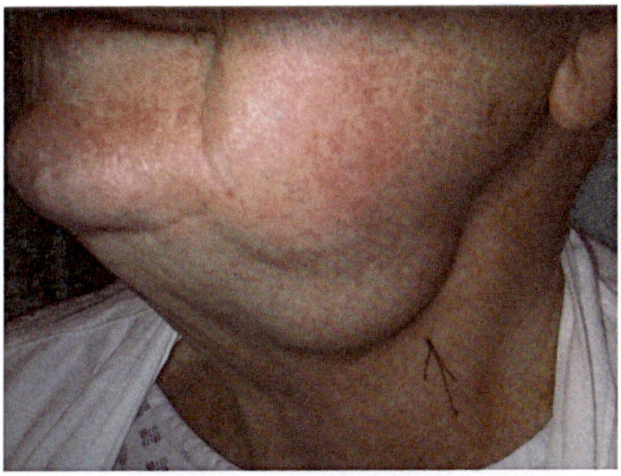

Figure 45.2 Enlarged submandibular gland due to a calculus.

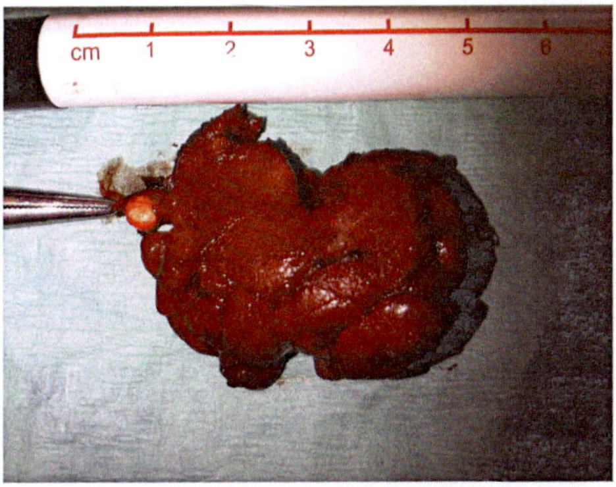

Figure 45.3 Submandibular gland with a large calculus.

Station 46

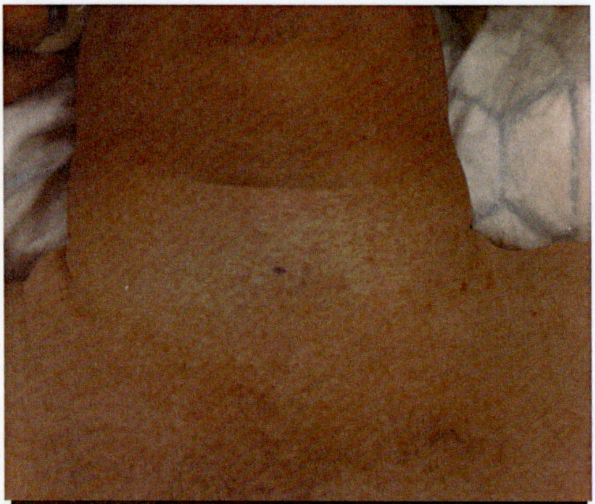

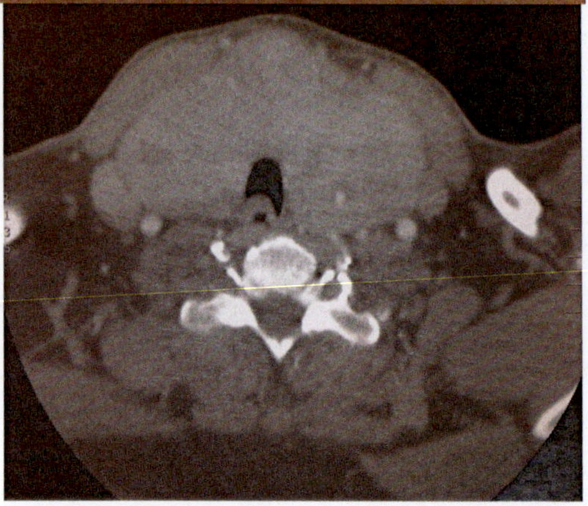

Questions

A. What is the abnormality present in both photographs?

B. List 5 possible causes for this condition.

C. List 5 symptoms this patient may complain of.

D. List 3 indications for surgery.

E. What are the possible complications of surgical treatment? List 5

Answers (Station 46)

Clinical picture of a huge goitre.

A. Goitre

B. Autoimmune causes such as Graves' Disease
Infective thyroiditis
Granulomatous disease such as Sarcoidosis
Iodine deficiency
Thyroid cancer

C. Neck lump
Dyspnoea
Dysphagia
Weak voice
Symptoms of hypo- or hyperthyroidism

E. Dyspnoea
Dysphagia causing reduced oral intake
Graves' uncontrolled by medical therapy

F. Bleeding
Infection
Hypocalcaemia
Recurrent laryngeal nerve palsy
Pneumothorax

Revision Notes

- Causes for goitre can be divided into subgroups as shown below:

  Physiological:
  Puberty, increased metabolic demand pregnancy

  Autoimmune:
  Graves' disease, Hashimoto's thyroiditis

  Thyroiditis:
  Subacute granulomatous/de Quervain's, subacute lymphocytic, silent Riedel's thyroiditis, acute infective (transient)

  Granulomatous diseases:
  Sarcoidosis, tuberculosis

Iodine deficiency
Idiopathic

- Symptoms of hypothyroidism include:
  Fatigue
  Depression
  Brittle hair
  Dry skin
  Bradycardia
  Cold intolerance
  Constipation
- Symptoms of hyperthyroidism are the opposite of above.
- Hypocalcaemia may occur post operatively as the parathyroid glands may be excised or may become transiently underactive post operatively.
  - Symptoms of hypocalcaemia include tingling in lips and tips of fingers, carpopedal spasm, ECG changes (prolonged QT), seizures and cardiac arrest.
  - Chvostek sign may be positive with hypocalcaemia (twitching of facial muscle ontapping on the side of the ear).
  - Patients with bilateral recurrent laryngeal nerve palsies will present immediately on extubation with stridor, respiratory distress and airway obstruction. These patients will need to be re-intubated immediately.

The recurrent laryngeal nerve is located in Beahr's triangle whilst the superior laryngeal nerve is found in Joll's triangle (Table 46.1).

Table 46.1 The borders of Joll's and Beahr's triangles.

Joll's triangle	Beahr's triangle
Midline Superior thyroid pedicle Strap muscle	Common carotid artery Trachea Inferior thyroid artery

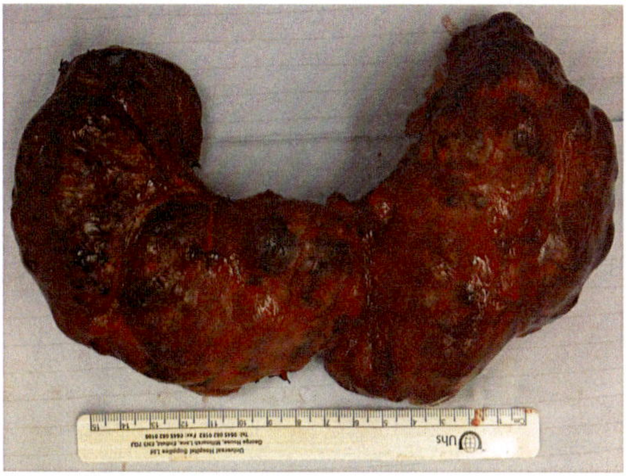

Figure 46.1 Thyroid specimen removed from above patient (with successful preservation of both RLNs and parathyroid glands).

Station 47

A 76-year-old man is referred to see you in clinic. He has a 3-month history of left-sided hearing loss, he describes it as muffled. He has no other otological complaints. On examination you note fluid in the left middle ear cleft, confirmed on tympanometry. His audiogram depicts conductive hearing loss on the left. Endoscopic examination of the post-nasal space is as shown.

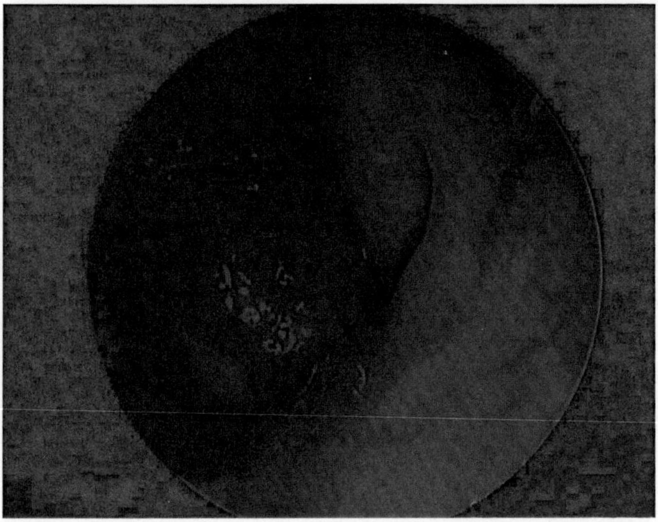

Questions

A. What is the most likely diagnosis?
B. What specific histological type is commonly found?
C. Where in the nasopharynx does it commonly arise?
D. What radiological investigation is most helpful?
E. Which ethnic group has a higher incidence of this condition?
F. What is the first step in surgical management for this patient?
G. What is the TNM classifiation if the lesion is confined to the post-nasal space and the patient has a 5cm neck node

above the supraclavicular fossa with no evidence of distant metastasis?

Answers (Station 47)

Picture of nasopharyngeal lesion

A. Nasopharyngeal carcinoma
B. Squamous cell carcinoma
C. Fossa of Rosenmuller
D. MRI
E. Oriental population (especially southern Chinese)
F. Biopsy of post nasal space and grommet insertions to reverse the conductive hearing loss (note that grommets may be associated with ear infection if the patient is subsequently treated with radiotherapy, for this reason some surgeons advocate hearing aids instead of grommets).
G. T1N1M0

Revision Notes

- Nasopharyngeal carcinoma is rare in the UK; however, it is the most common head and neck cancer in the oriental Chinese population.
- This condition is notoriously difficult to diagnose early as patients usually present later with a neck lump, unilateral hearing loss, recurrent epistaxis or even cranial nerve palsies.
- Other important aetiology of nasopharyngeal carcinoma to note is its association with Ebstein Barr Virus (EBV) and also genetic predisposition.
- It is classified into 3 subtypes by the World Health Organisation (WHO):
    - (i) Keratinising squamous cell carcinoma
    - (ii) Non-keratinising squamous cell carcinoma
    - (iii) Undifferentiated squamous cell carcinoma

- The mainstay of treatment for this condition is radiotherapy as most of its subtypes are sensitive to radiotherapy.
- There is also a role for complex salvage surgery (maxillary swing approach) where there is recurrence.

The TNM classification for nasopharyngeal system is unique (see Appendix Table 5)

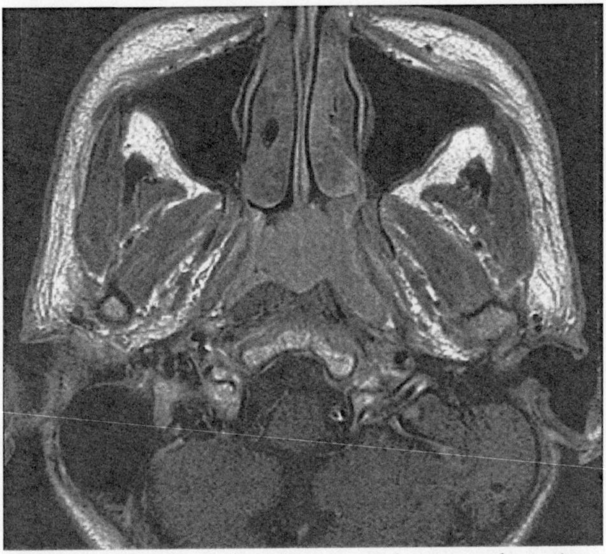

Figure 47.1 MRI scan showing nasopharyngeal carcinoma.

Station 48

You see a patient in clinic who has had a recent superficial parotidectomy. She complains of facial sweating of her face on the same side as the surgery.

Questions

A. What is this condition called?
B. Name 2 options for management of this condition
C. What 2 other complications would this patient been warned about pre-operatively?
D. Damage to which nerve causes a numb ear lobule?
E. Name 2 differential diagnoses of a parotid enlargement?

Answers (Station 48)

Complications of superficial parotidectomy.

A. Frey's syndrome
B. Aluminium based deodorant
Topical glycopyrrolate
Botox injection
Neuronectomy (Jacobson's nerve section in the middle ear)
C. Pain
Bleeding
Infection
Seroma
Facial nerve palsy
Numbness around ear lobule
D. Greater auricular nerve
E. Parotitis
Pleomorphic adenoma
Granulomatous disease

Revision Notes

- Frey's syndrome is also known as 'Gustatory sweating' related to parotid surgery or injury.

- During surgery, parasympathetic secretomotor fibres innervate the parotid gland may be transected. The fibres regenerate in the skin where they assume control of sweat gland activity because of the common neurotransmitter acetylcholine. This inappropriate innervation results in facial sweating in response to salivatory stimuli.
- The iodine starch test may be used to locate the affected regions (Figures 48.1a-d).
- Botulinum toxin (Botox) injection is now the gold standard treatment for Frey's syndrome. It works by blocking the release of acetylcholine from the cholinergic nerve end plates leading to inactivity of the glands or muscle innervated (for an evidence-based review of the use of Botox in non-cosmetic head and neck conditions, see Persaud *et al.* JRSM short report 2013; Feb 4 (2):10).
- Causes for parotid enlargement could be divided into:
  1. Infective: Mumps, HIV infection
  2. Autoimmune: Sjogren's syndrome
  3. Granulomatous diseases: Sarcoidosis, Tuberculosis
  4. Drugs: use mnemonic TOPIC: **T**hiouracil, **O**ral contraceptive pill, **P**henylbutazone, **I**soprenaline and **Co**-proxamol
  5. Neoplastic (Benign or malignant)
  6. Pseudo hypertrophy of masseter muscles

The following sequence of photographs illustrate the starch iodine test for gustatory sweating seen in Frey's syndrome.

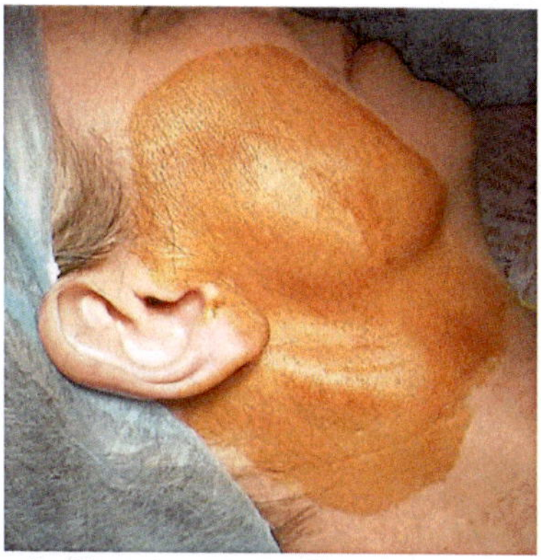

Figures 48.1a Iodine is painted onto the area affected by gustatory sweating (note that the patient is fully awake).

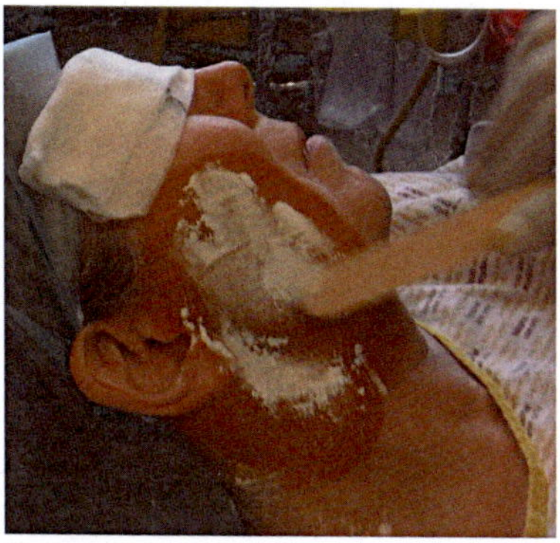

Figure 48.1b Starch is applied over the iodine.

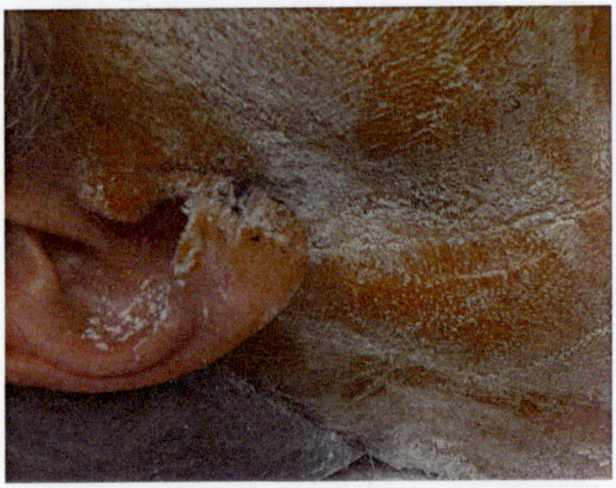

Figure 48.1c The patient is asked to eat something eg a few grapes.

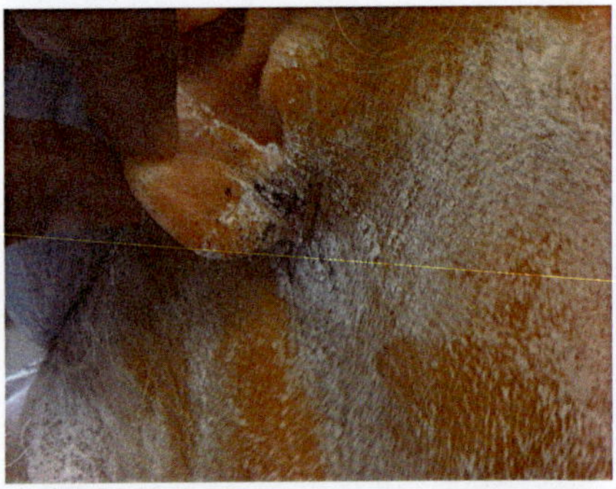

Figure 48.1d Evidence of gustatory sweating is seen near the ear lobe (this area can then be injected with Botox).

Station 49

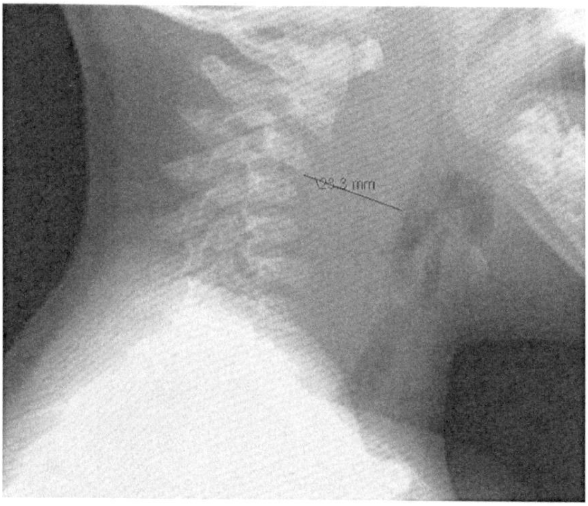

Questions

A. The above X-ray shows an increase in the thickness of the prevertebral soft tissue of the neck. Give 2 differential diagnoses?

B. List 5 likely symptoms on presentation.

C. Give one difference between the retropharyngeal space and the parapharyngeal space

D. List 5 complications of a deep neck space infection

E. What are the treatment options for this patient?

Answers (Station 49)

Clinical photograph of widened prevertebral soft tissue space of neck

A. Deep neck space infection (eg parapharyngeal or retropharyngeal abscess), a lodged sharp foreign body or a severe upper respiratory tract infection.

B. Pyrexia, poor feeding, irritability, drooling, stridor.

C. The retropharyngeal space by definition extends from the skull base to the lower border of the pharynx, however there is an inferior extension of the retropharyngeal space all the way to diaphragm (fortunately most retropharharyngeal abscesses are walled off in the superior mediastinium). The parapharyngeal space by definition extends from the skull base to the hyoid bone but communicates with the retropharyngeal space so a parapharyngeal abscess can also lead to mediastinial spread.

D. Septicaemia, endocarditis, thrombosis of the great vessels of the neck, pyopneumonitis, mediastinitis, purulent pericarditis, bronchial erosion, aspiration pneumonia and Grisel syndrome.

E. If the patient was unwell and drooling, then securing the airway in a controlled environment would be the initial management. This would require the paediatric anaesthetist and a Consultant ENT surgeon. In this case, the abscess would be incised and drained intra-orally, after aspiration to confirm pus. Note that the clinical picture is similar for acute epiglottis and severe tonsillitis.

Revision Notes

- Normal thickness of the prevertebral soft tissue between **C2 and C4** is 7mm maximum.
- Normal thickness of the prevertebral soft tisse between **C4 and T1** is 17mm maximum (this takes into account the oesophagus, retropharyngeal space and surrounding fascial layers (Figure 49.1).

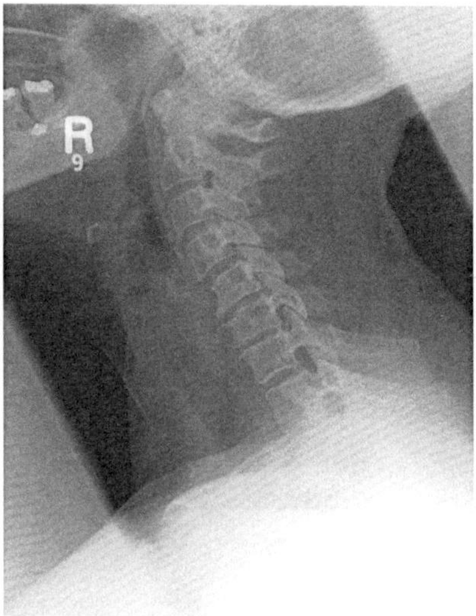

Figure 49.1 Lateral soft tissue neck x-ray showing normal thickness of the prevertebral soft tissue (7mm between C2-C4 and 17 mm between C4-T1).

- Neck infections may occur in the deep neck spaces or superficially (Figure 49.2).
  The key concern in patients who appear septic, drooling and having stridor, is the patient's airway and the help of an experienced anaesthetist should be sought immediately. When abscess is drained, samples should be sent for microbiology for culture and sensitivity.

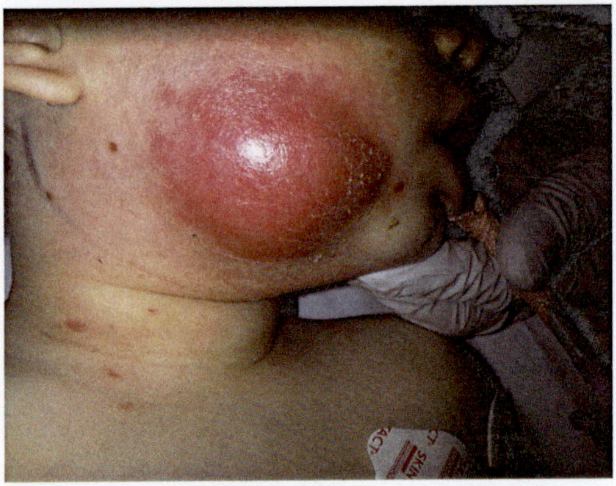

Figure 49.2 An example of a superficial neck space infection (this child required incision and drainage).

- Parapharyngeal abscess (Figure 49.3) may require cervical drainage.
- Superficial neck space infections are much easier to diagnosed and manage in comparison to deep neck space infection.

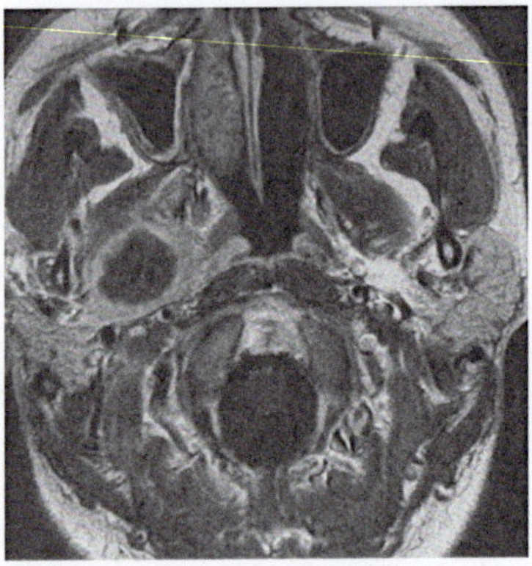

Figure 49.3 MRI of the suprahyoid neck showing a right parapharyngeal abscess

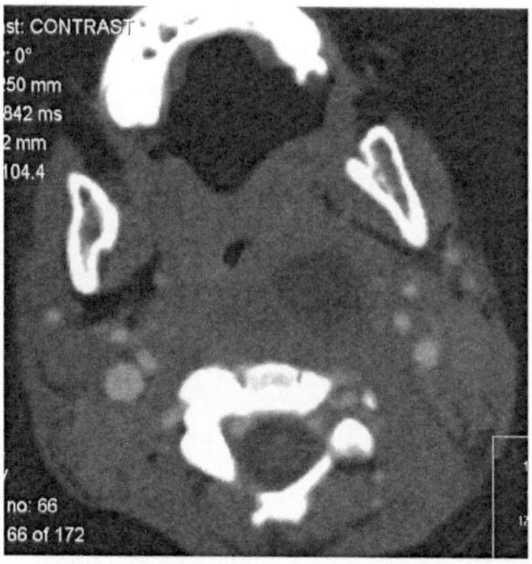

Figure 49.4 Contrast CT scan of the suprahyoid neck of a child showing a left parapharyngeal abscess

Station 50

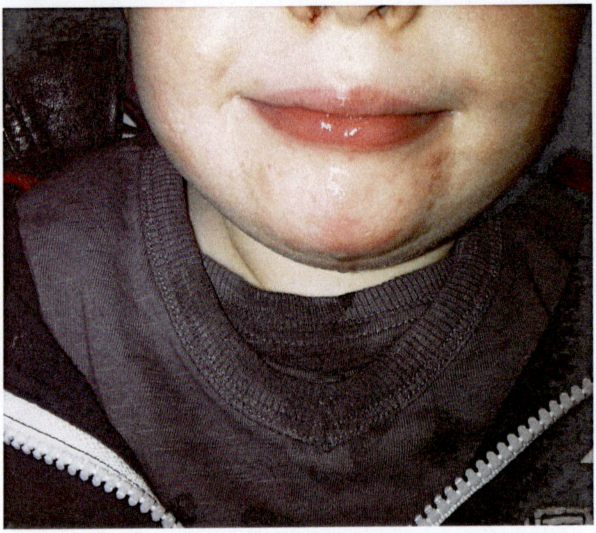

Questions

A. The mother of this child is concerned about excessive dribbling of saliva. What do we call this condition?

B. What is the underlying problem?

C. Name 2 syndromes associated with this condition.

D. Which of the three major salivary glands produces the most saliva whilst at rest.

E. Give 2 medical and 2 surgical options for managing this condition.

Answers (Station 50)

Clinical photograph of a child drooling.

A. Drooling.

B. Poor oro-motor control of saliva and not over production of saliva.

C. Cerebral palsy (because of poor neck posture) and Down (because large tongue results in poor lip seal).

D. Submandibular gland produces 70 percent of resting saliva.

E. **Medical**: Anticholinergic agents and Botox injections under ultrasound guidance.

Surgical: submandibular duct transposition, adenotonsillectomy and submandibular gland excision.

Revision Notes

- Most young children drool from time to time. Drooling is considered a problem after the age of 5.
- The problem can be monitored by the number of bibs or t-shirts changed over a specific period.
- It is generally due to poor oro-motor control of swallowing which is more commonly seen in children with developmental delay.
- Factors such as poor neck control, posture, nasal blockage (eg large adenoid) and dental factors may also contribute to drooling.
- Saliva overflow, rather than saliva over-production, is the main issue.
- Drooling may also present in acute conditions such as tonsillitis, acute epiglottis and food bolus obstruction.
- Certain drugs may also induce drooling eg anti- epileptic agents.
- Initial management is aimed at oro-motor exercises and improving posture usually with the help of the speech and language therapist.

Station 51

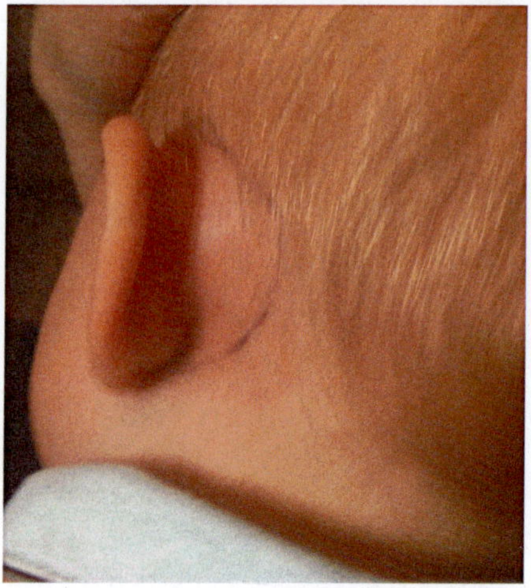

Questions

A. Give 2 differential diagnoses.

B. How would you differentiate between the 2 diagnoses?

C. In which childhood disease is the post auricular lymph gland commonly affected?

D. Assuming it was acute mastoiditis, which antibiotic would you use to treat the condition and why?

E. If the child is not getting better, despite intravenous antibiotic therapy, what would you do?

Answers (Station 51)

Clinical photograph of a child showing a swelling behind the left pinna.

A. Acute mastoiditis and post-auricular lymphadenopathy.

B. In contrast to post-auricular lymphadenopathy, acute mastoiditis is associated with corysal symptoms, fever, pain, red bulging tympanic membrane and lost of the post auricular skin crease.

C. Rubella.

D. If the patient is not allergic to penicillin, I would use co-amoxiclav (25mg/kg) because one of the 3 common bacteria responsible for this condition (*haemophilus influenza)* is resistant to amoxicillin.

E. Request an urgent CT brain with contrast to look for intracranial complication and sub-periosteal abscess. It is highly likely that the child would require cortical mastoidectomy +/- grommet insertion.

Revision Notes

- Acute mastoiditis is an infrequent complication of acute otitis media (see question 3).
- Children with acute mastoiditis usually presents with otalgia, fever, reduced oral intake, proptosis of the auricle, erythema and absence of the post-auricular sulcus.
- The tympanic membrane is commonly inflamed and thickened and may perforate releasing mucopurulent discharge.
- The causative organisms are *streptococcus pneumoniae, haemophilus influenzae* and *moraxella catarrhalis.*
- Computerised tomography (CT) scan with contrast is a useful tool to investigate for any intracranial complications of mastoiditis.
- There are usually mastoid lymph nodes (also known as retro-auricular or posterior auricular nodes) situated below the posterior auricular muscle.
- Although they are most commonly affected by rubella, the nodes can become enlarged by any localised infection (see Figure 55.1).
- Post auricular lymphadenopathy usually subsides once the underlying condition is treated.

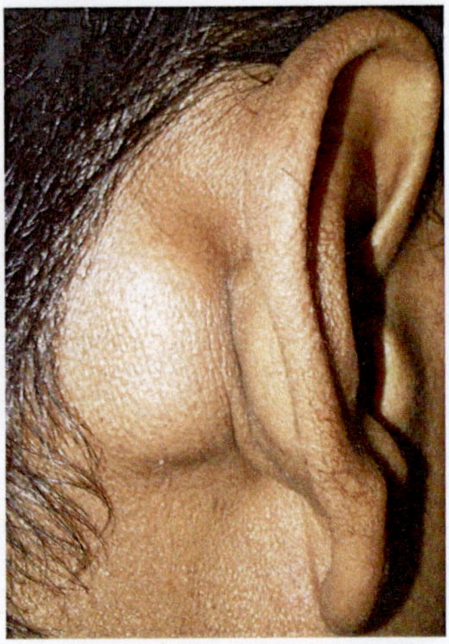

Figure 51.1 Post auricular lynphadenopathy due to a scalp infection.

Station 52

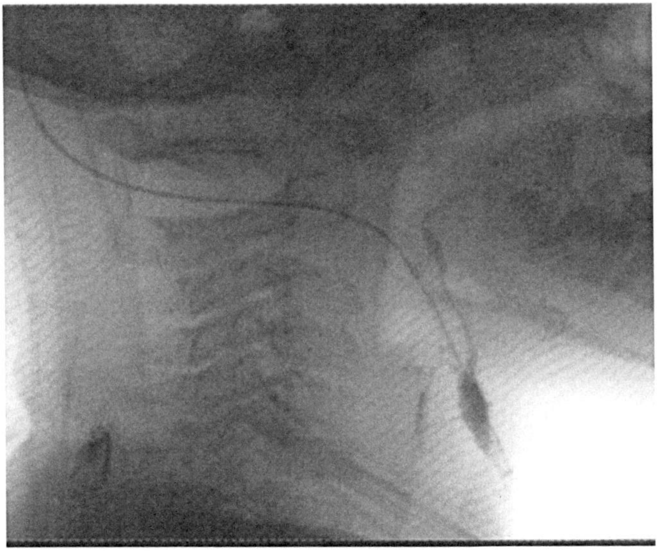

Questions

A. What type of imaging is shown here?
B. What abnormality is demonstrated?
C. Briefly described the course of the tract highlighted.
D. Which syndrome may be associated with this abnormality?

Answers (Station 52)

Clinical photograph of a fistulogram.

A. Fistulogram.
B. 2nd branchial apparatus fistula.
C. The fistula usually follows a path between internal carotid artery and the external carotid artery and over the hypoglossal nerve to open in the posterior pillar of tonsillar fossa.
D. Brachio-oto-renal syndrome

Revision Notes

- Branchial apparatus anomalies are usually due to failure of complete closure during embryological development.
- 2nd branchial apparatus anomaly is the commonest of all the branchial anomalies and manifest itself by weeping mucus on the neck. It may become infected and this may require analgesia and antibiotics.
- 1st branchial apparatus anomaly occur either anterior, posterior or inferior to conchal cartilage/pinna and above hyoid. It has a variable relationship with the facial nerve. Work classification: **Type 1** fistula has ectoderm only and is far from the facial nerve. **Type 2** fistula has both ectoderm and mesoderm and is closely related to the facial nerve. The fistula opens between angle of mandible and hyoid bone and may mimic parotid infection. Surgery for Type 2 fistula requires a lateral parotidectomy.
- 3rd branchial apparatus anomaly is rare and the tract runs through the thyrohyoid membrane and above superior laryngeal nerve to open in the lateral wall of the piriform fossa.
- 4th brancial apparatus anomaly is derived from the pharyngobranchial canal which connects the pharynx to the ultimobranchial body and superior parathyroid gland. The tract opens into the apex of the piriform fossa. It may lead to recurrent neck infection mimicking acute suppurative thyroiditis. Treatment involves endoscopic cautery to opening in piriform fossa.

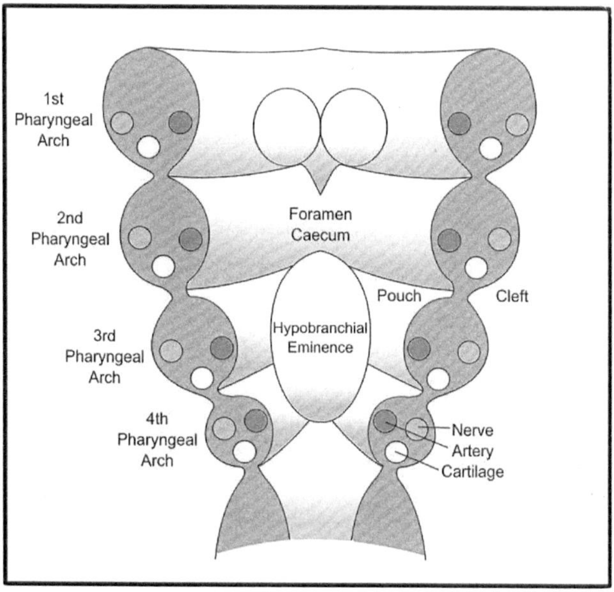

Figure 52.1 Early anatomical arrangements of the branchial apparatus during embryology.

Table 52.1 Derivatives of the branchial arches made easy.

Arch No.	Nerve	Artery	Associated structures
1	Trigeminal	Maxillary	Eustachian Tube (ET) (from pouch), tensor tympani muscle/tendon, Tensor Veli Palatini muscle (TVP).
2	Facial	Stapedial	Buccinator muscle, stapes, stapedius muscle/ tendon (from arch).
3	Glossopharyngeal	Carotid	Stylopharyngeus muscle (from arch).

4	Vagus (SLN)	Lt aorta Rt subclavian	Cricothyroid, all intrinsic muscles of soft palate, thyroid cartilage, epiglottis,Thymus (from pouch).
6	Vagus (RLN)	Pulmonary	Cricoid cartilage (from arch), intrinsic muscles larynx.

Table 52.2 Abnormalities arising from brachial apparatus.

Branchial apparatus	Abnormalities
1st cleft	Pathology/sinus/cyst above hyoid, type 1 close to EAC (atretic) and around the parotid, type II between angle of mandible and submandibular region (ant triangle neck), tracts may be close to facial nerve – deep or superficial to it.
1st arch	preauricular sinus/ deformed ears, downslanting palpabre fissures and webbed eye lids (Treacher-Collins).
2nd cleft	sinus anywhere below hyoid, usually ant lower 1/3 SCM; also consider checking for brachio-oto-renal syndrome.
2nd pouch	sinus tract to tonsil between great vessels.
2nd arch	long styloid +/- calcified stylohyoid ligament (Eagle's syndrome).
3rd pouch	sinus tract to lateral wall of piriform fossa; left sided neck absceses, mimic acute suppurative thyroiditis; anterior neck infection.
4th pouch	sinus tract to apex of piriform fossa;

	parallel RLN, absent thymus & PT glands.
4th arch	subglottic stenosis (may cause stridor); omega shaped epiglottis; asymmetrical larynx; chondromalacia; double aortic arches; subglottic stenosis.
6th arch	Subglottic narrowing secondary to underdevelopment of cricoid cartilage
Non-branchial structures	Tongue, Thyroglossal cyst and Thyroid

Station 53

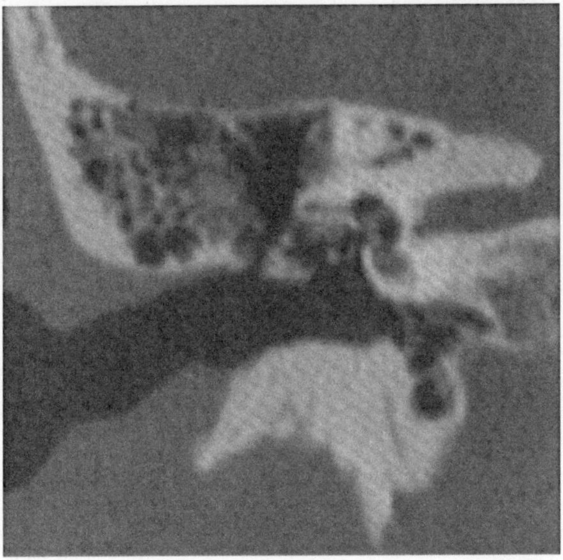

Questions

A. What is the imaging and view of the picture above?
B. What is the diagnosis?
C. What symptoms would the patient complain of? List 5.
D. What would this patients audiogram show?

Answers (Station 53)

Coronal CT scan of the temporal bone showing transverse temporal bone fracture.

A. Coronal Computerised Tomography of the right temporal bone.
B. Transverse fracture of the temporal bone with pneumolabyrinth indicative of a dead ear.
C. Bloody otorrhoea, headache, hearing loss, tinnitus, dizziness, facial nerve palsy.
D. Profound sensorineural hearing loss.

Revision Notes

- Head injury resulting in facial nerve palsy, profound hearing loss and nystagmus strongly suggests a temporal bone fracture.
- A haemotympanum (Figure 53.1) and/or Battle sign may suggest a temporal bone fracture.
- A transverse fracture (20%) of the temporal bone is not as common as a longitudinal fracture (80%) (Figure 53.2).
- Severe frontal or occipital force tends to lead to transverse fracture whilst a lateral force over the temporomastoid bone results in a longitudinal fracture.
- Cochlear and vestibular structures are usually damaged in a transverse fracture causing sensorineural hearing loss and vertigo.
- If facial nerve palsy occurs immediately after a longitudinal temporal bone fracture, it is often due to a segment of bone pressing on the nerve.
- Exploratory tympanomastoidectomy with facial nerve monitoring to decompress the facial nerve may reverse the nerve palsy.
- Transverse and longitudinal fractures of the temporal bone may occur simultaneously.

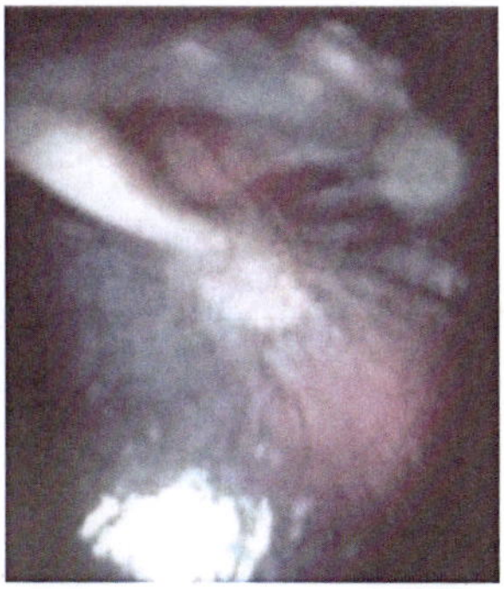

Figure 53.1 Haemotympanum following a horizontal fracture of the temporal bone.

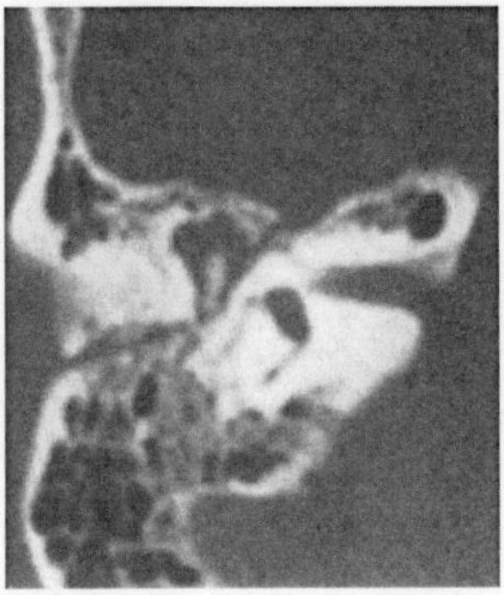

Figure 53.2 Axial CT scan showing a longitudinal fracture of the temporal bone.

Station 54

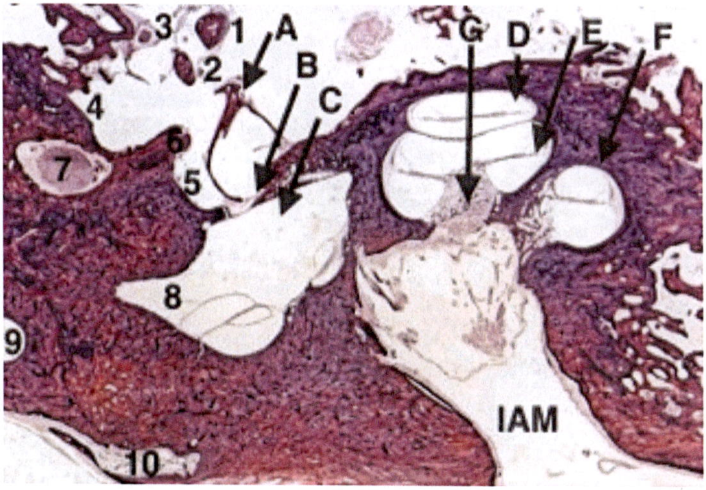

Questions

Label the arrows marked A-G

Answers (Station 54)

Temporal bone histology (Axial Section).

A Stapes
B Stapes footplate
C Labyrinth system (saccule)
D Reissner's membrane
E Basilar membrane
F Cochlea
G Cochlear nerve

Revision Notes

- Histology of the temporal bone is a popular past year question and after familiarising with the basic anatomy of the middle and inner ear, it is a very straightforward question.

- Dilatation of the scala media with or without rupture of Reissner's membrane suggests a diagnosis of endolymphatic hydrops (eg Meniere's disease).
- In terms of general anatomy the petrous part of the temporal bone is positioned obliquely (posterolateral to anteromedial); therefore in the coronal plane structures are sectioned obliquely and the cochlea (snail, Figure 54.1) is anterior to semi-circular canals (rabbit ears, figure 54.2).
- 1. Malleus, 2. Incus, 3. Chorda Tympani, 4. Facial Recess (posterolateral mesotympanum), 5. Sinus Tympani (posteromedial mesotympanum), 6. Pyramidal Process (separates sinus tympani medially from facial recess laterally), 7. Facial nerve, 8. Utricle, 9. Posterior Semi-Circular Canal, 10. Vestibular Aquaduct.

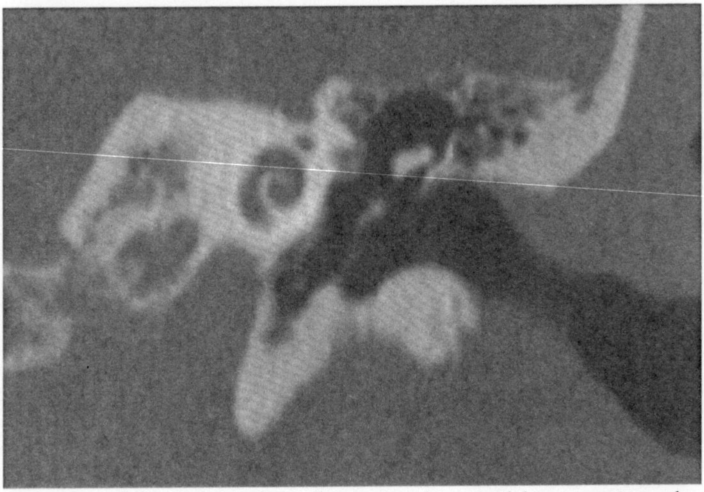

Figure 54.1 CT image through the cochlea (notice the snail's eyes representing the labyrinthine and horizontal portions of the facial nerve)

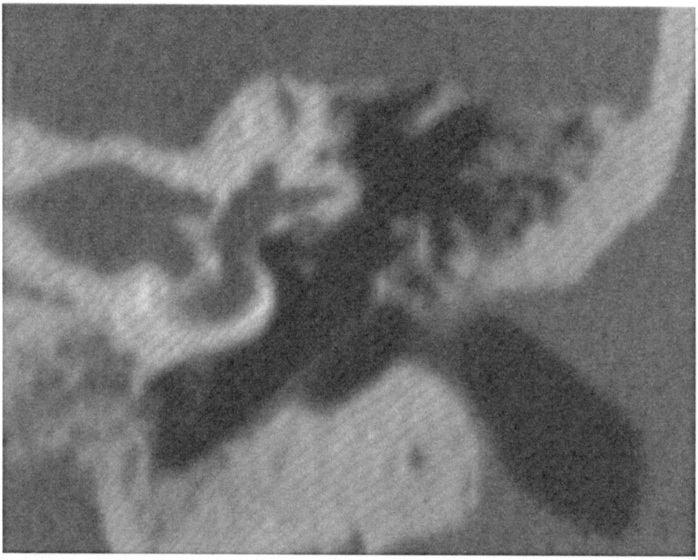

Figure 54.2 A CT image through the semicircular canal canals (notice the rabbit ears representing the superior semi-circular canal and the lateral semi-circular canal).

Station 55

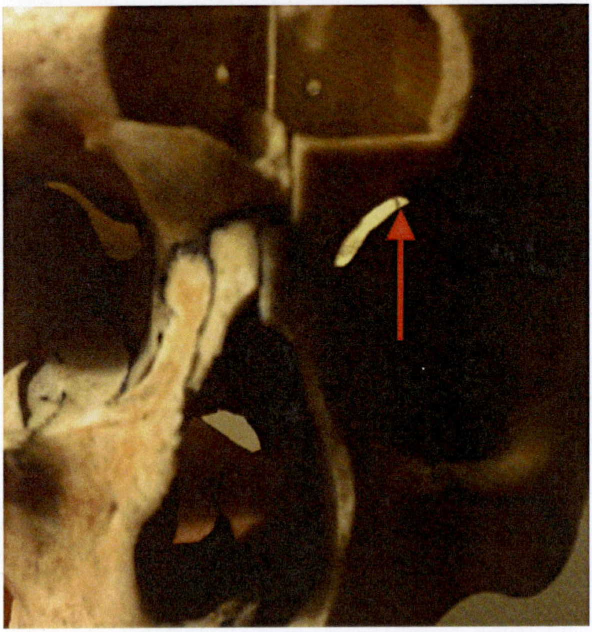

Questions

A. What is the name of the fissure shown at the back of the orbit?

B. In which bone is this fissure formed?

C. List 5 structures which pass through this fissure.

D. Name 3 symptoms that can occur if the content of the fissure is disturbed.

E. List 3 causes for the above syndrome.

Answers (Station 55)

Superior orbital fissure.

A. Superior orbital fissure

B. Sphenoid bone

C. Branches of trigeminal (V1): lacrimal, frontal & nasociliary, cranial nerves III, IV, VI (for eye movements), sympathetics, superior ophthalmic vein, branches of middle meningeal artery and lacrimal artery.

D. **Double vision** due to dysfunctional eye movement, **ptosis** due to 3rd nerve dysfunction and **numbness** above the upper eye lid due to superior orbital nerve dysfunction (collective referred to as the superior orbital fissure syndrome).

E. **Trauma** mainly (eg blow out fracture) but may also be due to **infection**, **inflammatory** condition and **neoplasia** (benign or malignant).

Revision Notes

- The cleft like superior orbital fissure is formed between the greater and lesser wings of the sphenoid bone.
- Blindness coupled with triad of superior orbital fissure syndrome is known as orbital apex syndrome as the orbital apex is involved.
- The inferior orbital fissure is formed by the sphenoid bone and the maxilla.
- The inferior orbital fissure transmits the maxillary nerve, parasympathetic branches from the pterygopalatine (hayfever) ganglion, inferior ophthalmic vein and infraorbital vessels.

Station 56

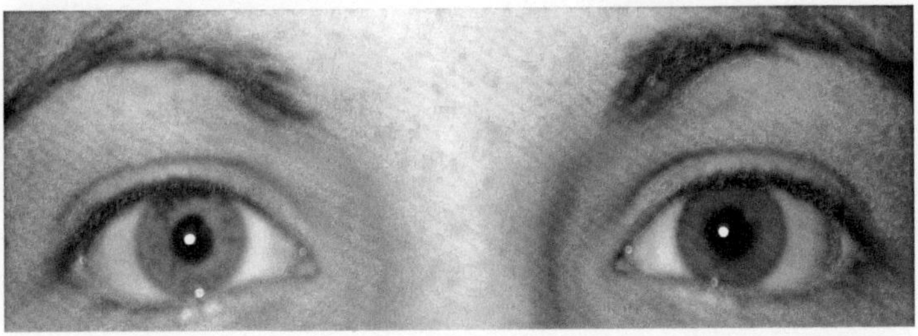

Questions

A. Which sign is shown in this clinical photograph (patient is not wearing contact lens)?
B. Name the syndrome in which this sign is present
C. List 3 other features of the named syndrome
D. How is the condition inherited?

Answers (Station 56)

Clinical photograph of heterochromia irides

A. Heterochromia irides
B. Waardenburg syndrome
C. Hearing loss
White forelock
Skin pigmentory changes
D. Autosomal dominant

Revision Notes

- At least 4 types of Waardenburg syndrome have been described.
- Types I and II are the more common ones and thet are distinguished by the presence of dystopia canthorum, which refers to the lateral displacement of the inner canthi.
- Type IV is associated with Hirschsprung disease.
- Dystopia canthorum is present in Type I.

- Hypertelorism (ie the width of between the medial canthi) results from the presence of dystopia canthorum.
- The syndrome is associated with congenital non-progressive hearing loss, either unilateral (70%) or bilateral (30%).
- Rehabilitation of hearing loss involves an air conduction hearing aid; if hearing aid is inadequate then a cochlear implant may be suitable.

Station 57

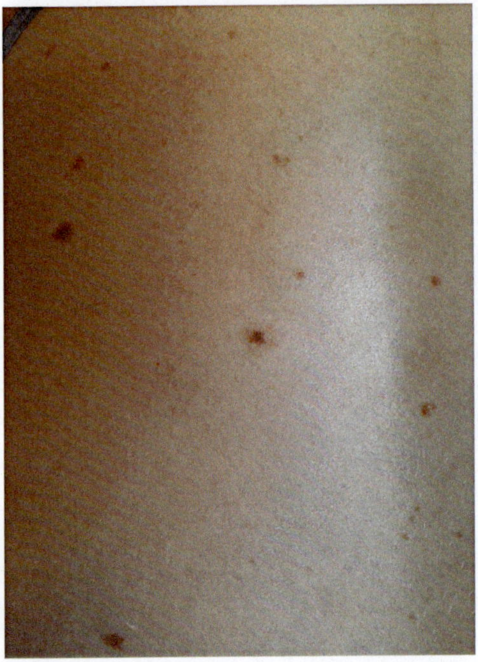

Questions

A. List the 4 suspicious features of the above skin lesion that may be consistent with the diagnosis of a malignant melanoma.

B. List 3 types of malignant melanomas.

C. Name 2 histological staging systems for cutaneous melanomas.

D. On which part of the body is cutaneous melanoma most commonly found?

E. What is the best modality for the treatment of malignant melanoma?

Answers (Station 57)

Clinical photograph of a suspicious looking skin lesion

A. The ABCD warning features in any naevus or mole are: **A**symmetry, **B**order irregular, **C**olour and **D**iameter greater than 6mm.
B. Superficial spreading, acral lentiginous and lentigo maligna.
C. Clark and Breslow
D. Trunk
E. Surgery

Revision Notes

- Malignant melanomas arise from either benign epidermal melanocytes or from fields of hyperplasia/dysplasia of the skin.
- According to the National Cancer Institute, the ABCD warning features in any naevus or mole are Asymmetry, Border, Colour and Diameter.
- Other red flag signs are development of itching, burning, swelling, pain in a pre-existing mole, development of a raised area in a previously flat mole, a change in the consistency of the mole, a change in the surface characteristics such as bleeding, scaling, ulceration or crusting and the development of satellite lesions. New moles on an elderly person should also ring alarm bells.
- Types of malignant melanomas:
    - acral lentiginous
    - superficial spreading
    - lentigo maligna
    - nodular.
    - dysplastic naevi
- The different staging options for cutaneous malignant melanomas are shown in Table 1.

Table 57.1 Staging of cutaneous malignant melanomas

STAGING OF CUTANEOUS MALIGNANT MELANOMAS	
AJC Clinical staging	**Features**
Stage I and II	Local
Stage III	Regional spread
Stage IV	Distant metastasis
Clark's clinical staging	
Stage I	Local disease
Stage II	Local plus regional nodal disease
Stage III	Distant metastases present
Breslow's histological staging	
<0.76mm	Thin
0.76-1.49	Intermediate
1.50-4.00	Intermediate
>4.00	Thick
Clark's histological staging	
Level I	Above the basement membrane (*in situ*)
Level II	Through the basement membrane
Level III	Spread to the papillary or reticular interface
Level IV	Spread to the reticular dermis
Level V	Spread to subcutaneous tissue

- Cutaneous melanomas are often seen on the trunk but there is no true correlation between the site of a mole and its tendency to become malignant.
- Surgery is the best modality for treating melanoma for a possible curative outcome. Other modalities are either palliative or experimental and includes radiation therapy, chemotherapy, immunotherapypt and gene therapy. Primary cutaneous lesions should be excised with the following margins:
  - For lesions <1mm 1cm margin of excision
  - For lesions 1-4mm 2cm margin of excision
  - For lesion > 4mm 3 cm margin of excision

All depth should include underlying muscular fascia.

Station 58

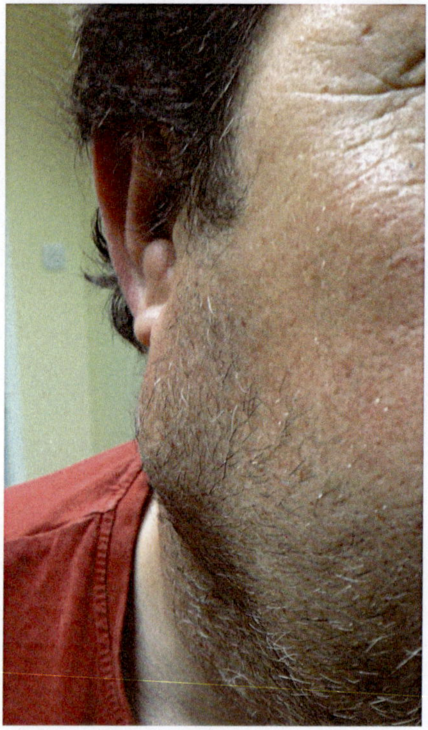

Questions

A. What is the differential diagnosis for the lump shown above?

B. What investigations would you request to help with the diagnosis?

C. List 3 ways to identify the facial nerve during parotid surgery.

D. Name 4 cancers associated with the salivary gland other than adenoid cystic carcinoma.

E. Why might the FNAC of the lump suggests pleomorphic adenoma whilst the histology of the specimen suggest adenoid cystic carcinoma?

Answers (Station 58)

Clinical photograph of a right parotid lump.

A. **Non-salivary**: (eg masseter hypertrophy) and **salivary**: inflammatory, neoplastic [benign or malignant (primary or secondary)].

B. Ultrasound scan, FNAC and MRI scan.

C. Tympanomastoid suture, posterior belly of the digastrics muscle, tragal pointer.

D. Mucoepidermoid, accinic, metastatic lesions (eg malingnant melanoma) and lymphoma.

E. Pleomorphic adenomas arise from myoepithelial and intercalated duct cells whilst adenoid cystic carcinomas arise from the latter only. Therefore the two tumours have similar cytological profiles.

Revision Notes

- A benign tumour arising from just one type of salivary cell is called monomorphic.
- Pleomorphic adenoma is the commonest benign salivary tumour, and tends to arise from the tail of the parotid gland.
- 80% Rule pertaining to the parotid gland:
  - 80% of parotid tumours are benign
  - 80% of parotid tumours are pleomorphic adenomas
  - 80% of salivary gland pleomorphic adenomas occur in parotid
  - 80% of parotid pleomorphic adenomas occur in the superficial lobe
  - 80% of untreated pleomorphic adenomas remain benign
- The salivary unit is made up of 5 different type of cells (mnemonic MAISE): myoepithelial, accinic, intercalated duct, secretory and excretory.
- Retrograde dissection of a branch of the facial nerve may also help to identify the main trunk.

- During parotid surgery it is important to be aware of the stylomastoid artery (branch of posterior auricular artery) exiting stylomastoid foramen along with the facial nerve.
- Pleomorphic adenoma have a pseudocapsule of compressed parotid tissue into which the tumour has many fingerlike projections and rupture of this capsule during surgery may lead to recurrence.
- Parotidectomy may be performed using the modified Blair incision (Figure 58.2) or a face-lift incision (Figures 58.3a-b).

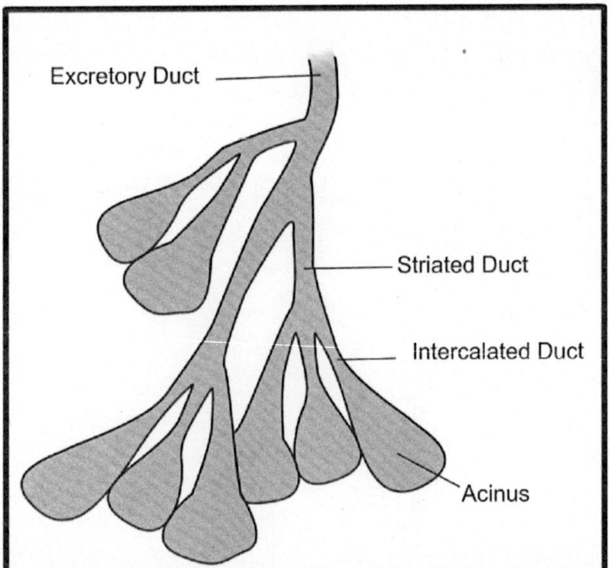

Figure 58.1 Schematic diagram showing the anatomy of a salivary gland unit (myoepithelial cells not shown).

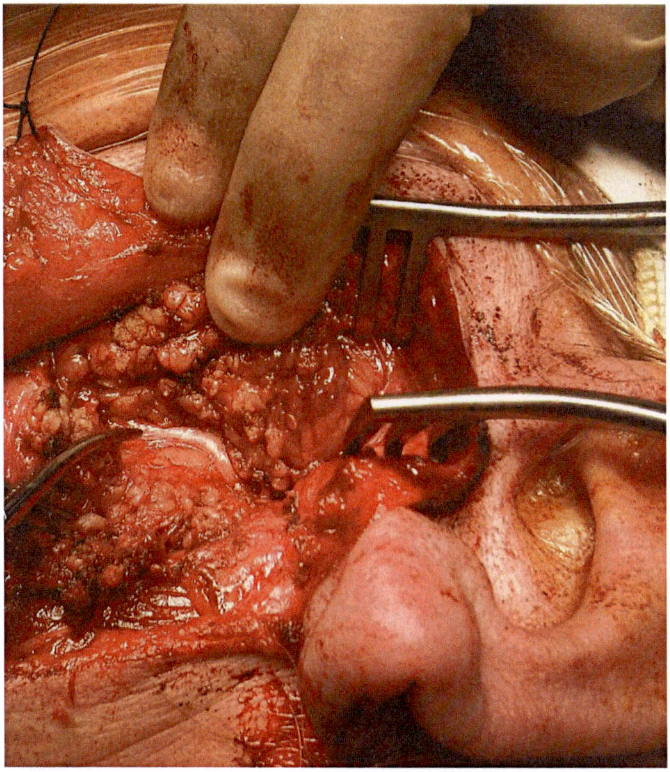

Figure 58.2 Intraoperative photograph showing the trunk and lower main branch of the facial nerve (Modified Blair incision used).

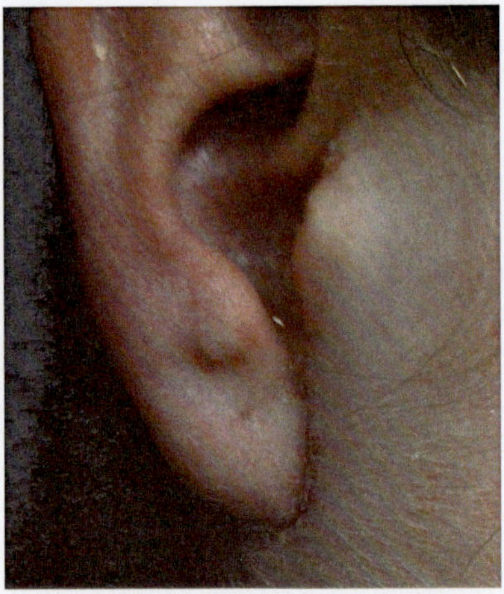

Figure 58.3a Modified face-lift incision for parotidectomy.

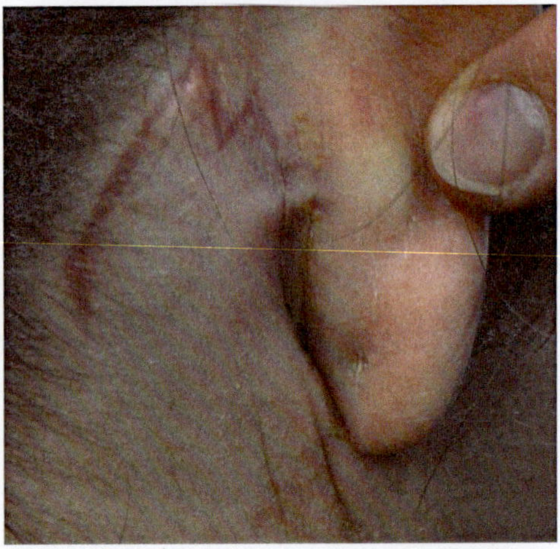

Figure 58.3b Modified face-lift incision for parotidectomy.

Station 59

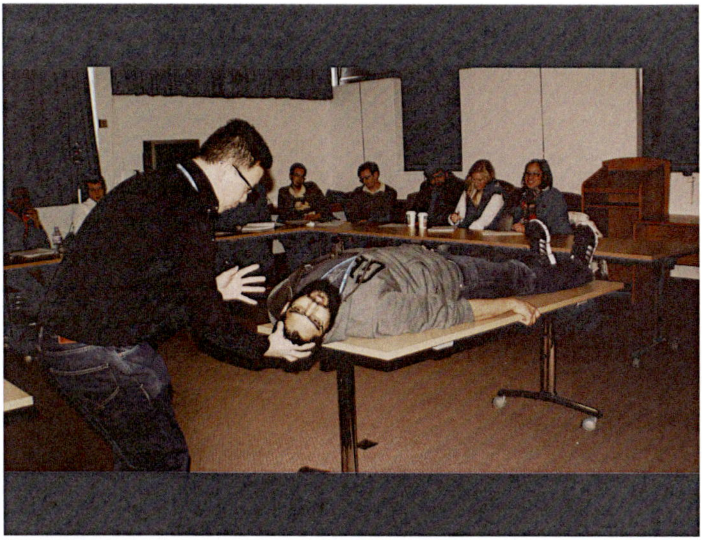

Questions

A. What test is being performed?

B. What is this test used to diagnose?

C. What is the manoeuvre used to treat the condition above?

D. How often can the manoeuvre used to treat the condition above be repeated?

E. List 4 instructions for the patient post procedure to treat the condition.

Answers (Station 59)

Clinical photograph of Dix-Hallpike Test being performed.

A. Dix-Hallpike Test.

B. Benign Paroxysmal Positional Vertigo (BPPV).

C. Epley's manoeuvre.

D. As often as needed if the patient is symptomatic.

E. Avoid driving, avoid lying flat for 48 hours, avoid bending forwards and avoid lying on the affected side.

Revision Notes

- BPPV is the most common peripheral vestibular condition that usually occurs after a head injury or an upper respiratory tract infection.
- BPPV predominantly affects middle aged women.
- Patients with BPPV may present with
  - o Sudden onset of vertigo induced by certain head movements
  - o Symptoms lasting seconds
  - o Nausea and vomiting
  - o There will be no other otological symptoms.
- The Dix-Halpike test is used to diagnose BPPV which involves turning the patients head 45^0 towards the affected side and laid backwards with the head below the edge of the bed. The eyes are observed for geotrophic rotatory nystagmus.
- The treatment of BPPV could be divided into:
  - o Conservative: most BPPV resolves spontaneously.
  - o Medical: Symptomatic relief of vertigo with vestibular sedatives such as Prochlorperazine.
  - o Epley's manouvre.
  - o Surgical: Labyrinthectomy, transtympanic gentamicin, vestibular nerve section.

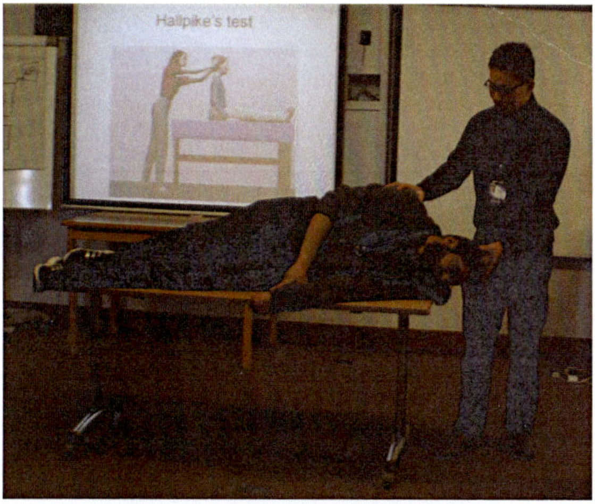

Figure 59.1a Epley manoeuvre in progress.

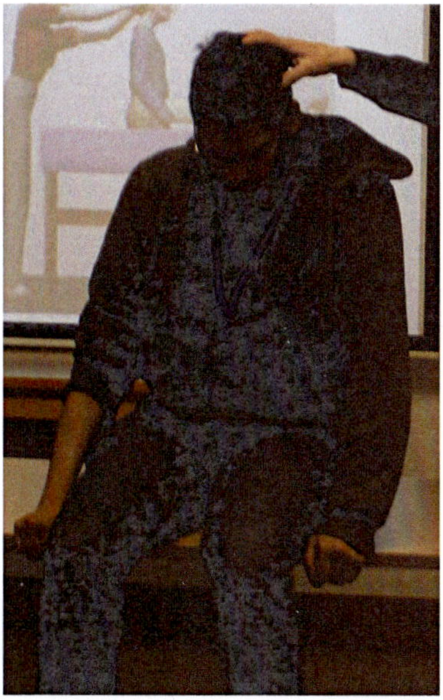

Figure 59.1b Epley manoeuvre final position.

Station 60

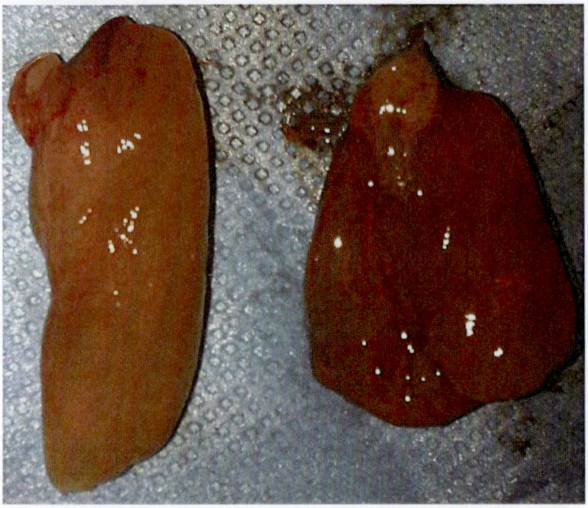

Questions

A. Give the most likely diagnosis and 5 differential diagnoses of a solid nasal lesion.

B. List 3 symptoms which may be present.

C. What is the first line medical treatment?

D. What is the surgical treatment?

E. Which condition should be considered in a 5 year old boy with bilateral lesions?

Answers (Station 60)

Clinical photograph showing nasal polyps.

A. Nasal polyps

Differential diagnoses:

Inverted papilloma
Antrochoanal polyp
Glioma
Pyogenic granuloma
Adenocarcinoma
Squamous cell carcimoma

B. Nasal blockage
Discharge

Anosmia

C. Intranasal or oral corticosteroids.

D. Functional Endoscopic Sinonasal surgery (FESS).

E. Cystic fibrosis (diagnosed by a sweat test).

Revision Notes

- Nasal polyposis is a sinonasal condition which severely interferes with quality of life. It is usually bilateral as a result of a generalised inflammatory reaction involving the mucous membranes of the nose, paranasal sinuses and the lower airways.
- The trigger of this inflammatory response may be allergy, intrinsic rhinitis, chronic infection or idiopathic.
- It is important to note Samter's triad of recurrent nasal polyposis, asthma and aspirin (or NSAID) hypersensitivity as these patients may need a more aggressive intervention.
- Patients with nasal polyposis usually present with nasal obstruction, discharge, anosmia and postnasal drip.
- A skin prick test or Radioallergosorbent test (RAST) can be performed to identify any allergic cause. A common cause is the faeces from house dust mites (Figure 60.1).

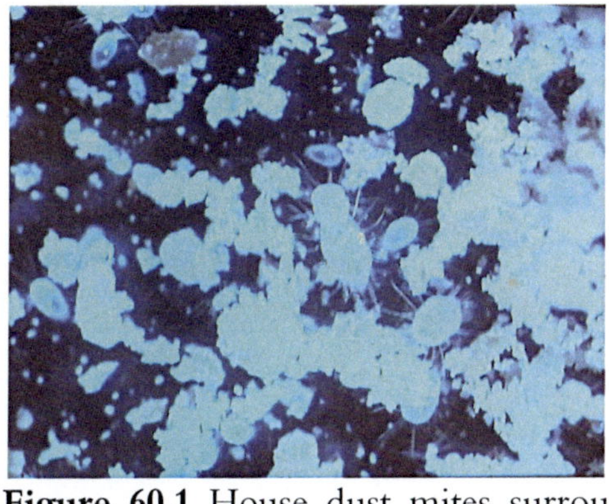

Figure 60.1 House dust mites surrounded by faeces and food material.

- Patients are initially treated medically with nasal decongestants, topical steroids and oral prednisolone. In patients who are refractory to medical treatment, surgical intervention is indicated.
- In recurrent cases and where Functional Endoscopic Sinus Surgery (FESS) is being planned, a CT scan of the sinuses would be appropriate to rule out any secondary pathology and as a road map to surgery. Any polyps that are removed should be sent for histological diagnosis, especially if they are unilateral.

Table 60.1 Differential diagnosis of nasal polyps.

BENIGN	MALIGNANT
Nasal polyp	Squamous cell carcinoma
Inverted papilloma	Malignant melanoma
Antrochoanal polyp (Figure	Adenocarcinoma
Rhinosporidiosis	Transitional cell carcinoma
Other: Meningocoele, encephalocoele, Hamartoma, Glioma, Chordoma, Teratoma, pyogenic granuloma (Figure 60.2a-c)	Metastasis

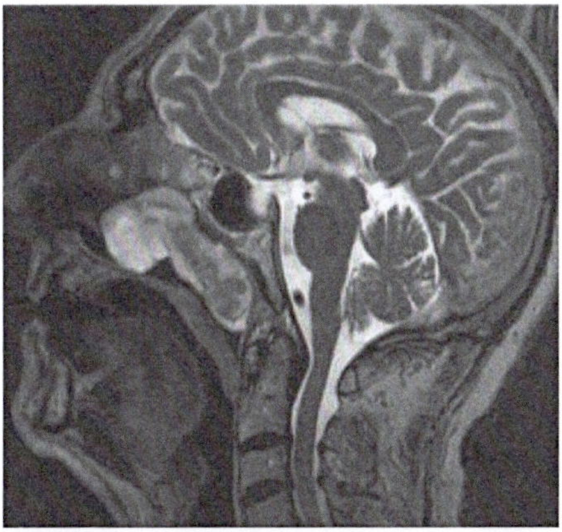

Figure 60.2 T2 weighted MRI of an antrochoanal polyp.

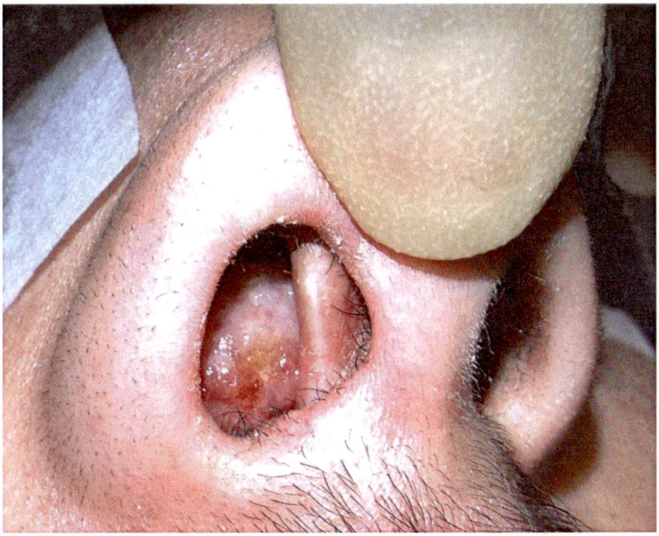

Figure 60.3a Pyogenic granuloma in situ (attached to the lateral nasal vestibule skin).

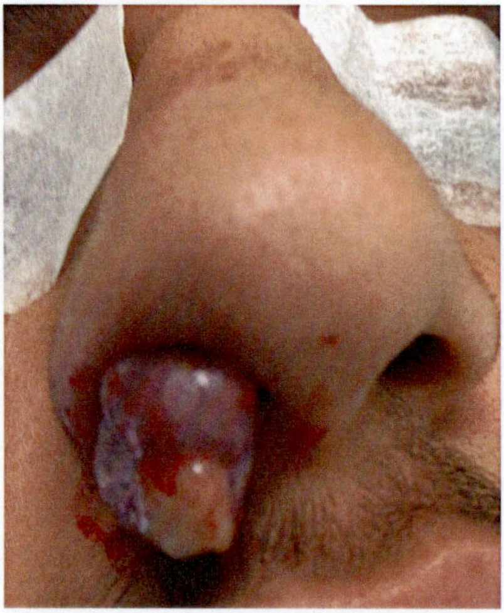

Figure 60.3b Pyogenic granuloma lifted out of the nasal vestibule.

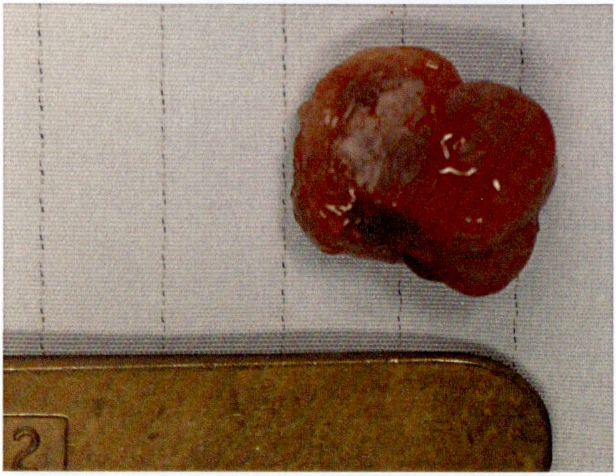

Figure 60.3c Pyogenic granuloma specimen.

Station 61

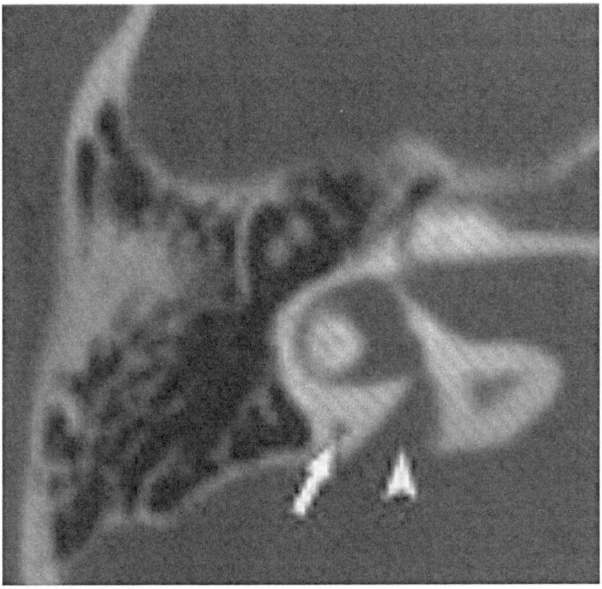

The arrow head on this CT image of the temporal bone points to the commonest radiographic abnormality of the inner ear. The presenting complaint was progressive hearing loss.

Questions

A. What is the plane of the CT scan?
B. In which window is this CT scan shown?
C. What is the abnormality indicated by the arrow head?
D. What type of hearing loss is associated with this abnormality?
E. Name one syndrome associated with this finding.
F. What advice would you give to this patient regarding sports?

Answers (Station 61)

A. Axial
B. Bone window

C. Enlarged vestibular aqueduct
[note (1) this large aqueduct may be easily confused with the IAM which, in contrast to the cochlear aqueduct, is on the same level and (2) the normal size of the aqueduct should be the same as the diameter of the space indicated by the complete arrow].

D. Progressive sensori-neural hearing loss (SNHL)

E. Pendred syndrome

F. Avoid contact sports and head injury may speed up the progression of SNHL.

Revision Notes

- The inner ear is essentially made up of a bony labyrinth lined by a membranous labyrinth and connecting aqueducts (Figures 61.1a and b).
- Therefore inner ear abnormality associated with hearing loss may occur in the:
  1. Membraneous labyrinth
  2. Bony labyrinth or
  3. Aqueducts

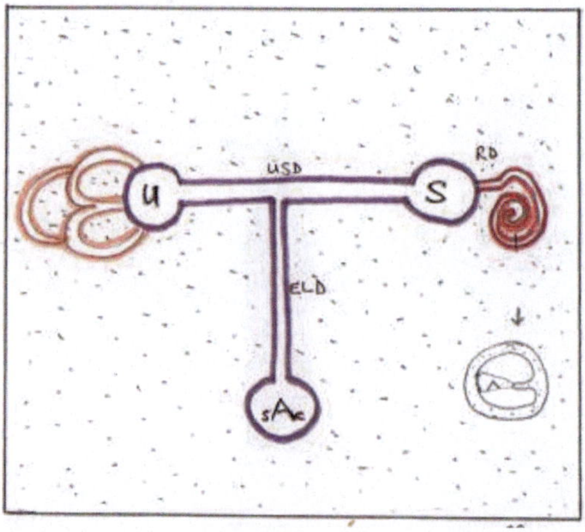

Figure 61.1a Schematic diagram of the labyrinth (**U** utricle, **S** saccule, s**A**c sac of endolymphatic, RD reunion ductus, ELD endolymphatic duct, USD utriculosaccule duct.

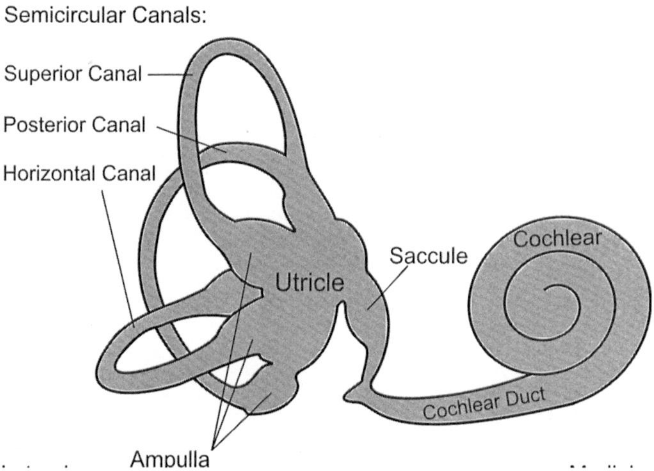

Figure 61.1b Diagram of the labyrinth for comparison with Figure 61.1a.

1. **Membraneous labyrinth dysplasia**
   - ***Limited*** abnormality (commonest is saccular/cochlear, ***Sc****heibe*)
   - ***Complete*** abnormality (rare, *Usher, Jarvell & Lange-Nelson,* ***Bind-Seebenman)***

   Sensori-neural HL, rehabilited with Cochlear Implants.

2. **Bony labyrinth dysplasia**
   - ***Limited*** (1.5 turn vs 2.5, *Mondini – 50% of cochlear abnormality*)
   - ***Complete*** (no cochlea, *Michel,* absolute contraindication to Cochlear Implant; requires brainstem implant).

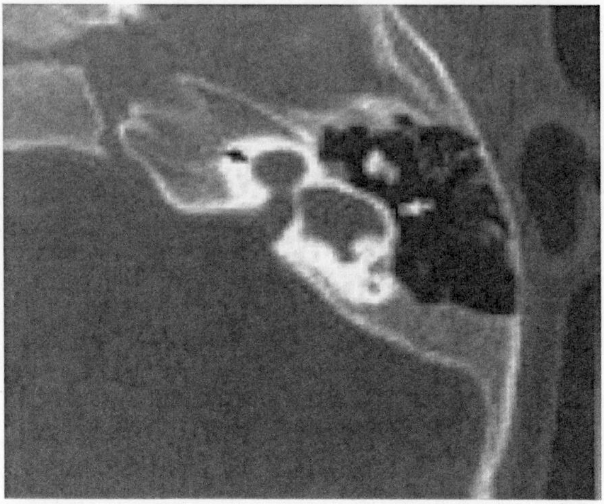

Figure 61. Axial CT image illustrating a Mondini deformity.

Pendred syndrome

- First described by Englishman Dr.Vaughan Pendred (described family in Durham, 1896).
- Bilateral SNHL and Goitre.
- Auto Recessive & accounts for 7.5% of all congenital deafness.
- Mutation in Pendrin genes (codes for an iodine/chloride transporter protein, chromosome 7).
- Associated with Enlarged Vestibular Aquaduct (EVAs,) enlarged endolymph system & Mondini deformity.
- CSF Rhinorhoea (CSF may flow from ear to eustachian tube to post-nasal space to nose).

Management: Multidisciplinary team, cochlear implants, thyroxine, no contact sport.

Station 62

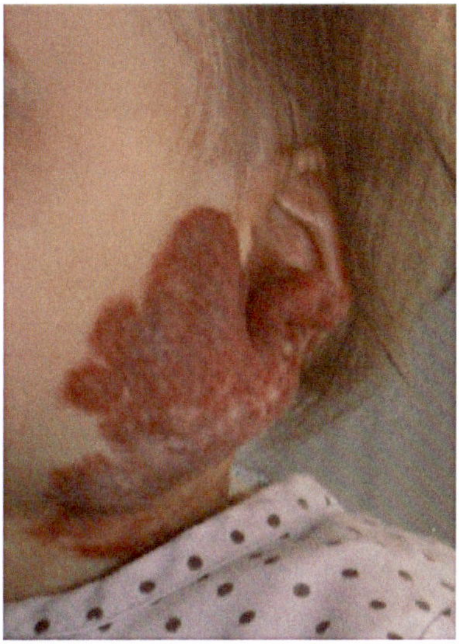

Photograph A

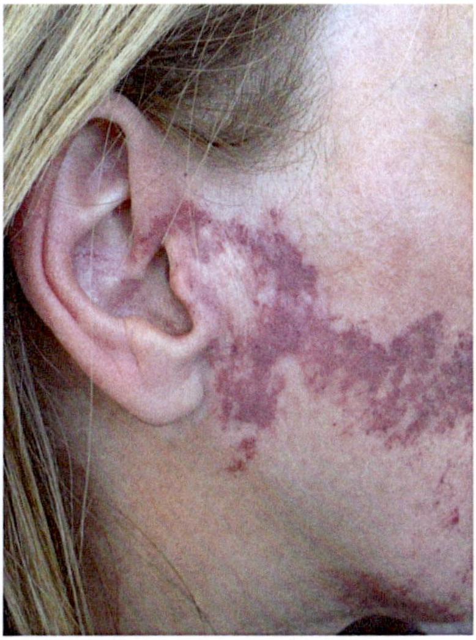

Photograph B

Questions

A. What clinical conditions are seen in Photograph A and B?

B. List 3 differences between the 2 conditions.

C. List 3 complications of condition A.

D. List 2 medical treatment options for the condition shown in photograph A.

E. List 2 treatment options for the condition shown in photograph B.

Answers (Station 62)

A. Haemangiomas and vascular malformations.

B. In contrast to vascular malformations, haemangiomas are usually abscent at birth but grows rapidly and then involute spontaneously by 18 months.

C. Bleeding, infection and platelet depletion (Kasabach-Merritt syndrome).

D. Beta-blockers (eg propanolol) and steroids.

E. Camouflage with make-up and laser therapy.

Revision Notes

- Congenital vascular anomalies may be classified as
  - Haemangiomas
  - Vascular malformations
- Haemangiomas
  - Develops after birth
  - Expands rapidly under the influence of self-secreting fibroblast derived growth factors
  - Often mistaken for malignancy especially in the parotid region
  - May cause stridor due to airway obstruction at the level of the subglottis
  - Involutes with time by apoptosis; therefore management is conservative unless causing functional problems such as visual field defects.

- Vascular malformations
  - High-flow Arteriovenous malformations; these are dealt with by the neurosurgeons
  - Low-flow Venous malformation; these are dealt with by ENT surgeons
    - Lymphatic malformation
    - Lymphatic-venous malformation (cystic hygroma)
    - Capillary (or venular) malformation (Portwine stain)

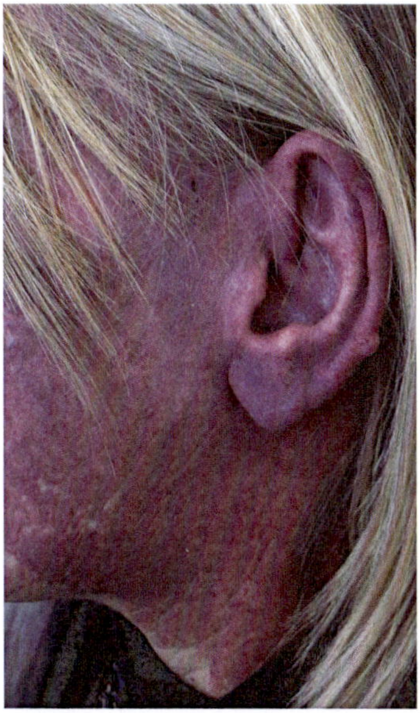

Figure 62.1 Extensive capillary vascular malformation – a low flow vascular malformation

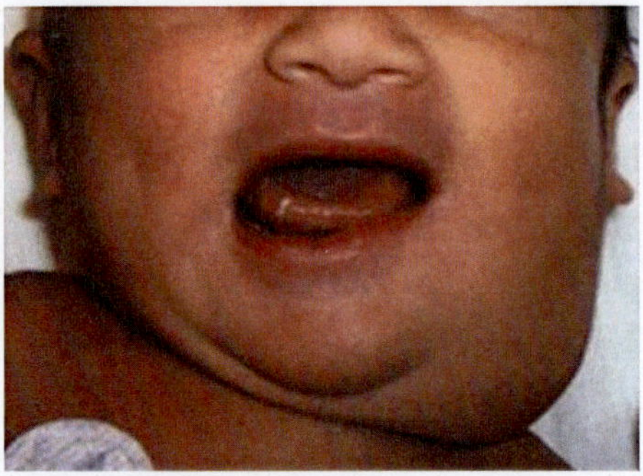

Figure 62.2 Clinical photograph of a left cystic hygroma – a low flow vascular malformation.

Chapter 2

Operation Notes

2.1 Introduction

Writing operation notes are important and may be tested in the DO-HNS exam. Although we may be writing this on a daily basis, it is important to remember that there are only 7 minutes for this station and there is a lot to cover during that time. You need to remember that in the station, they may just give you a blank piece of paper and you need to fill in ALL headings and details. The description for the station is usually short and includes the patient's name and what operation you have done. In this chapter a suggested template, including the main headings, is provided. A few examples have also been included for completeness.

Top tips

- Learn the headings for writing operation notes.
- Make sure you time yourself in writing the operation notes of some common procedures – it's harder than you think!
- See below for a guide to writing operation notes and the headings you should consider including.

2.2 Template for operation notes

NAME OF OPERATION
X Hospital
DATE TIME
PATIENT NAME
DOB
HOSPITAL NUMBER (HN)
THEATRE 2
SURGEON,

ASSISTANT
ANAESTHETIST,
SCRUB NURSE

INDICATION
ANTIBIOTICS
ANAESTHESIA (GA/LA)
STANDARD DRAPE

FINDINGS
PROCEDURE

POST-OP INSTRUCTIONS

Signature: (and print)
CT2 to Mr Smith (consultant ENT surgeon)
GMC XXXXXXX
Bleep 246

2.3 Adenotonsillectomy

Instructions

You have just done an adeno-tonsillectomy on a 5 year old girl called Anne Jones. The anaesthetist is happy for the patient to be discharged the same day. Please write an operation note for this patient.

<u>ADENO-TONSILLECTOMY</u>
London Hospital

DATE 23.05.2013 **TIME** 12:00
PATIENT NAME Anne Jones
DOB 12.02.2008
HOSPITAL No. 23113677

THEATRE 2
SURGEON Miss A. Hart
ASISTANT: Dr John Spiliotis
ANAESTHETIST Dr Gas
SCRUB NURSE Miss Ford

INDICATION Obstructive sleep apnoea
ANTIBIOTICS none
ANAESTHESIA GA
STANDARD DRAPE
FINDINGS Moderate adenoid, Grade 4 tonsils

PROCEDURE

Boyle davis gag and draffin rods
Adenoids curetted
Haemostasis with PNS pack and adrenaline (1:10,000)
Bilateral cold Steel dissection of tonsils with 2.0 silk ties to each lower pole
Haemostasis using bipolar diathermy (12W)

Swab count correct, PNS suctioned, teeth ok, TMJ, lips ok at end of procedure

POST-OP INSTRUCTIONS

Airway and saturation monitoring
Regular observations: 15 min observations in recovery, 30min observations on ward
Analgesia regularly
Encourage eating and drinking
Home later if well and no signs of bleeding

Doctor to review prior to discharge
No routine follow up
Information sheet given to patient

Miss A Hart
CT2 to Mr Smith (Consultant ENT surgeon)
GMC 123456
Bleep 246

2.4 Questions and answers

Instructions

A three year old boy has come in for an elective operation for bilateral grommet insertion due to glue ear. You proceed with the operation. During the operation you note that on the right side, the tympanic membrane was dull with some middle ear fluid. On the left, you also notice a dull tympanic membrane with a large middle ear effusion. There were no complications. Please write an operation note for this patient who will be discharged the same day.

BILATERAL MYRINGOTOMIES AND GROMMET INSERTIONS

LONDON HOSPITAL

DATE 23.05.2013 **TIME** 14:00

PATIENT NAME William Thomas
DOB 23.01.2000
HOSPITAL No. 2111455

THEATRE 2
SURGEON Miss A. Hart
ANAESTHETIST Dr Gas
SCRUB NURSE Miss Ford

INDICATION Bilateral glue ear
ANTIBIOTICS none
ANAESTHESIA GA
STANDARD DRAPE

FINDINGS Right – flat, dull TM with small quantity of middle ear fluid
Left – dull TM with large middle ear effusion

PROCEDURE

Ear canal – suctioned of wax atraumatically
Antero-inferior myringotomies performed
Effusions aspirated, Shah grommets inserted
Attics clear on right and left sides

POST-OP INSTRUCTIONS

Airway and saturation monitoring
Regular observations: 15 min observations in recovery, 30min observations on ward
Analgesia regularly
Eat and drink as able
Home today when comfortable
Doctor to review prior to discharge
Follow up – 2 months with audiology
Information sheet given to patient

Miss A Hart
CT2 to Mr Smith (Consultant ENT surgeon)
GMC 123456
Bleep 246

2.5 Microlaryngoscopy and biopsy

Instructions

Please write an operation note for a patient you have just done a microlaryngoscopy and biopsy for hoarseness of voice.

MICROLARYNGOSCOPY AND BIOPSY

LONDON HOSPITAL

DATE 23.05.2013 **TIME** 15:00

PATIENT NAME Laurie Williams
DOB 24.03.1965
HOSPITAL No. 1284737

THEATRE 2
SURGEON Miss A. Hart
ASSISTANT Dr John Spiliotis
ANAESTHETIST Dr Gas
SCRUB NURSE Miss Ford

INDICATION Hoarseness
ANTIBIOTICS none given
ANAESTHESIA GA
STANDARD DRAPE

FINDINGS Small vocal cord polyp on right ant 1/3 and 2/3 border

PROCEDURE

Mouthguard inserted
Laryngoscopy performed
Laryngoscope in suspension
Microscope used to inspect cords
Microdissection of vocal cord polyp

Haemostasis with 1:1000 adrenaline patty
Teeth, TMJ, lips ok at end of procedure
Specimen sent to histology

POST-OP INSTRUCTIONS

Airway and saturation monitoring
Regular observations: 15 min observations in recovery, 30min observations on ward
Analgesia regularly
Eat and drink as able
24 hours voice rest
Home tomorrow if well
Doctor to review prior to discharge
Follow up in Mr Smith's outpatient clinic – 2 weeks with histology
Information sheet given to patient

Miss A Hart
CT2 to Mr Smith (Consultant ENT surgeon)
GMC 123456
Bleep 246 **date** 23.05 13

Chapter 3

Discharge Summaries

3.1 Introduction

All patients in the UK require a discharge summary before they can be discharged from hospital. This gives a summary of what has happened in hospital, any tests, investigations or operations that have been done and any follow up plan that is required. A copy is usually given to the patient and one is sent to their GP. This chapter includes a discharge summary template with a few completed examples.

Top tips:

- Read the question carefully
- Time yourself writing a discharge summary
- Make sure you have included any relevant information given to you in the question
- See below for a guide to writing a discharge summary. Usually you will only be given a blank sheet of paper.

3.2 Template for discharge summary

HOSPITAL

DATE TIME

PATIENT NAME
DOB
HOSPTIAL No.
ADDRESS

GP DETAILS
CONSULTANT
WARD

DATE OF ARRIVAL (DOA)
DATE OF DISCHARGE

PRIMARY DIAGNOSIS
PRESENTING COMPLAINT (PC)
CO- MORBIDITY (this is particularly relevant to clinical coding)

INVESTIGATIONS
OPERATION/ SURGEON
COMPLICATION

DISCHARGING MEDICATIONS/ALLERGIES

ADVICE

FOLLOW UP

SIGN AND PRINT NAME
DESIGNATION
BLEEP or contact number
DATE

3.3 Endoscopic nasal polypectomy

Instructions

Write a discharge summary for a patient who underwent an endoscopic nasal polypectomy.

DISCHARGE SUMMARY

HOSPITAL	London
DATE TIME	5th April 2013 16:00hrs
PATIENT NAME	Mr Daniels
DOB	1st Jan 1966
HOSPTIAL No.	L124536
ADDRESS	20 Kent Way, London, SE21 9LA.
GP DETAILS	Dr Siva Sundar, Gloucester Garden Practice
CONSULTANT	Mr Ronald Smith
WARD	Toynbee Ward
DATE OF ARRIVAL	21st Feb 2013
DATE OF DISCHARGE	21st Feb 2013
PRIMARY DIAGNOSIS	Nasal polyposis
PRESENTING COMPLAINT	Nasal obstruction ongoing for 2 years
Co-MORBIDITY	Diabetic and Hypertensive
INVESTIGATIONS	CT sinuses – bilat nasal polyposis, all other sinuses

	ventilated with minimal mucosal thickening
OPERATION	Endoscopic nasal polypectomy
SURGEON	Mr Smith
COMPLICATION	No intra-operative or post-operative complications
MEDICATIONS	4 weeks nasal douche Continue Flixonase spray 200mcg BD No other changes to medications
ADVICE	Nasal packing removed prior to discharge Crusting and dry blood can cause nasal obstruction for 1-2 weeks Larger bleed requires readmission to hospital One week off work
FOLLOW UP:	Mr Smith's out-patient clinic in 4-6 weeks (with histology) Nasal splints out in 1 week time in OPD clinic
SIGN AND PRINT NAME	Signature, S.Patel, SUNIL PATEL
DESIGNATION	Registrar to Mr Smith, Consultant ENT Surgeon

BLEEP or contact number ***234*** *DATE* ***21st Feb 2013***

3.4 Submandibular gland excision

Instructions

Write a discharge summary for a patient who underwent a right submandibular gland excision.

<u>DISCHARGE SUMMARY</u>

HOSPITAL	London
DATE TIME	5th April 2013 16:00hrs
PATIENT NAME	Mr Smith
DOB	1st Jan 1966
HOSPTIAL NUMBER	L124536
ADDRESS	20 Kent Way, London, SE21 9LA.
GP DETAILS `	Dr Siva Sundar, Gloucester Garden Practice
CONSULTANT	Mr John Smith
WARD	Toynbee Ward
DATE OF ARRIVAL	21st Feb 2013
DATE OF DISCHARGE	21st Feb 2013
PRIMARY DIAGNOSIS	Submandibular calculus (right side)

PRESENTING COMPLAINT	Lump at floor of mouth, painful eating
Co-MORBIDITY	Diabetic and Hypertensive
INVESTIGATIONS	Sialogram – submandibular stone
OPERATION	Right submandibular gland excision
SURGEON	Mr Smith
COMPLICATION	Nil
MEDICATIONS	Co-codamol 30/500 2 tablets four times a day as required
ADVICE	Pain killers as able, off work for one week, if notice temperature, pain and swelling in the neck or difficulty to breathe please come to A+E immediately. Any concerns seek medical advice from GP or A&E .
FOLLOW UP	3 weeks
SIGN AND PRINT NAME	Signature, SUNIL PATEL
DESIGNATION	Registrar to Mr Smith, Consultant ENT Surgeon.
BLEEP or contact number	234 DATE 21st Feb 2013.

Chapter 4

ENT Instruments, Devices, Prostheses and Materials

4.1 Introduction

One or more of the non-interactive stations assesses your knowledge of instruments, devices and materials pertaining to Otolaryngology. This may take the form of a matching exercise or simply identification and description. In this chapter we present and describe some of the ENT apparatus which are likely to appear in the examination. The following list of surgical, outpatient and audiological apparatus is by no means exhaustive, but is a good representation of what has appeared in previous examination. A top tip is to look at the inventory sheet that comes with each theatre set that is used in common ENT operations, such as tonsillectomy, grommet insertion, septoplasty, FESS, myringoplasty, parotidectomy and thyroidectomy.

4.2 Oral apparatus

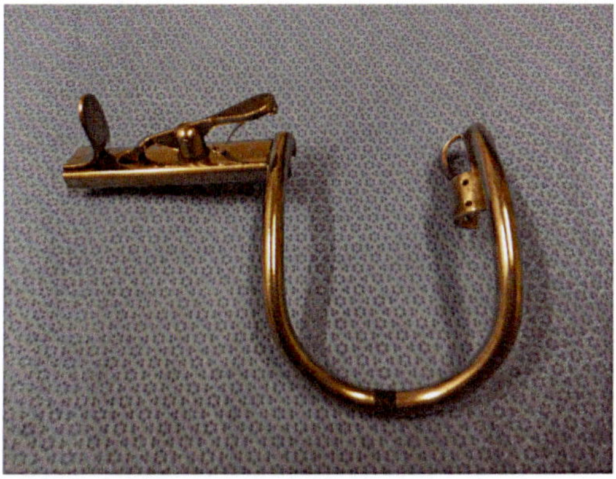

Figure 4.1 Boyle Davis mouth gag

This instrument is used in oral and oropharyngeal surgeries to keep the mouth open. Common ENT procedures where it is used include tonsillectomy, adenoidectomy and palatal surgery (such as UPPP). It comes in adult and paediatric sizes. It has a mouth guard which protects the teeth and gum from trauma.

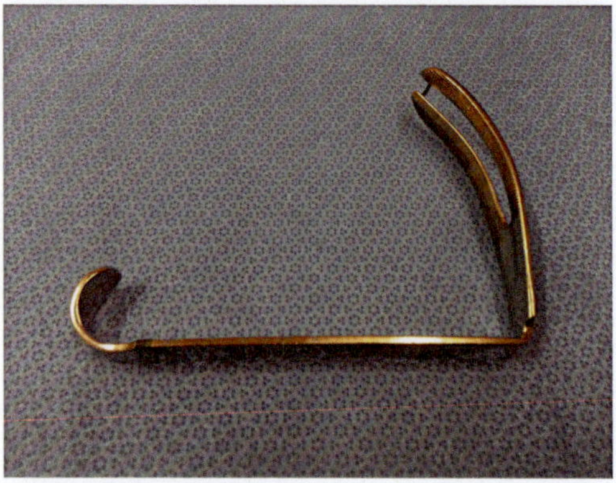

Figure 4.2 Doughty blade

This instrument slides through the Boyle Davis mouth gag to keep the mouth open in oral and oropharyngeal surgeries. It comes in a variety of sizes. The appropriate size to be used can be estimated by placing the blade across the chin and back of tongue. Care must be taken when removing this Doughty blade from the patient in order to prevent accidental extubation of the patient as the ET tube may get stuck in the groove.

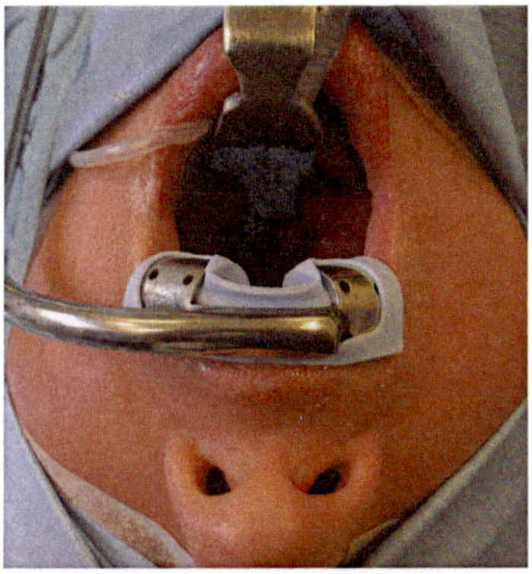

Figure 4.2a A Boyle Davis gag and a Doughty blade in position for tonsillectomy

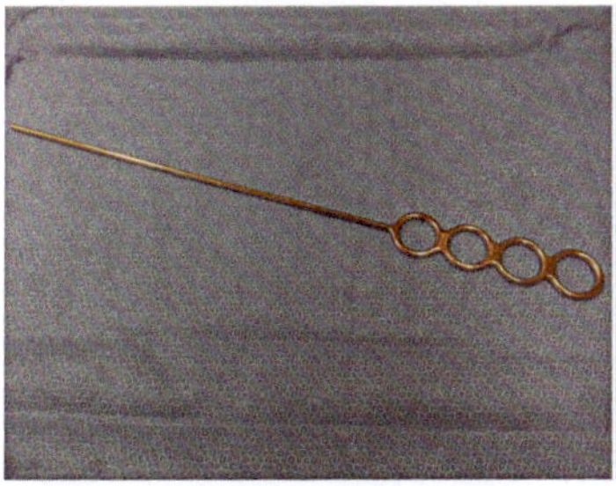

Figure 4.3 Draffin rods

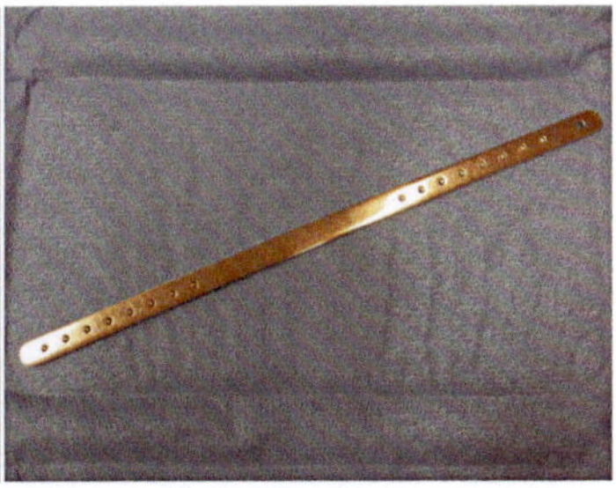

Figure 4.4 Magauran plate

Draffin rods (picture 3) are used in pairs in a crossed position to keep the Boyle Davis mouth gag in place. In order to prevent the Draffin rods from slipping during surgery, the ends of the rods are rested in the holes of a Magauran plate (picture 4). The plate itself lies under the patient's scapula. Together, the Draffin rods and Magauran plate stabilise the Boyle Davis mouth gag (Figure 4.a).

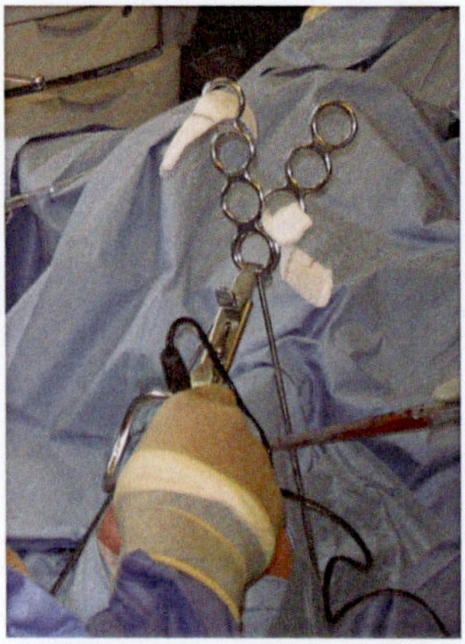

Figure 4.4a Draffin rods in position during tonsillectomy.

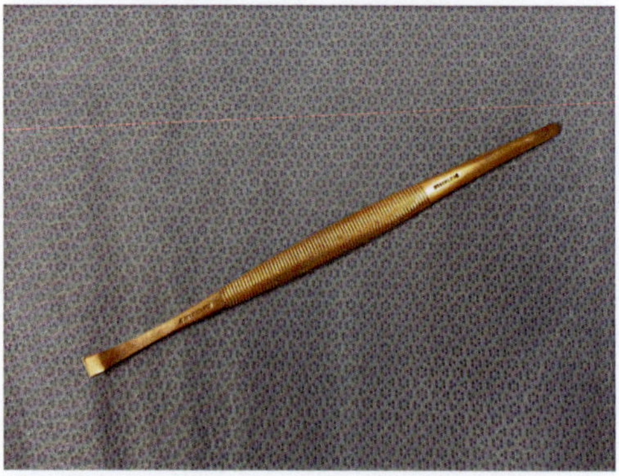

Figure 4.5 Gwynne Evans tonsils dissector

This instrument is used in tonsillectomy to bluntly peel the tonsillar capsule from the surrounding superior constrictor. An incision is made superolaterally on the anterior pillar (palatoglossus) and the tonsillar capsule is found. The dissector is used to peel the fibres of the muscle off the tonsillar capsule. This method of cold-steel tonsillectomy is associated with a higher primary haemorrhage rate but a smaller secondary haemorrhage rate (as seen in the national tonsillectomy audit).

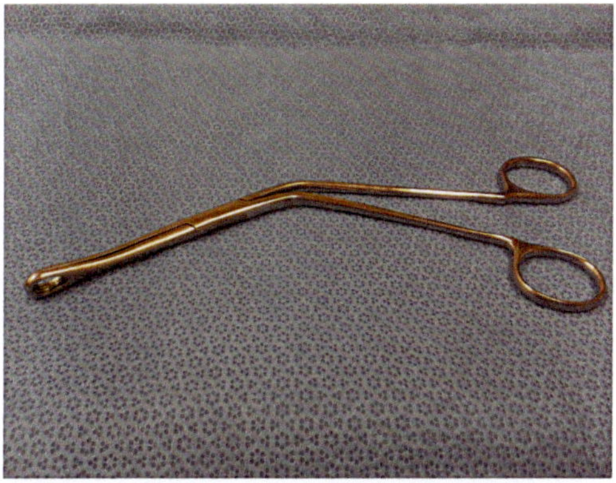

Figure 4.6 Denis Brown Tonsil holding forceps

This instrument is used in tonsillectomy to apply traction on the tonsil in order to identify the dissection plane. The Denis Brown forceps is usually held with the surgeon's non-dominant hand while the dissector with the dominant hand.

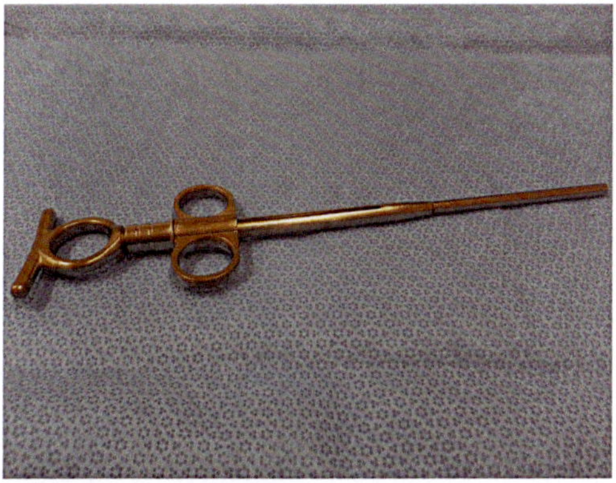

Figure 4.7 Eve Tonsil Snare

This instrument is used to snare the tonsil (i.e. section the inferior pole of the tonsil after the other parts have been dissected). A metallic wire protrudes from its inferior end. This wire is looped around the tonsil pedicle. When the top end of the instrument is pressed, the metallic wire snares the tonsil. This crushes the pedicle to reduce the bleeding. The Eve's tonsil snare is not used as often as in the past because bleeding can be sometimes difficult to control. Surgeons now prefer to tie off the inferior pole or use diathermy.

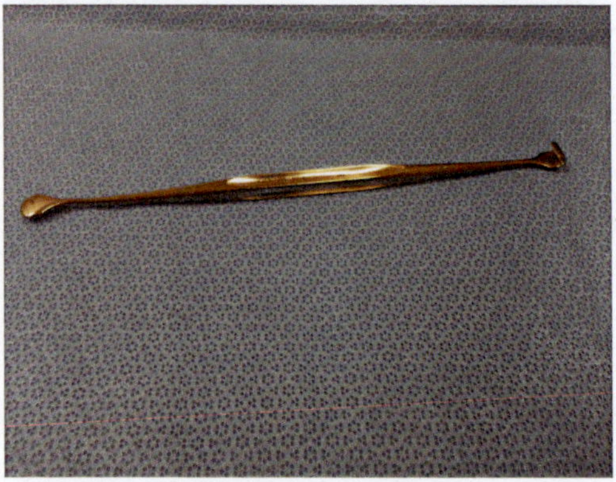

Figure 4.8 Mollison's pillar retractor

This instrument is used after tonsils have been dissected away to retract the anterior pillar. This allows careful examination of the tonsillar fossa to identify bleeding points for haemostasis. The retractor has two ends: the hook-like end is used to retract the superior pole while the flatter curved end is used to retract elsewhere.

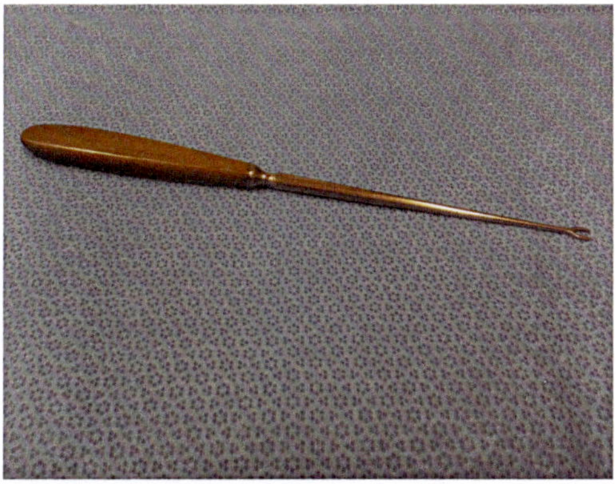

Figure 4.9 Negus knot pusher

This instrument is used to tie a knot around the inferior pole of the tonsil after the tonsil has been dissected. Using this instrument makes it easier to tie at depth and tighten the knot to prevent bleeding. Silk is the common choice of material for the tie.

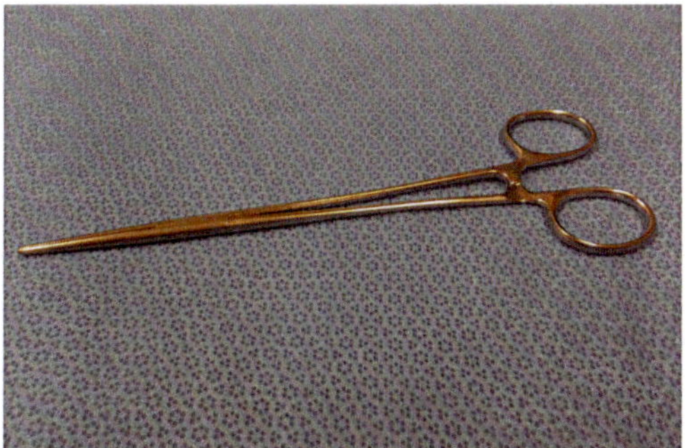

Figure 4.10 Straight Birkett forceps

Straight Birkett forceps is used to catch bleeding points on the tonsillar fossa. Once tightened around the bleeder, the straight Birkett forceps is gently lifted off the tonsillar bed before applying the Curved Negus forceps. This is followed by tying a knot to achieve haemostasis.

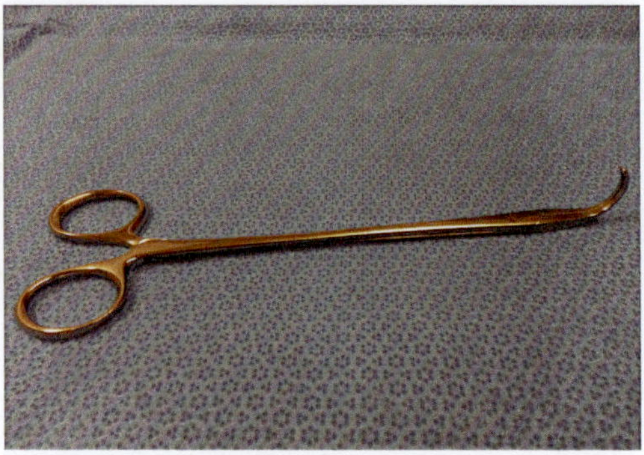

Figure 4.11 Curved Negus forceps

The curved Negus forceps is also commonly used to clamp the inferior pole of the tonsil just before removing it. Silk tie is then used to tie a knot around the tonsil pedicle to prevent it from bleeding.

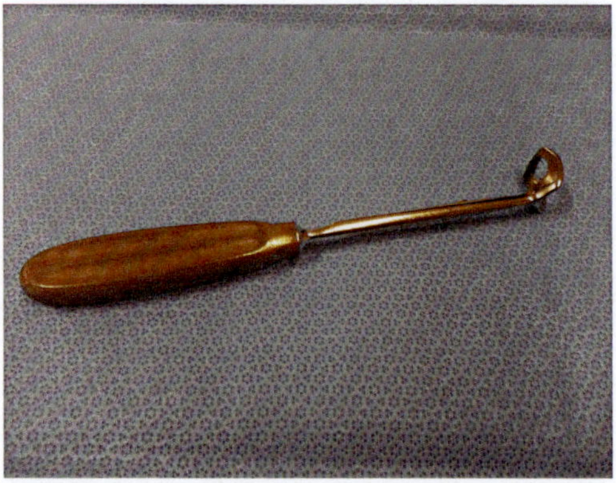

Figure 4.12 St Clair Thomson adenoid curette

This instrument is used to curette the adenoid from the post nasal space. This is a blind procedure. Adenoidectomy is indicated in adenoid hypertrophy causing symptoms of nasal obstruction, recurrent Otitis Media with Effusion (OME) and obstructive sleep apnoea. Adenoid curettage has higher risk of bleeding than suction diathermy (1% vs 0.5%).

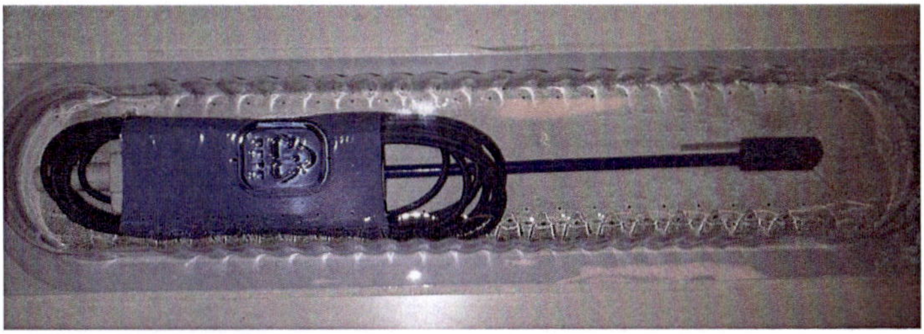

Figure 4.13 Monopolar Suction Diathermy

This instrument is used for adenoidectomy and is gradually becoming the method of choice. It is set at about 30 watts and the adenoid is removed layer by layer under direct vision. The risk of post –op bleeding with suction diathermy is approximately 0.5 % (with curette it is about 1%). However, there is an increase risk of infection because of the residual dead tissue, which may be associated with halitosis a few days after the procedure.

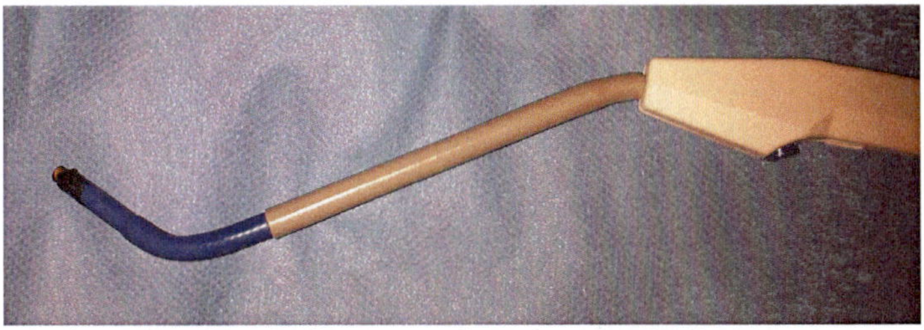

Figure 4.13a A used monopolar suction diathermy (notice how the bend to allow easy access to the post nasal space).

4.3 Ear apparatus

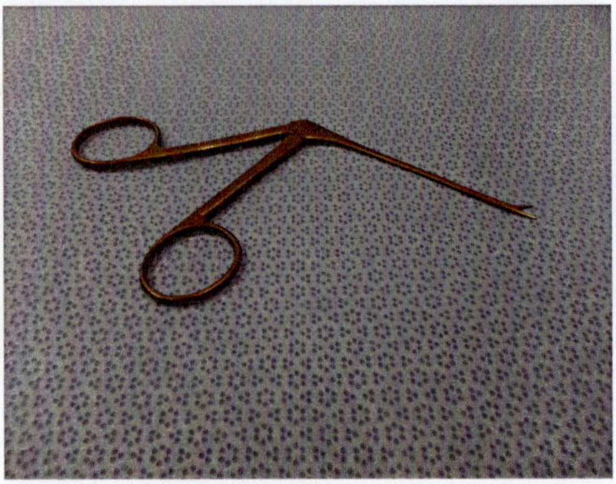

Figure 4.13 Crocodile forceps

This instrument is commonly used in surgery and procedures involving the ear. Its fine shape and small jaws allow good access to areas of the ear canal and also middle ear. It can be used to remove foreign bodies from the ear canal such as cotton wool. It is also used to insert grommets and ear wick.

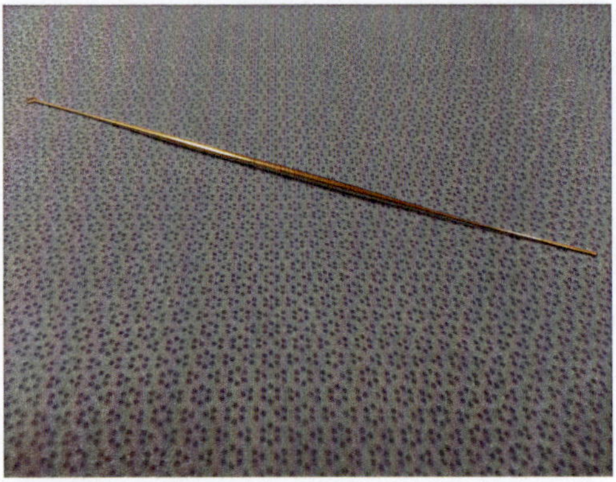

Figure 4.14 Jobson Horne probe

Curette loop

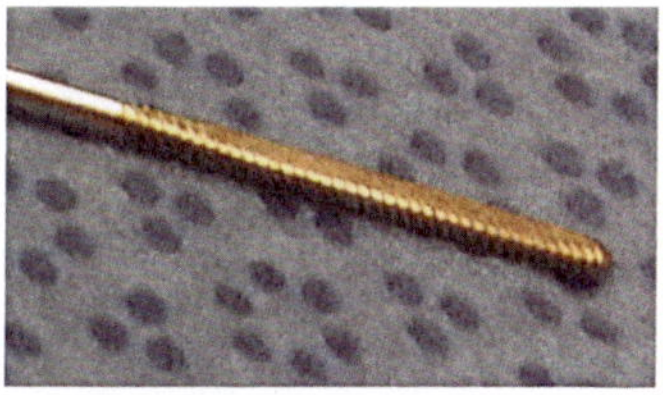

Serrated end

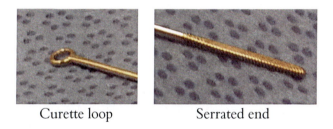

This instrument has a curette loop at one end and a serrated section at the other end. The curette loop end is used to remove wax and round foreign bodies from the ear canal. The serrated end holds cotton wool which is often used to mop ear discharge.

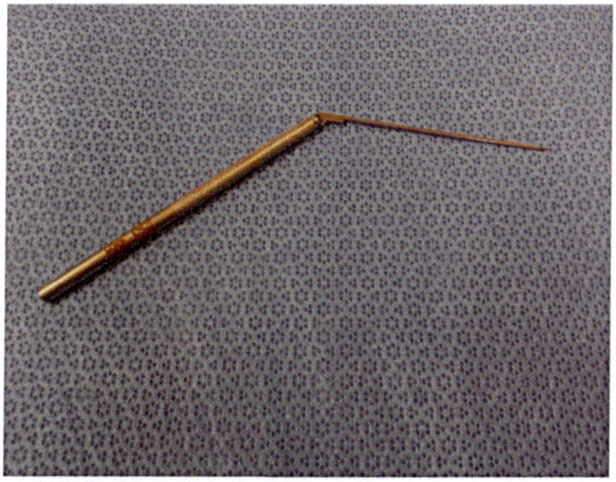

Figure 4.15 Agnew myringotome

This instrument is used in the surgical management of glue ear. It is used to make a radial incision in the anteroinferior segment of the tympanic membrane before the effusion is aspirated and a ventilation tube (such as Shah grommet) inserted. Myringotomy is usually performed under general anaesthetic in children but can be done under local anaesthetic in adults. Common local anaesthetic agent used before myringotomy is EMLA cream.

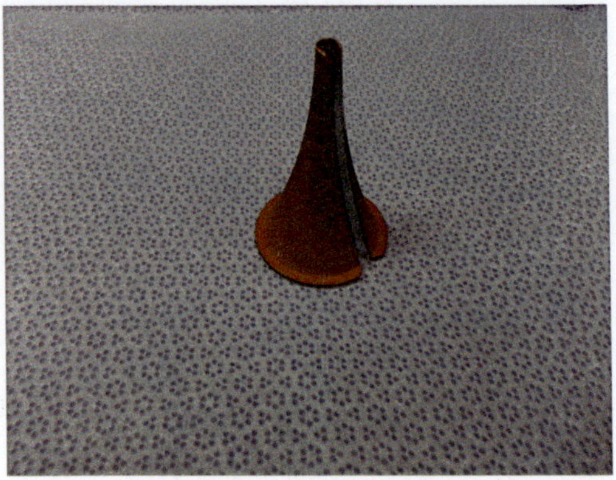

Figure 4.16 Tumarkin aural speculum

This instrument is used in ear surgery and simple otological procedures to straighten the ear canal in order to obtain adequate view of the tympanic membrane. It is dark coloured to prevent reflection of light when using the microscope. As shown in the picture above, it has a slot which makes the use of instruments such as the Agnew Myringotome and Zoellner sucker easier. It comes in a variety of sizes. Usually, the largest size that fits the patient's ear canal is used to give the best view and also allow easier use of instruments.

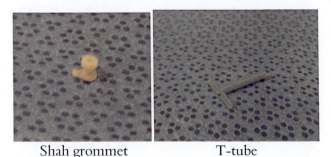

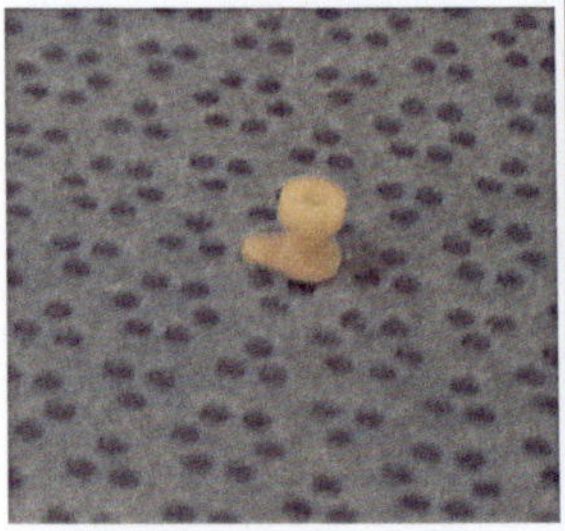

Shah grommet

T-tube

Figure 4.17 Ventilation tubes

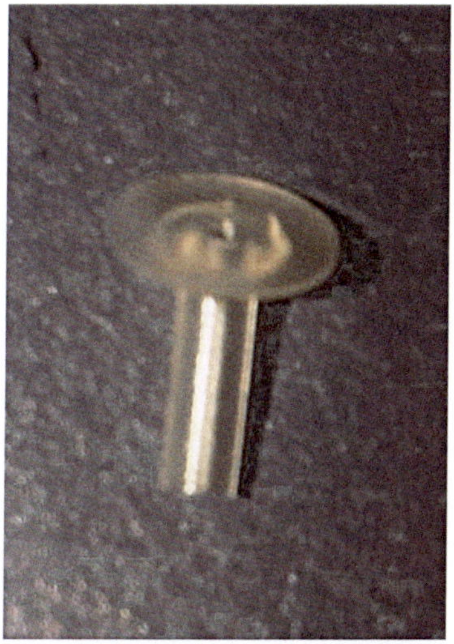

Shephard permavent tube

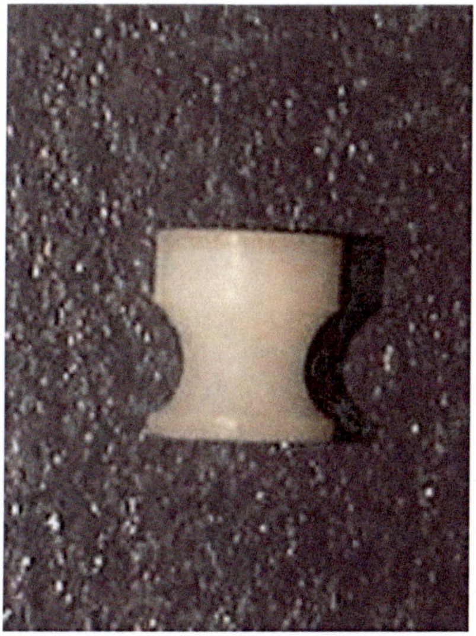

Shepherd grommet

Ventilation tubes are inserted into the tympanic membrane to allowing air entry into the middle ear, thereby equalizing pressure between the middle ear and outside. There are many types of ventilation tubes avaible on today eg Shah and Shepherd. In general they can be divided into short term and long term tubes. Short term grommets usually stay in for about 6-12 months and fall on their own. When they do, the tympanic membrane heals up by scarring. However, in about 2 % of patients, there is a persistent perforation which may require further surgery. Long term grommets usually stay in for 1-2 years. They are used when longer period of benefits of ventilation is required. However, they have a higher risk of perforation than short term grommets. NICE guidelines recommend grommets for surgical management of persistent otitis media with effusion (OME) associated with hearing loss greater than 25 dBHL, after 3 months of watchful waiting. The evidence based on TARGET supports performing adenoidectomy at the time of grommet insertion.

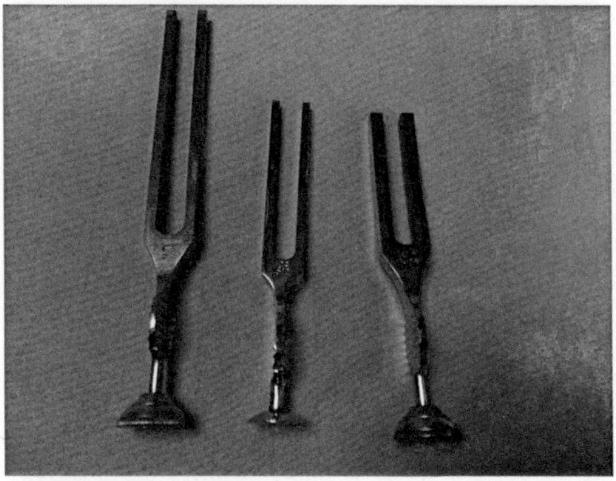

Figure 4.18 Tuning forks

Tuning forks come in various frequencies. The frequency which is used in hearing evaluation (Rinne's and Weber's tests) is 512 Hz because it produces sound for sufficiently long time without being perceived by vibration. It is important to note that there should be an air bone gap greater than 20 dB to obtain a negative Rinne's test with a standard 512 Hz tuning fork.

Tuning fork tests as still a reliable method of assessing hearing loss in the clinic setting. A 256 or 512 Hz tuning fork is commonly used. Weber's tests places a vibrating tuning fork on the forehead and asks the patient where the noise is heard loudest. It is therefore a test of asymmetry. If there is asymmetry the sound lateralizes towards conductive loss or away from sensorineural loss. Rinne's test assesses for a differential perception when the same sound is presented to the mastoid tip (bone conduction) verus the ear canal (air conduction). Sound should be perceived louder through air conduction. However, if there is a conductive problem, bone conduction will seem louder, giving a negative Rinne result. A false negative can be achieved when there is a complete dead test ear and a functioning non test ear. When the tuning fork is presented to the mastoid tip of the dead ear, the sound will travel through the skull to the functioning ear and be perceived as louder than sound presented to the ear canal of the dead ear

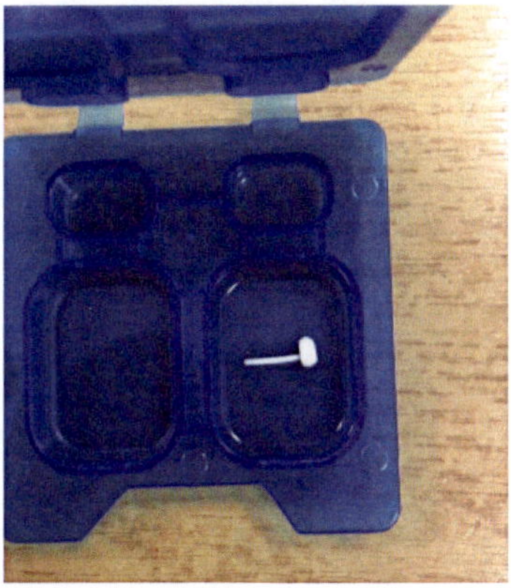

Figure 4.19 Total ossicular reconstruction prosthesis (TORP)

This prosthesis is used to reconstruct the ossicular chain when the incus and arch of the stapes are eroded, or when the malleus, incus and arch of the stapes is absent. The prosthesis has two components; the disc and cylinder unit and secondly the shaft. The prosthesis usually made of titanium and is placed during an ossiculoplasty or tympanoplasty procedure. Majority of TORP prosthesis are MRI safe.

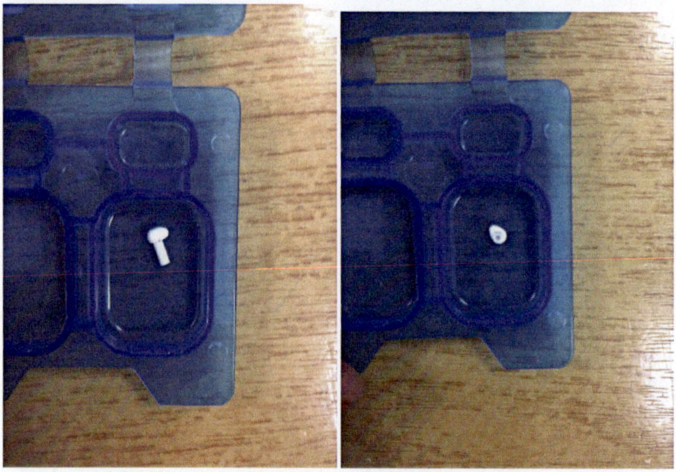

4.20 Partial ossicular reconstruction prosthesis (PORP)

This prosthesis is used to reconstruct the ossicular chain when the malleus and incus are absent in the presence of an intact stapes. It is similar to the TORP but the stem is thicker so that it can sit on the stapes. The prosthesis is often made of titanium and is placed during an ossiculoplasty or tympanoplasty procedure. Majority of PORP prosthesis are MRI safe.

Figure 4.21 Stapes piston

A stapes piston is a prosthesis that is used to replace the stapes arch as part of a stapedotomy. The procedure is performed for the treatment of otosclerosis and can be performed under a general or local anaesthetic. Following removal of the stapes arch, a small hole is drilled in the stapes footplate through which the piston is inserted and the hook aspect of the prosthesis is attached to the incus.

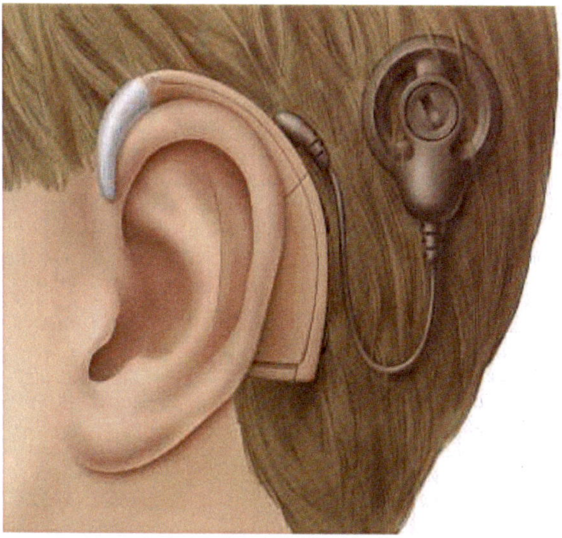

Figure 4.21 Cochlear implant

Cochlear implants, often known as bionic ears, are electronic devices that are surgically implanted under the skin behind the ear to provide a sense of sound to an individual who has profound sensorineural hearing loss in both ears who fail to cope with at least 3 months of hearing aids.

In the UK, NICE recommends bilateral cochlear implants for children and visually impaired adults.

The cochlear implant is not suitable for single sided deafness because the other ear is hearing sounds normally and the perceptions with a cochlear implant would only cause confusion. Cochlear implant is also unsuitable for rehabilitation of hearing loss after acoustic neuroma surgery because the cochlear nerve is damaged. A brainstem implant should be considered especially if there is no hearing in the other ear.

The basic components of a cochlear implant are:

External components

- Microphone – picks up sound from the environment and converts it into an analog electrical signal
- Speech processor – this prioritises audible speech and transmits the analog electrical signal to the transmitter via a thin cable
- Transmitter – placed behind the external ear and held in position by a magnet, the transmitter sends the processed electrical signals through the skin to the implanted receiver-stimulator device by radiofrequency or electromagnetic induction

Internal components

- Receiver-stimulator – implanted in bone beneath the skin, this converts the signals into electrical impulses and transmits them to electrodes via an internal cable

- Electrodes – there can be up to 22 electrodes which are placed in the cochlea, send the electrical impulses to the brain via the auditory nerve

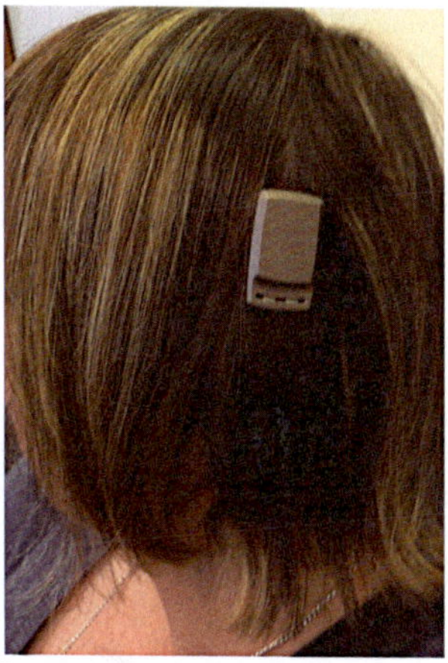

Figure 4.22a Processor attached to Titanium screw osteointegrated within the skull for the bone anchored hearing aid (BAHA).

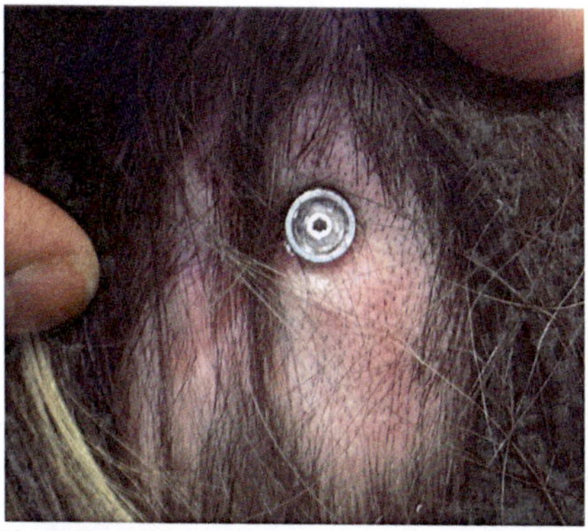

Figure 4.22b Titanium screw osteointegrated within the skull for bone anchored hearing aid (BAHA).

The bone anchored hearing aid (BAHA) is based on bone conduction. Indications for this device include:

- Chronic ear disease – continuous or intermittent ear drainage can make wearing conventional hearing aids difficult.
- External ear canal abnormalities – for example microtia, chronic infection.
- Single sided deafness of any sort.
- Congenital malformations – patients with Down's syndrome can have narrowed ear canal and/or middle ear malformation.

The device consists of a titanium prosthesis that is surgically implanted in the skull with a small abutment exposed through the skin onto which a sound processor is fitted. The implant receives sounds vibrations from the processor and vibrates the skull and inner ear. These stimulate the inner ear directly.

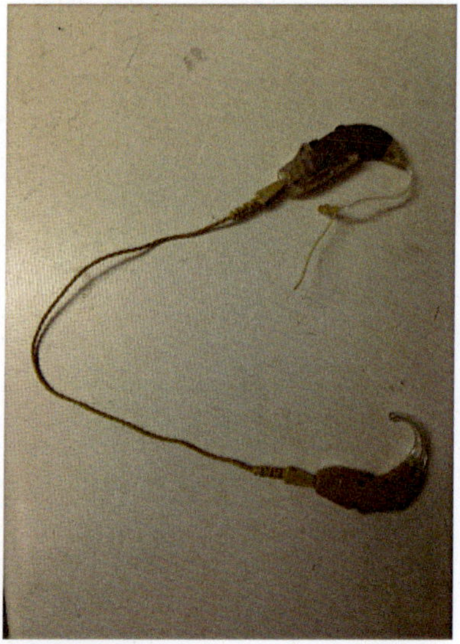

Figure 4.23 CROS aid

CROS stands for Contralateral Routing of Signal. A CROS hearing aid is used to treat unilateral deafness. It consists of a microphone (transmitter) in the deaf ear and the hearing aid (receiver) in the better hearing ear. Sound is transmitted via a wire connecting the two units. The main advantage is that sound from the patient's deaf side does not get lost but instead is heard in the good ear. The CROS aid is particularly useful in children with unilateral deafness because they can have a trial period to see the benefits before considering the surgical option of a Bone Anchored Hearing Aid (BAHA).

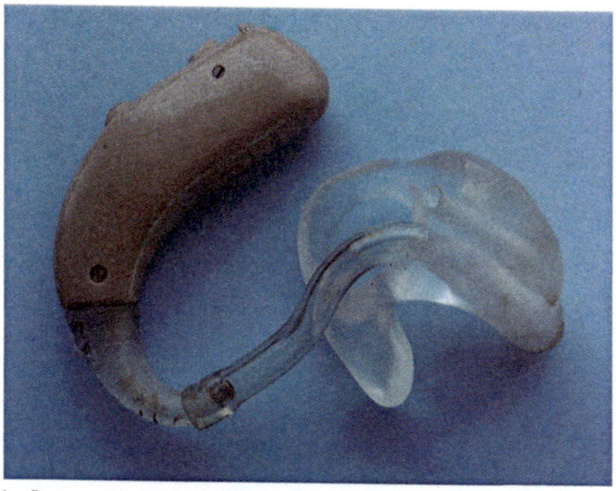

Figure 4.24 An air conduction hearing aid

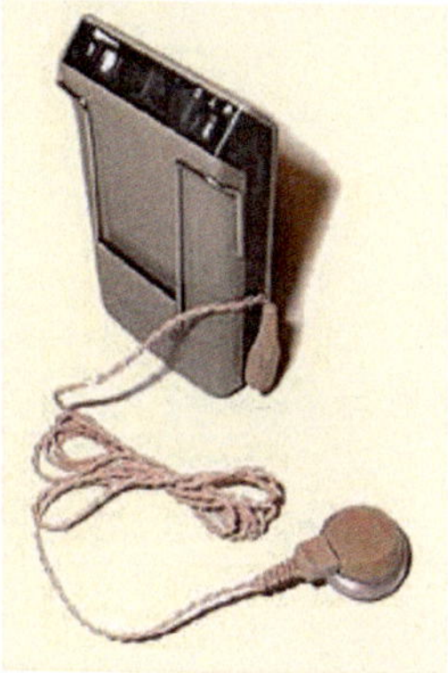

Figure 4.26 A body worn air conduction hearing aid

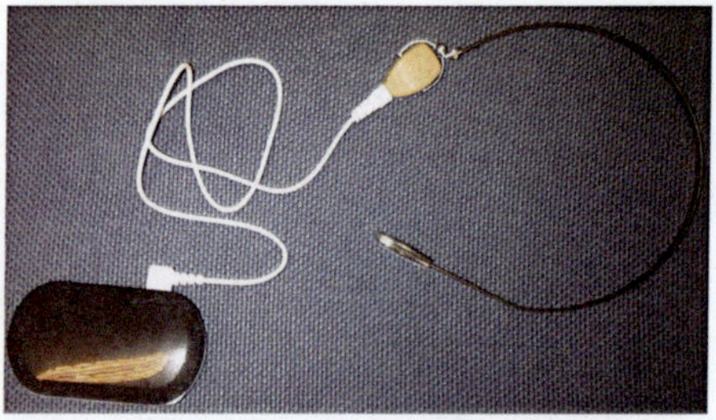

Figure 4.25 A body worn bone conduction hearing aid

Hearing aids are devices that are usually worn within the ear canal or behind the ear. They are used to amplify and modulate sounds for the patients on the affected hearing side. They consist of 4 basic parts:

- Microphone – picks up the sound, converts it into an electrical signal and sends it to the amplifier.
- Amplifier – increases the volume of the sounds and sends it to the receiver.
- Receiver/speaker – changes the electrical signals back into sounds and sends it into the ear.
- Battery – provide power to the hearing aid. These are button batteries and commonly contain zinc or mercury.

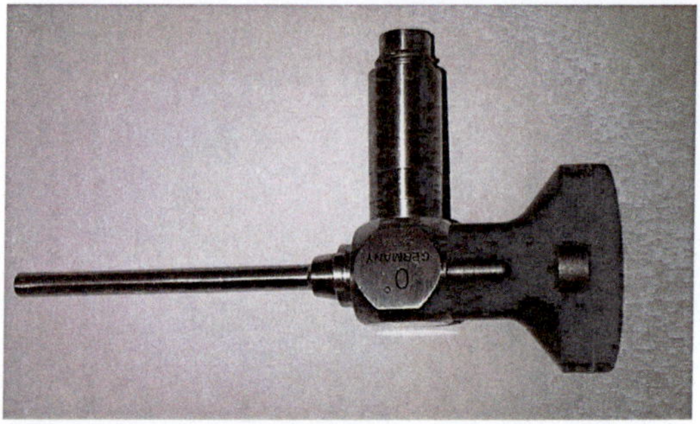

Figure 4.26 An otoendoscope

This is very useful for taking photograph and for projecting the examination on the ear onto a a screen so that the patient can also see the pathology and be part of the decision process.

4.4 Nose apparatus

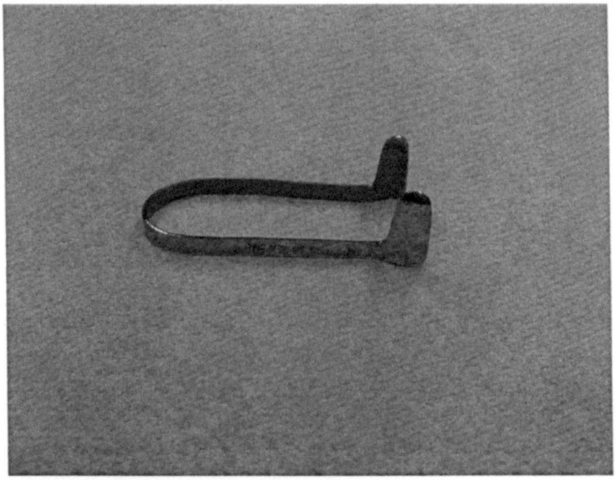

Figure 4.26 Thudicum speculum

This instrument is used in anterior rhinoscopy to examine the nasal cavity and for procedures such as cauterisation in the outpatient setting. It comes in a variety of sizes. It takes a bit of practicing to be able to use it properly.

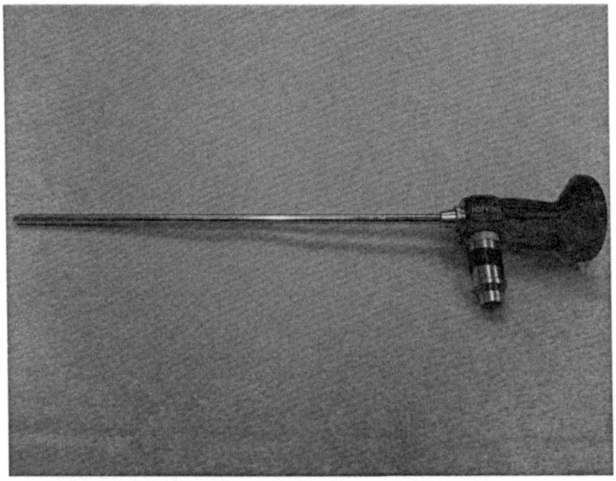

Figure 4.27 Hopkins rigid nasendoscope

This instrument is used both in the outpatient and theatre setting to examine the nasopharynx and sinuses for diagnostic purposes and minimally invasive surgery. It has attachments for an external light source and a camera. The nasendoscopes are available with various angled lenses (0^0, 30^0, 45^0, 70^0) to allow better visualisation of the maxillary, ethmoidal and frontal sinuses as well as the skull base. A smaller version is available for examining the ear (otoscope).

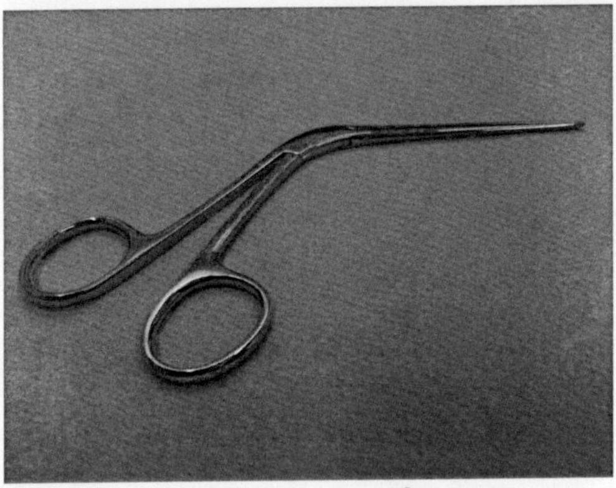

Figure 4.28 Tilley nasal dressing forceps

This instrument's shape allows easy access to the nasal cavity. It is therefore used to pack the nose in epistaxis or post-operatively. A shorter version (Tilley aural forceps) is available for packing the ear.

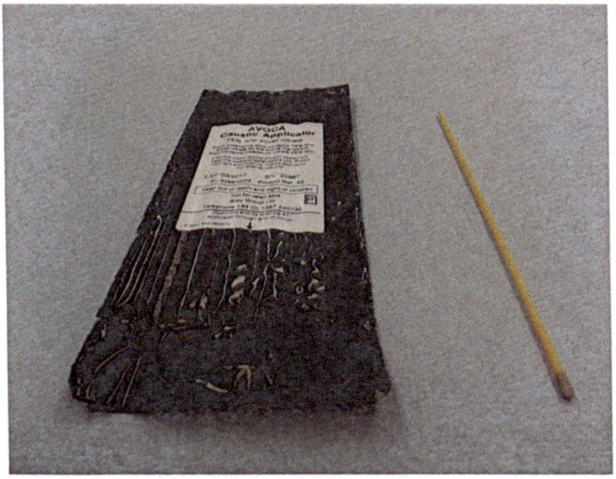

Figure 4.29 Silver nitrate stick

Silver nitrate is a form of chemical cautery. The sticks are used to cauterise bleeding points on the nasal septum to stop epistaxis. Before silver nitrate is applied on the nasal septum, topical local anaesthetic (such as cophenylcaine which also contains adrenaline) is used on the nasal septum. The best way to achieve haemostasis using silver nitrate sticks is to cauterise on the periphery of the bleeding point and then the bleeding point itself. This reduces the risk of brisk bleeding which would wash away the cautery resulting in unsuccessful cauterisation.

Silver nitrate works in a moist environment by producing free radical silver ions which denature proteins. The freee radical may be neutralised with normal saline.

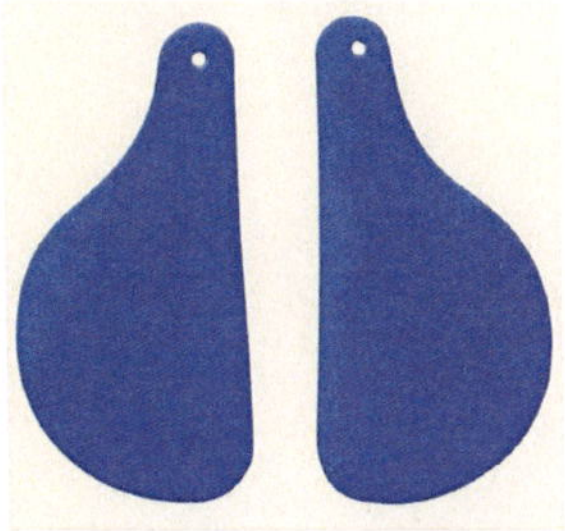

Figure 4.30 Intranasal silastic splint

Intranasal silastic splint is used in procedures such as septorhinoplasty, septoplasty, FESS and polypectomy to provide support and to prevent adhesions. Adhesions can form when two moist surfaces heal together with collagen causing scar formation. An example is following nasal septal in which post-operative oedema can lead to mucosal linings to come into contact each other and lead to adhesion formation. Intraoperatively, the splint is inserted lengthways in the nasal cavity with the larger end of the splint introduced first using Tilleys dressing forceps. The splint is secured to the nasal septum by suturing through the small holes on the smaller end of the splints with a silk suture. The splint is removed in outpatient clinic after about a week.

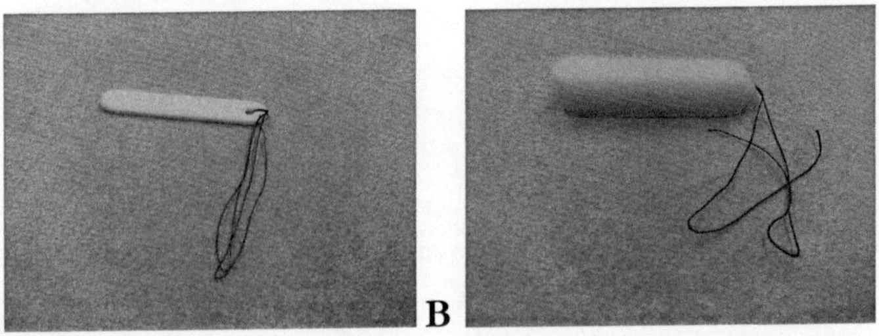
A B

Figure 4.31 Merocel nasal pack
(a) A dry merocel **(b) A wet merocel**

This is used in the management of anterior epistaxis that has not responded to conservative measures or cautery with silver nitrate. It is inserted horizontally in the nasal cavity. The proximal end has a thread that is taped to the patient's cheek to prevent the pack from falling posteriorly potentially causing aspiration. The thread also aid in removal of the merocel pack from the nasal cavity. Merocels are available in multiple sizes although the 10cm merocel is most commonly used in epistaxis management as a nasal packing device by applying direct pressure over the bleeding point. As seen in the picture on the above right, the merocel pack expands when in contact with saline or water. The pack is usually left for at least 24 hours. It stops bleeding by applying pressure on the nasal septum. It is often used in pairs, one in each nostril. Oral antiobiotics (such as co-amoxiclav) should be given to patients who have the nasal pack for more than 48 hours to reduce the risk of infection.

The merocel pack is inserted dry and will inflate following absorption of the patient's blood or the application of water.

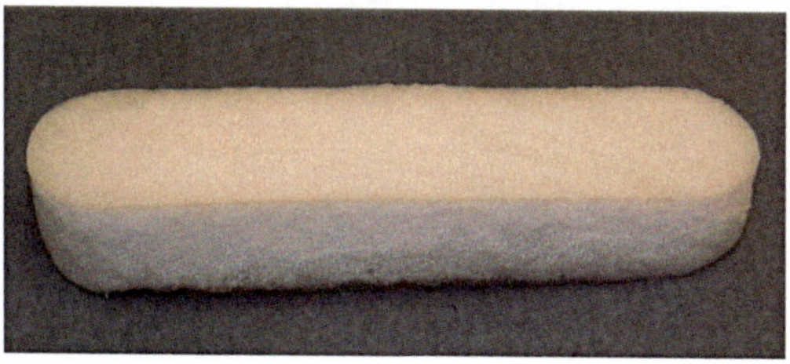

Figure 4.32 Nasopore

Nasopore nasal dressing is a fully synthetic biodegradable fragmentable foam. It is used in multiple ENT procedures including FESS surgery, septoplasty and, in the management of epistaxis. It is a biologically inert substance that can absorb fluid rapidly and up to 25 times its weight due to its high porous structure. It also provides pressure to and supports the surrounding structures as well as preventing adhesion formation.

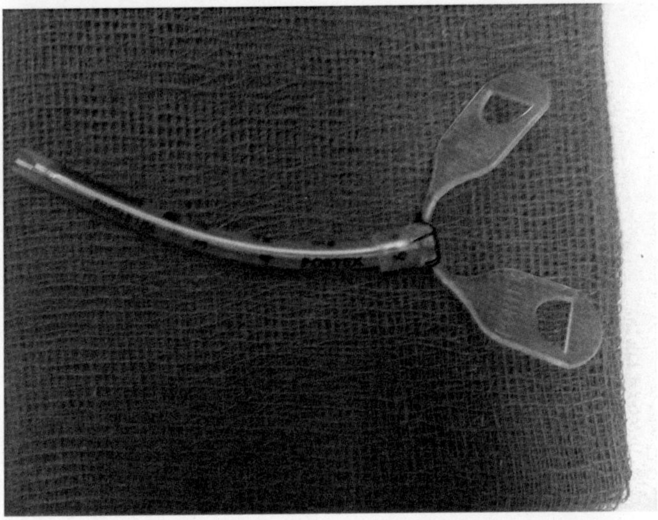

Figure 4.33 A nasal prong

A nasal prong may be necessary to manage obstructive sleep apnoea in children or when large adenoid is causing nasal obstruction in the presence of a large tongue. This is very relevant when surgery is delayed or contraindicated. This above nasal prong was custom made to fit the child below.

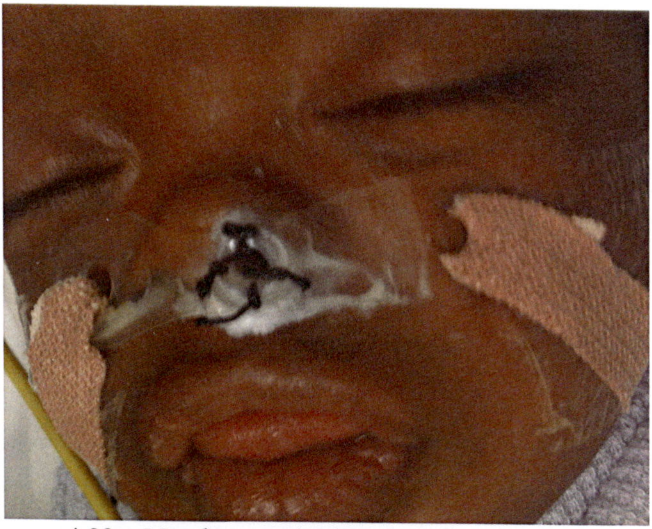

Figure 4.33a Nasal prong *in situ*.

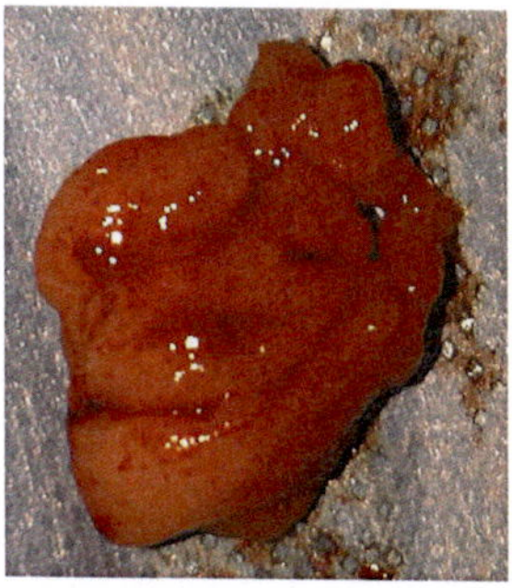

Figure 4.33b Large obstructive adenoid removed from above patient.

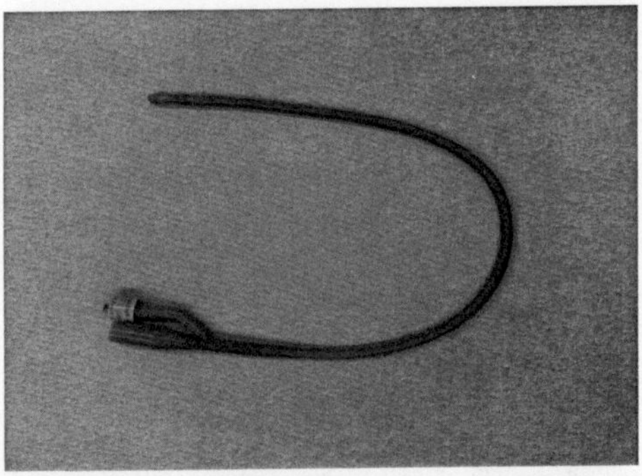

Figure 4.34a Foley catheter

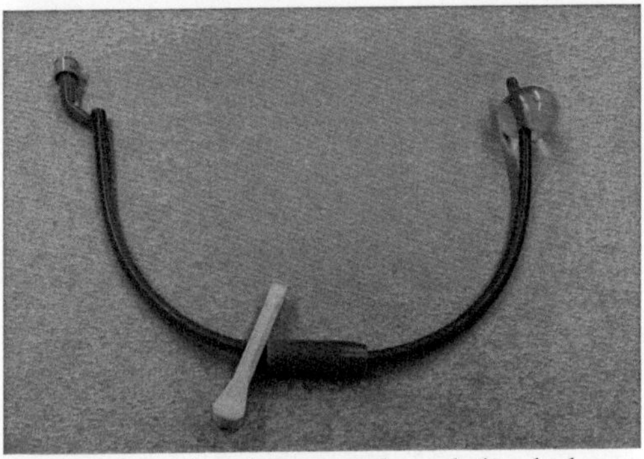

Figure 4.34b Inflated catheter and umbilical clamp

This is a normal urinary catheter that is used in the management of posterior epistaxis. The catheter is introduced through the nasal cavity until the end is visualized in the oral cavity just behind the soft palate. The catheter is then pulled up while inflating it with sterile water or air (not saline). The inflated balloon rests against the posterior choana thereby stopping bleeding by pressure. While the anterior end of the catheter is held in tension, the anterior nasal cavity is packed with BIPP or tri-adcortyl impregnated ribbon gauze. The anterior end of the catheter is then secured by an umbilical clamp. Care should be taken to protect the alar cartilage of the nose from excessive pressure as this may result in necrosis.

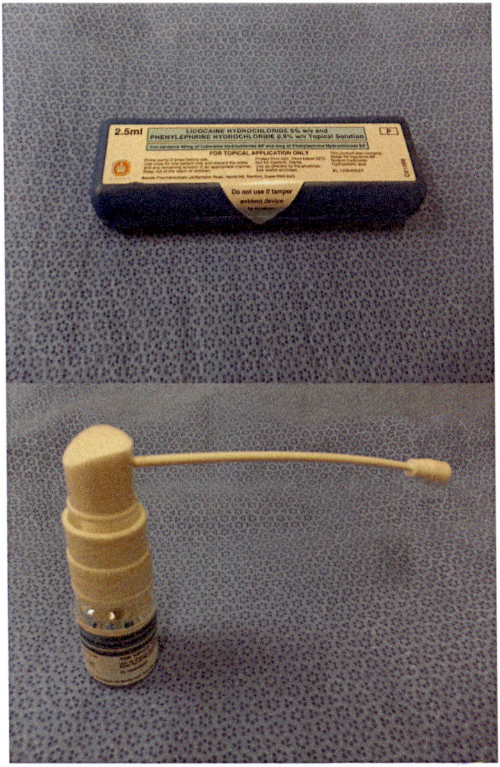

Figure 4.35 Co-phenylcaine spray

Co-phenylcaine contains both an anaesthetic (5% lidocaine) and a vasoconstrictor (0.5% phenylephrine). It is used topically in the nasal cavity before cauterising bleeding points on the nasal septum. Not only does it reduce the patient's discomfort, it also vasoconstricts blood vessels minimising bleeding which would wash away the silver nitrate cautery. Methods of topical administration include spraying on the septum directly or using a cotton wool soaked in the solution.

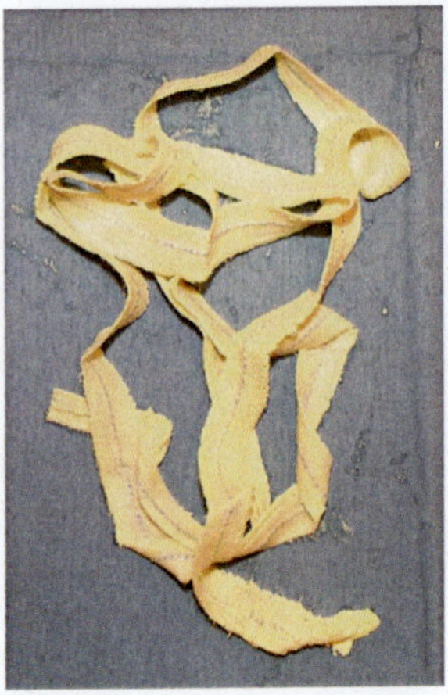

Figure 4.36 BIPP pack

BIPP stands for **B**ismuth **I**odoform **P**arrafin **P**aste. The BIPP pack is a sterile ribbon gauze impregnated with bismuth subnitrate, iodoform and sterile liquid paraffin in the ratio 1:2:1. BIPP pack is used to pack the nose or ear after surgery. Bismuth subnitrate is antiseptic and has antibacterial properties. Iodoform converts to iodine which is also an antiseptic. Paraffin serves as lubrication and therefore reduces trauma to the area packed. Rare complications from the use of BIPP during repeated packing or packing large areas include iodine toxicity and neurotoxicity from the bismuth.

4.5 Head and neck apparatus

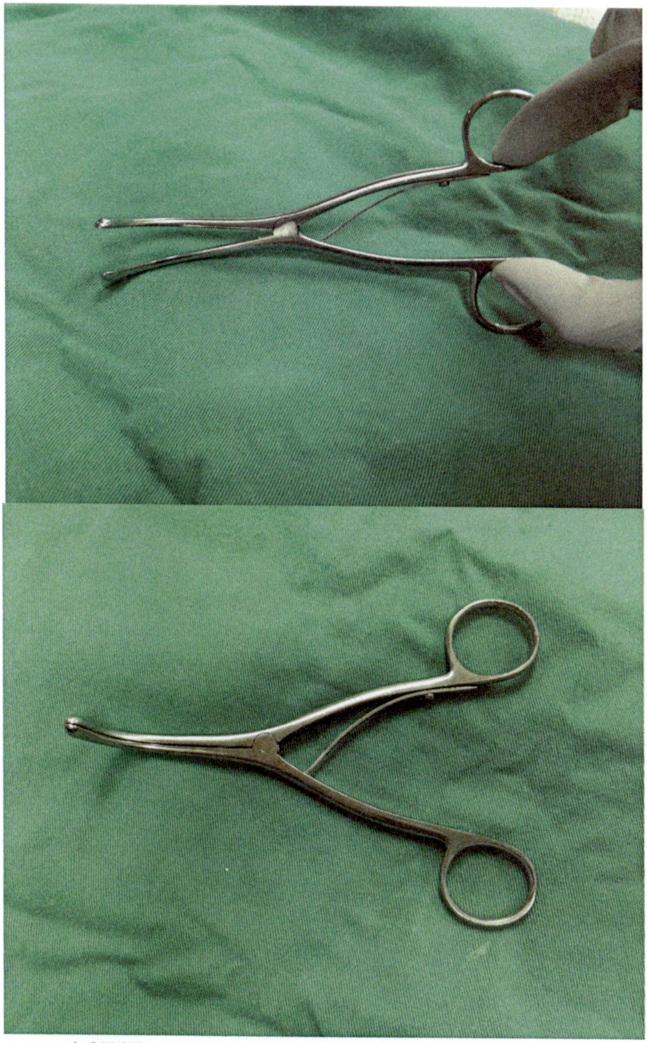

Figure 4.37 Trousseau tracheal dilator

This instrument dilates tissue planes as its handles are compressed. It is used when inserting a tracheostomy tube proves difficult. When a tracheostomy is made a series of holes are made in different tissue planes. These holes when lined up make a tunnel for the tracheostomy tube to fit through. In the first week when a tract is not yet formed, if the tube falls out or is removed, replacement can prove difficult as the holes may not necessarily line up. The dilators are used to open each tissue plane hole in turn until the trachea is reached. The tube can then be placed through the 2 arms of the dilator into the trachea.

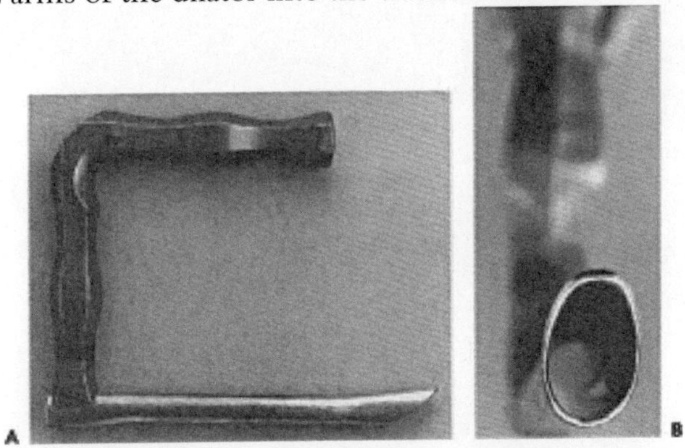

Figure 4.38 Anterior commissure scope

This instrument is used for laryngoscopy (A). This ideal position for laryngoscopy is head extended and neck flexed. This helps line up the oropharynx with the larynx. The most difficult anatomical landmark to see is the anterior commissure. When a view proves difficult the neck and head position can be altered, and pressure can be placed on the trachea from the external neck. Difficulties are faced when the patient has cervical osteoarthritis, teeth and limited mouth opening. In these cases if patient position does not help then an anterior commissure scope can be used. This instrument has a beaked end which gives a better view of the anterior commissure (B).

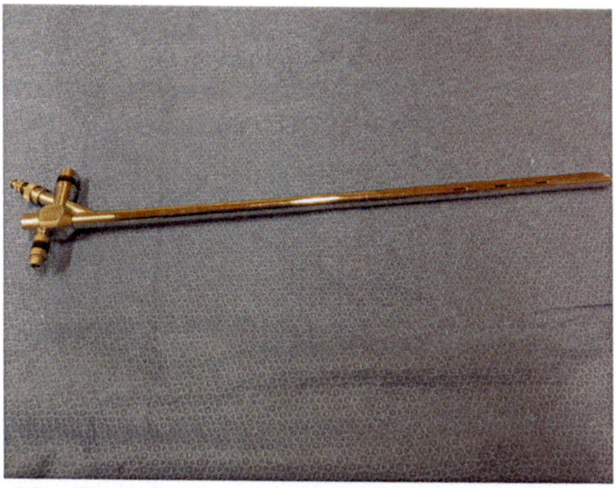

Figure 4.39a Rigid ventilating bronchoscope

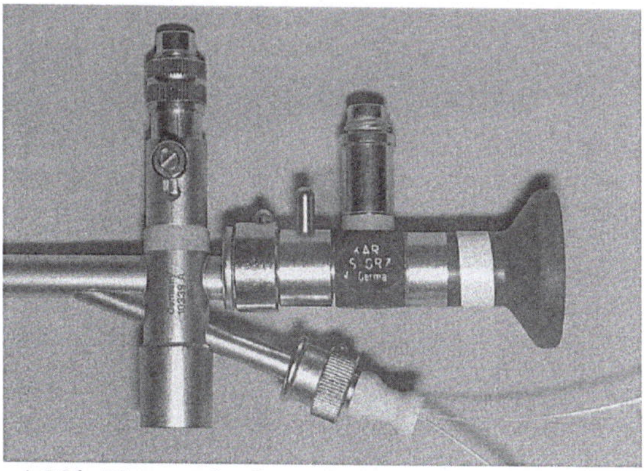

Figure 4.39b Top end of a ventilating bronchoscope (try to work out the function of each part)

This instrument is used to remove foreign bodies from the airway, particularly in children. It is a potentially life saving instrument and every ENT surgeon should know how to assemble the ventilating bronchoscope. As seen in the above picture, the bronchoscope has various attachments: light lead, suction catheter, Hopkins rod with or without optical grasping forceps. Of note are the three holes on the side of the bronchoscope at the other end which assist in ventilating the patient while instruments are being used.

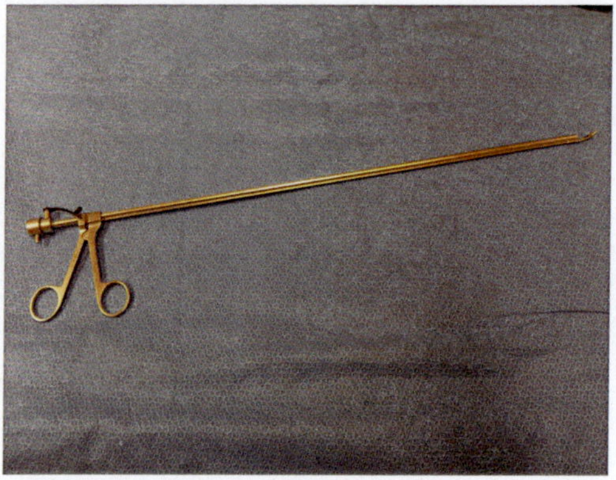

Figure 4.40 Optical grasping forceps

This instrument is used in conjunction with the rigid ventilating bronchoscope to remove foreign bodies from the airway. See above picture for its attachment in the ventilating bronchoscope.

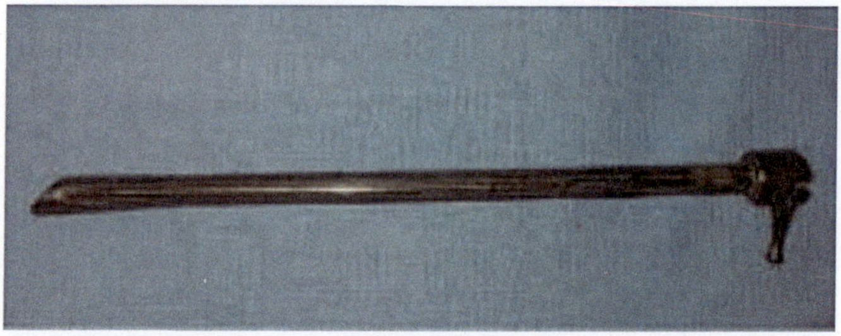

Figure 4.41 Rigid oesophagoscope

This instrument is used to remove oesophageal foreign bodies, examination of the oesophagus for diagnostic purposes and treatment of pharyngeal pouch. Rigid oesophagoscopy is usually performed under a general anaesthetic. The main risks are oesophageal perforation, mediastinitis and damage to lips, gums and teeth.

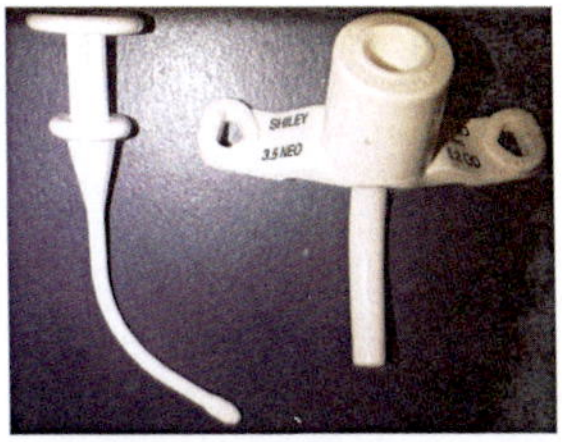

Figure 4.42 Tracheostomy tubes

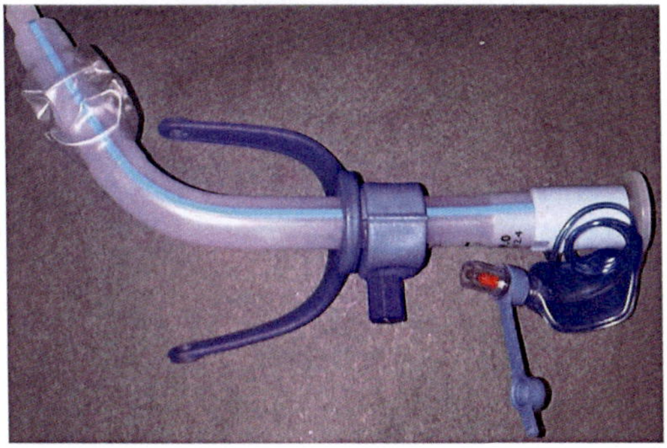

Figure 4.42a Neonate tracheostomy tube.

Figure 4.42b Cuffed adjustable flange tube (air is used in cuff).

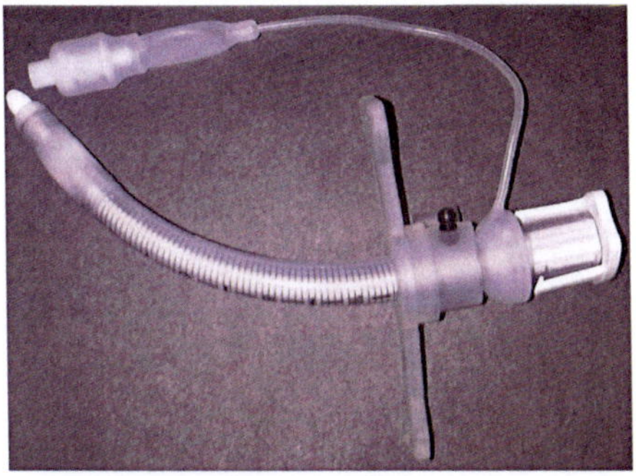

Figure 4.42c Cuffed Bivona tracheostomy tube (water is used in cuff).

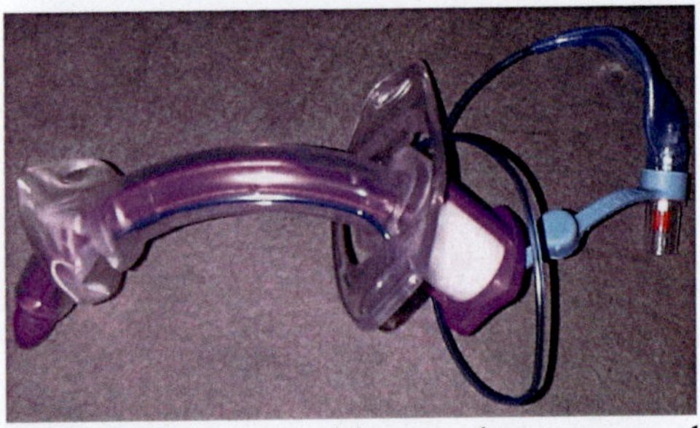

Figure 4.42d Cuffed Portex blue tracheostomy tube.

A tracheostomy tube is a curved tube which is inserted into a tracheostomy stoma. Tracheostomy tubes can be cuffed or uncuffed and fenestrated or non-fenestrated. They can be made of metal or more lightweight materials like plastic which are becoming increasingly common. Cuffed tracheostomy tubes are used in patients with new formed stoma or are at risk of aspiration and need protection of the tracheobronchial tree. It is however contraindicated in children under age of 12 due to the risk of subglottic stenosis. Uncuffed tracheostomy tubes are used in children and patients with a stable stoma.

The indications for a tracheostomy include:

- Acute airway obstruction
- Severe facial or laryngeal trauma prohibiting access for endotracheal intubation
- Bilateral vocal fold paralysis
- Long-term ventilatory support
- Lung toilet
- Obstructive sleep apnoea

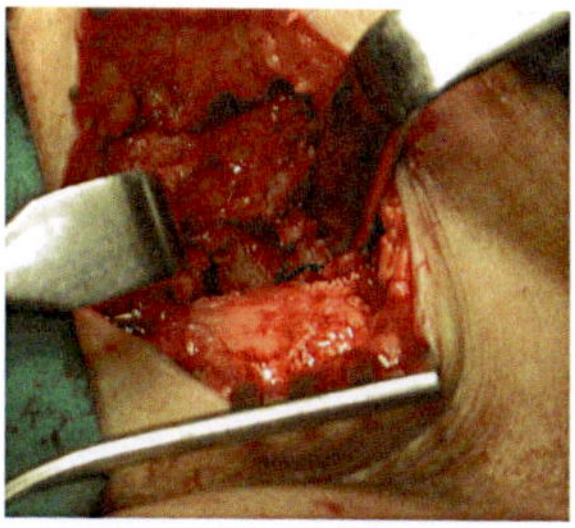

Figure 4.43 Inter-operative photograph from an emergency tracheostomy showing the trachea after dividing the isthmus.

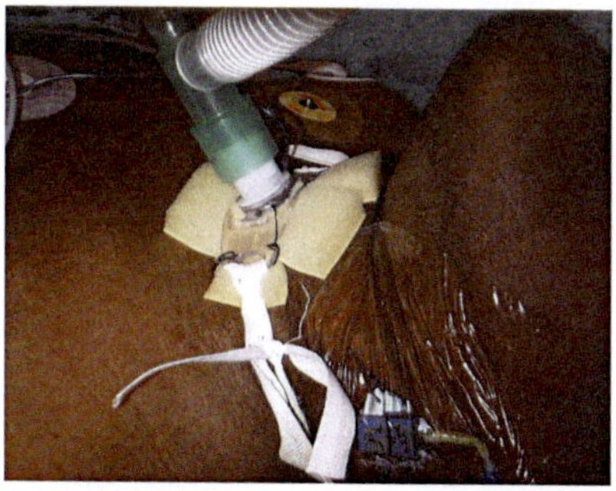

Figure 4.44 An adult patient with an elective tracheostomy for long term ventilatory support.

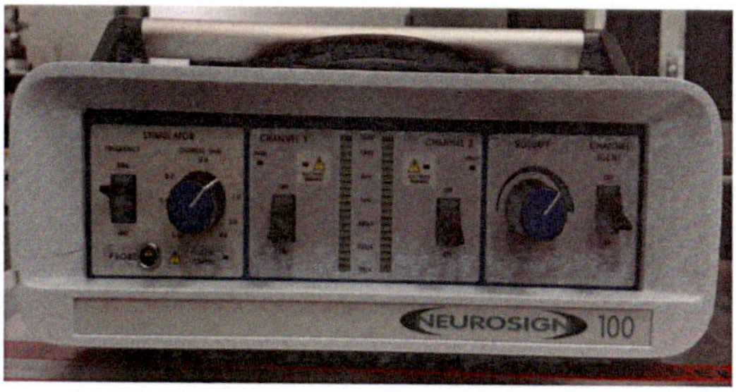

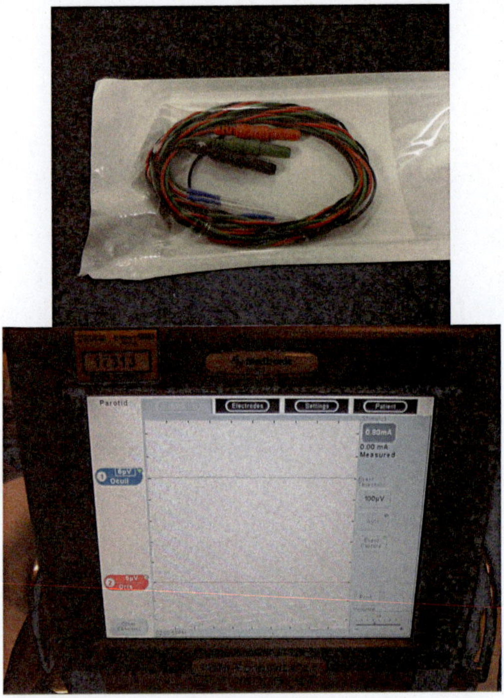

Figure 4.45 Nerve monitor system

A nerve monitor system is used in ENT in procedures such as thyroid and parotid surgery where the recurrent laryngeal and facial nerves are at risk of injury. It helps identify the nerves so that they are preserved and not accidentally injured intraoperatively. The electrodes (above right picture) are connected to the monitor via leads. The electrodes are applied to the relevant muscles groups (facial muscles in parotid surgery, vocal cords in thyroid surgery). A nerve stimulator is connected to the monitor unit. A small amount of current passes through it to tissues causing depolarization. When the stimulator is used on a nerve, it causes contraction of the muscle and a loud fast beeping sound from the monitor unit. This helps identify the nerve during surgery.

Chapter 5

Fundamentals of Clinical Audiology

5.1 Introduction

A basic understanding of clinical audiology is important for everyday clinical practice in Otolaryngology. The subject is poorly taught and one is expected to learn by pattern recognition. In the first section of this chapter we aim to address this problem by highlighting the essential foundation information pertaining to audiograms, tympanograms and speech audiograms. In order to reinforce some of the key issues, and in keeping with our principle of retrograde learning, we have included an exercise involving matching audiograms with clinical situations in the second part of this chapter.

5.2 Audiograms

An audiogram is a graph with frequency (Hz) plotted on the x-axis and intensity (dBHL) on the Y-axis (Figure 5.1). However, unlike most graphs the Y-axis is plotted from the lowest intensity at the top of the graph to the highest intensity at the bottom. Frequency is listed either at the top or bottom of the graph (Figure 5.1).

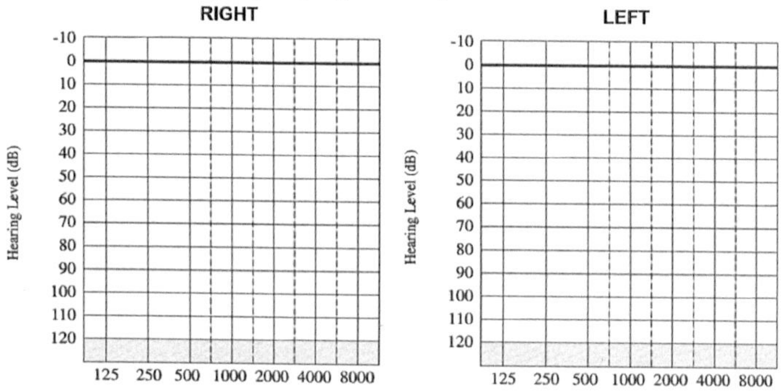

Figure 5.1 The audiogram (blank template).

Pure tone audiogram

- A pure tone audiogram (PTA) is the main behavioural hearing test for adults and children from around developmental age of four years.
- The thresholds of hearing for a range of tones (250Hz - 8000Hz) are deduced for each ear by the patient responding to the each tone that is heard (threshold is defined as the softest intensity detected 50% of the time).
- Air and bone conduction thresholds enable initial differentiation between conductive, mixed and sensorineural.
- If noise induced hearing loss is suspected or the gap between thresholds at the higher frequencies (2-8kHz) is greater than 20dBHL, then 3kHz and/or 6kHz are/is tested.
- Bone conduction audiometry (500Hz -4kHz) is only required if any thresholds fall outside the normal range.
- Any asymmetry needs investigating with masking (air-conduction or bone conduction) so that the function of each cochlea can be determined.

Table 5.1. The main symbols used in Clinical Audiology in the UK

	Right		Left
Air conduction, masked if necessary	O		×
Bone conduction, not masked		Δ	
Bone conduction, masked	[		]

How to do a PTA

- Otoscopy and explanation
- Start AC in better ear
- Start at 1000Hz at 60dB
- Down 10dB until no response

- Up 5dB until response (3 out of 5)
- Up and down frequencies
- Repeat 1000Hz
- Same for BC

Contraindications to PTA

- Too young age (under 4 years old)
- Consent/Non-compliance
- Occluding or excessive wax
- Blood in EAM
- Active infection

Average threshold dB	Hearing loss
0-20	None (normal)
20-40	Mild
40-70	Moderate
70-90	Severe
> 90	Profound

Table 5.2. Degrees of hearing loss (a rough guide)

Masking

- Masking is needed whenever the signal presented to the test ear could be detected by the non-test ear rather than the test ear.
- Masking involves temporarily elevating the hearing threshold of the non-test ear (usually the 'good hearing ear') by a known amount of sound in order to accurately assess the threshold of the test ear.
- Masking is always through air conduction (never bone conduction).
- Unmasked bone-conduction thresholds will reflect the threshold of the better ear, not necessarily the intended test ear.

- It is usually unnecessary to mask at all frequencies to gain an accurate representation of the audiometric configuration.
- There are 3 rules of masking which are simplified in Tables 5.3a and 5.3b.
- As aid memoire is shown in Figure 5.2 (ENTTZAR's Triangle)
- The text describing the rules are as follows:
  1. Masking is needed at any frequency where the air conduction between the left and the right ear is 40dB or more (will be simplified later). The worse ear will become the test ear and the good ear (i.e. non-test ear) will need to be masked.

  2. Masking is needed at any frequency when the bone conduction threshold of the worse ear is 40dB or more than the air conduction of same ear (will be simplified later). Again the good ear (i.e. non-test ear) will need to be masked.

  3. Masking is needed when the bone conduction threshold is 10 dB or more than the worse ear air conduction threshold (will be simplified later). Here the worse ear (by air conduction) is the test ear and therefore the better ear is masked.

	Symbol under investigation	Application of masking noise (non-test ear)	Symbol after masking
Rule 1 (because of O)	X	Right	⧖ or ⧗
Rule 2	Δ	Right	]
Rule 3 (because of Δ)	X	Right ***(must have a CHL)***	⧖ or ⧗

Table 5.3a Three rules of masking simplified in a table format (non-test ear is the RIGHT ear).

	Symbol under investigation	Application of masking noise (non-test ear)	Symbol after masking
Rule 1 (because of X)	O	Left	◒ or ●
Rule 2	Δ	Left	[
Rule 3 (because of Δ)	O	Left ***(must have a CHL)***	◒ or ●

Table 5.3b. Three rules of masking simplified in a table format (non-test ear is the LEFT ear).

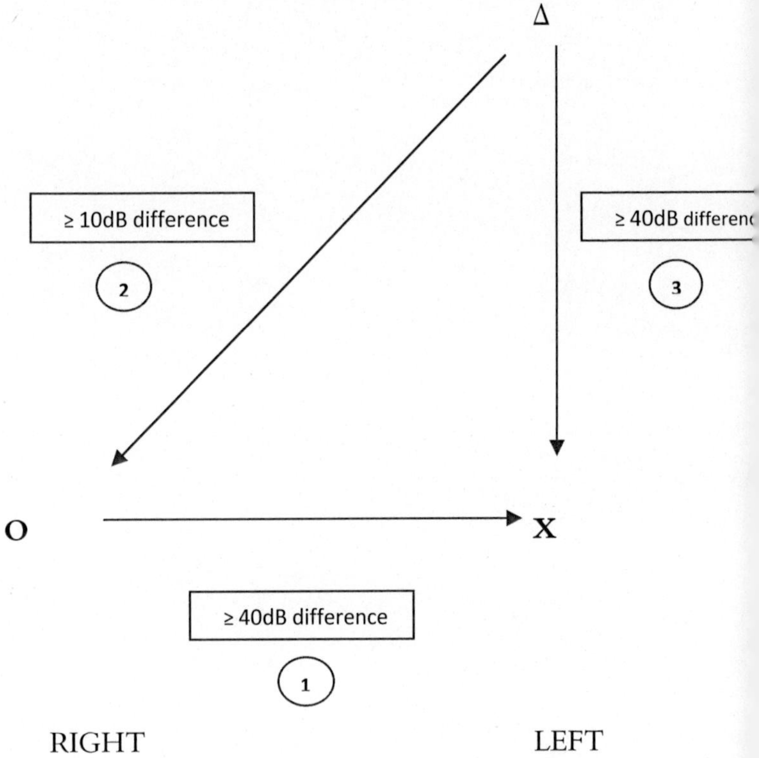

Figure 5.2 Three rules of masking simplified as a triangle (ENTTZAR's triangle).

Top tips

- If thresholds are beyond the maximum output limits of the audiometer, a downward pointing arrow is used to indicate the absence of response.
- Sound-field testing uses air-conduction pathway and is performed through speakers (rather than earphones) on each side of the patient, usually placed at 45 degrees angle. It is used in young children who cannot be tested with earphones.

- Sound-field testing can also be done with and without hearing aids; each 'aided' threshold is marked 'A'

5.3 Tympanograms

A tympanogram is a graph of acoustic admittance/impedance (or of related quantities such as acoustic compliance) as a function of ear canal pressure, which is varied from positive to negative. Acoustic admittance is the amount of sound transmitted through the middle ear system and is the reciprocal of impedance, which is the amount of sound that is not transmitted or is reflected back from the tympanic membrane. Please note that the term 'immittance' (currently depreciated) is a more general term that means either admittance or impedance.

For tympanometry, a pure-tone signal (usually at 226Hz) is introduced into an acoustically sealed ear canal and the acoustic admittance is recorded whilst varying the ear canal pressures. The soft probe sits in the outer third of the ear canal and has three components: (i) a phone to give the tone, (ii) a microphone to measure the reflected sound and (iii) a pressure transducer to vary the pressure within the ear canal.

Three variables are of particular interest in tympanometry: (1) ear canal volume, (2) peak acoustic admittance and (3) middle ear pressure.
Tympanometry is an indirect measure of the middle ear status. Although an airtight seal is required, no behavioural response of the patient is required. The patient sits quietly during the investigation.

Quantity	Traditional unit	Recommended unit
Impedance	ohms (cgs)	cm3 equivalent vol or ml (per equivalent air vol)
Admittance	mho (cgs)	cm3 equivalent vol or ml (per equivalent air vol)
Compliance	cm3 equivalent vol or ml (per equivalent air volume	cm3 equivalent vol or ml (per equivalent air vol)
Air pressure *Note: a pressure of 1mm water is equivalent to 0.98daPa.*	mm water	daPa

Table 5.4 Units of tympanograms (old and new units).

Normal values

There is no agreed standard on normal values for middle ear pressure and admittance. The following is a guide:

Admittance or Compliance

The normal ranges for admittance or compliance is **0.3 - 1.6** ml (per equiv. air vol.) with a mean of **0.7ml** (per equiv. air vol.).

The peak will occur when the pressure in the middle ear is equal to the pressure in the ear canal. The normal pressure in the middle ear is atmospheric pressure (0) because the Eustachian Tube (ET) periodically ventilates the middle ear to keep it at that pressure. A shallow peak at or near atmospheric pressure is seen when the tympanic membrane is scarred or thickened or when the middle ear system is stiff, such as in otosclerosis or OME; the resulting tympanogram is known as type As. On the other hand, if the ear drum is flaccid or the middle ear system is hypermobile, eg in ossicular discontinuity, the peak will be high or even off the chart; this is know as a type Ad tympanogram (because it is 'deep').

Middle-ear pressure

Adults	+50 to -50 daPa
Children	+50 to -150 daPa

Table 5.5 Normal ranges of middle ear pressure

The normal canal volume is **1 - 1.5 ml (per equivalent volume of air).**

Note: If the tip of the probe is occluded, for example, by the wall of the canal or wax, a seemingly small canal volume will be indicated. If a perforation is present the middle ear volume will be added to the canal volume giving an abnormally large result. Both situations will result in flat tympanograms.

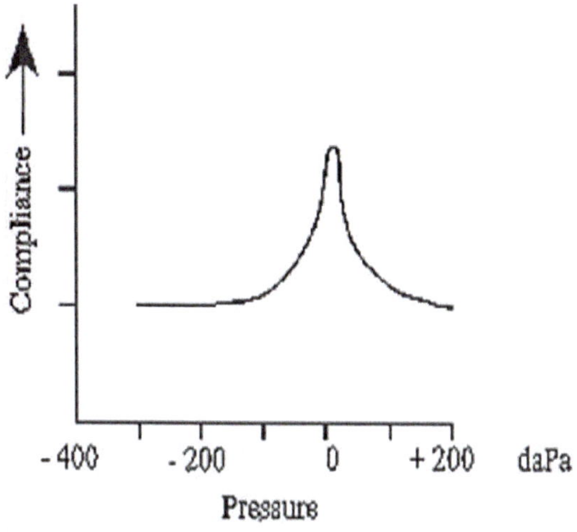

Figure 5.3 A normal tympanogram.

5.4. Speech audiograms

- Measures:
  - The speech reception/recognition threshold (SRT) in dBs
  - The ability to understand speech (word/speech discrimination)
- Subjective, behavioural test
  - Repeating what is heard at varying intensities
- Uses sentences or more commonly, word lists (eg AB word list)
- Good rehabilitation tool

Speech Recognition Threshold

- Determines the softest level at which the patient begins to recognise speech (ie lowest intensity level to repeat 50% bi-syllabic words - words that have equal stress on each syllable)
- Results should mirror PTA (?Non Organic Hearing Loss present)
- Ear specific

Speech discrimination

- Determines how well the patient hears and understands speech when the volume is set at their most comfortable level (typically read at 40 decibels above SRT level)
- Scores over 90% are considered to be normal. Scores below 90% indicate a problem with word recognition.
- If the score is under 50%, word discrimination is poor.

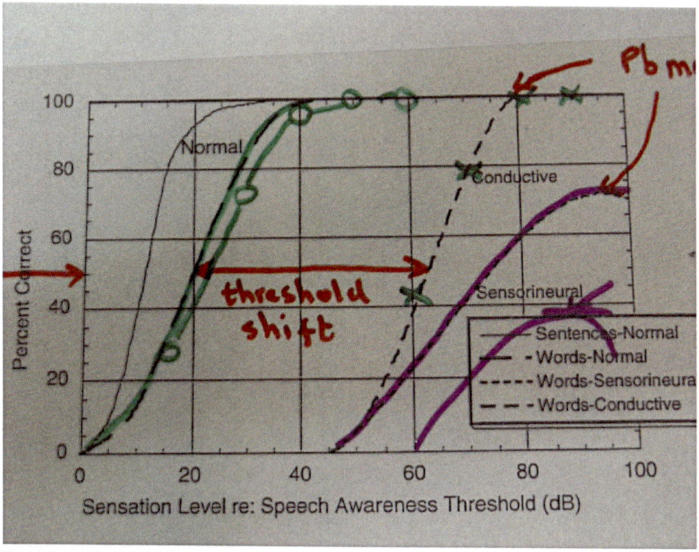

Figure 5.4 A Speech Audiogram.

Summary:

Pure Tone Audiometry

- Subjective, behavioural test
- Ear specific
- Compare AC & BC pathways

Tympanometry

- Objective
- Helps support PTA & diagnosis of SNHL or CHL

Speech Audiometry

- Subjective, behavioural test
- Ear specific
- SRT results should reflect PTA thresholds
- Speech discrimination scores are good indicator of disability

5.5. A matching exercise on audiograms in clinical practice

Please select which one of the following options corresponds with the audiograms (there are 20 audiograms labelled 5.1-5.20) shown below *(if you want to test yourself, use a sheet of paper to cover the answer written below each audiogram).*

A. A retrocochlear lesion
B. Cochlear conductive presbyacusis
C. Congenital hearing losses
D. Drug-induced hearing loss
E. Free field testing
F. Intermediate presbyacusis
G. Masking dilemma
H. Masking rule 1 is necessary
I. Masking rule 2 is necessary
J. Masking rule 3 is necessary
K. Meniere's syndrome
L. Mixed presbyacusis
M. Neural presbyacusis
N. Noise-induced hearing loss
O. Non-organic hearing loss
P. Occlusion effect
Q. Otosclerosis
R. Sensory presbyacusis
S. Strial presbyacusis
T. Sudden sensory neural profound hearing loss

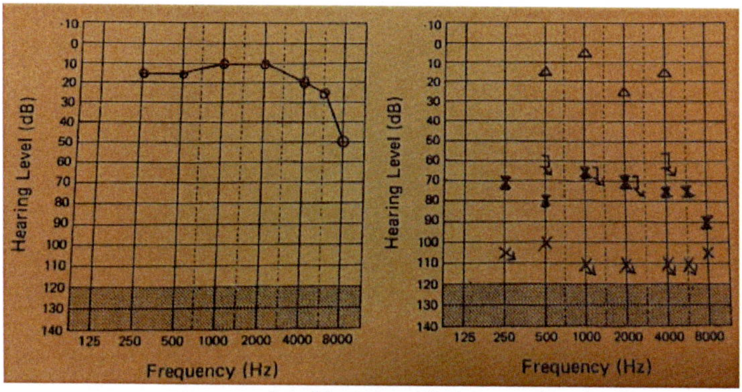

Audiogram 5.1

(T) Sudden sensorineural hearing loss

Revision Notes

- Sudden sensory neural hearing loss is defined as a hearing loss greater than 30dB HL in at least three frequencies over a period of less than three day.
- The cause may be congenital, trauma, infection, tumour, meniere's disease, iatrogenic or idiopathetic.
- Sudden SNHL is an ENT emergency condition and some otologists advocate early intratympanic steroid injection.
- Investigations includes MRI (CPA/IAM), FBC, U&Es, ESR, glucose, cholesterol, triglycerides, TFTs, clotting, HIV, lymes serology, Syphilis (FTA-Abs, VDRL), ANA and RF.
- **Hearing loss rehabilitation (if no recovery)**: CROS aid or BAHA to reduce the head shadow effect.

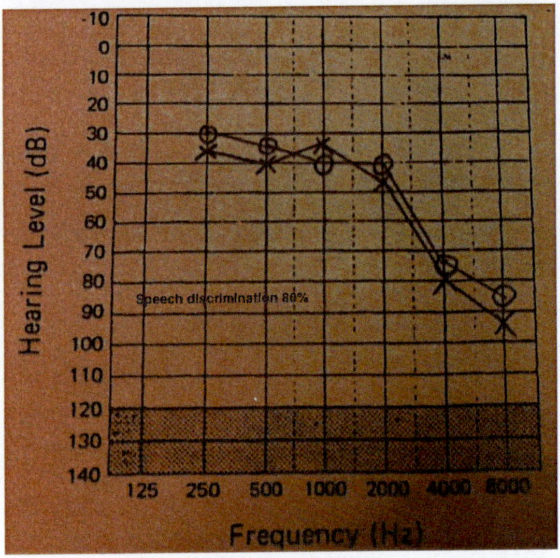

Audiogram 5.2

(R) Sensory presbyacusis

Revision Notes

- Presbyacusis may be defined as the inevitable process of aging of the entire auditory system; it is a complex disorder caused by environmental and genetic factors. It is the 4th commonest non-infective disease in the world.
- In sensory presbyacusis there is atrophy of the neurosensory and/or supporting cells of the basal turn of the cochlea.
- The outer hair cells are the first to be affected followed by the inner hair cells.
- The deposition of lipofuscin (aging pigment) may be involved in the process.
- Other causes include noise exposure and co-morbidities such as renal failure and cardiovascular disease.
- The abnormal perception of sound with small increase in intensity (recruitment) occurs in sensory presbyacusis (typically the patient says 'speak up doc I cannot hear

you' and then when you raise your voice the patient says 'don't shout I am not deaf.'

- Since sensory presbyacusis involves bilateral high frequency SNHL, and not the speech frequency area, speech discrimination is generally good.
- **Hearing loss rehabilitation**: An air conduction hearing aid

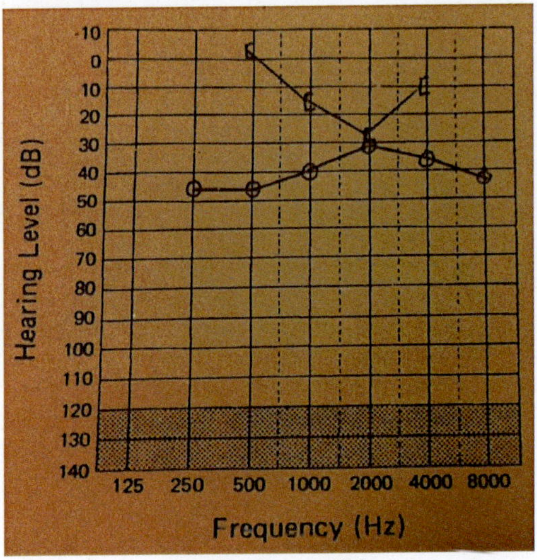

Audiogram 5.3

(Q) Otosclerosis

Revision Notes

- Audiogram shows a conductive hearing loss with a typical carhart notch.
- Differential diagnoses of an audiogram with a carhart notch include any pathology affecting the sound transmission mechanism of the middle ear as well as superior semicircular canal dehiscence.
- A carhart notch may therefore be present in otitis media with effusion.
- A trick question relevant here is to show a post-op audiogram with air conduction thresholds better than bone conduction threshold! This is only possible if the pre-op bone thresholds are used with post-op air conduction thresholds.
- **Hearing loss rehabilitation**: A bone conduction hearing aid (eg BAHA)

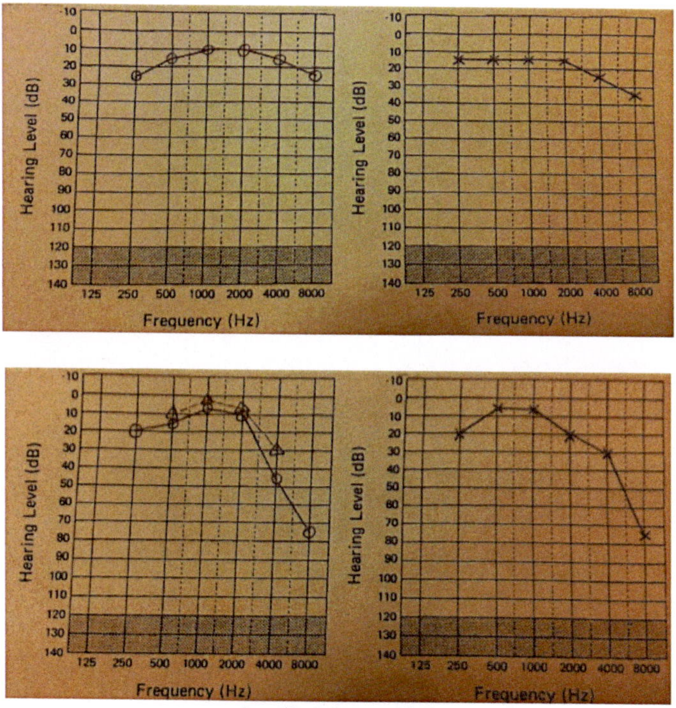

Audiograms 5.4
(audiograms taken 1mth apart)

(D) Drug induced sensori-neural hearing loss

- Bilateral symmetrical symptoms of hearing loss, vertigo and tinnitus are typical of ototoxicity; if symptoms are asymmetrical, it is likely that the less affected ear will develop symptoms at a later time.
- Ototoxic drugs include antibiotic (eg aminoglycoside), loop diuretics (eg frusemide) and platinum-based chemotherapy (eg cisplatin).
- The most cochleotoxic aminoglycoside agent is neomycin followed by amikacin (which is what this patient was taking for resistant tuberculosis)

- Drug-induced hearing loss may be may be temporary or permanent.
- Ototoxicity from aminoglycoside and platinum containing chemotherapeutic agents may be due to oxygen free radicals which damage cells in the cochlea; the effect may be permanent;. Co-administration of N-acetylcysteine and amifostine may be protective.
- Reversible ototoxicity, eg with the macrolide antibiotics or may involve impairment of ion transport in the stria vascularis as a result of recent organ transplantation or renal and hepatic impairment.
- There is no specific treatment for ototoxicity apart from stopping the drug, if this is possible.
- The vestibulotoxicity of gentamicin may be exploited to treat vertigo in patients with Meniere's disease.
- **Hearing loss rehabilitation (if irreversible)**: Air conduction hearing aids.

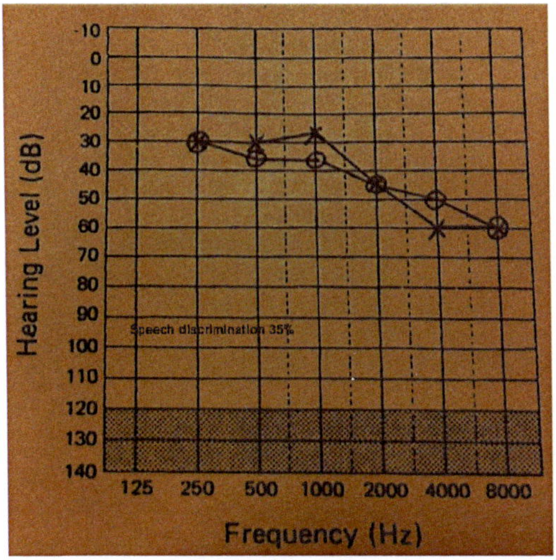

Audiogram 5.5

(M) Neural presbyacusis

Revision Notes

- Involves central auditory pathway degeneration.
- Only results when the neural units fall below the minimum level required for acoustic message processing (usually not until 90% neuronal loss).
- Audiogram shows bilateral moderate high frequency hearing loss.
- Speech discrimination is poor.
- Recruitment is not present in neural presbyacusis.
- Hearing loss rehabilitation: An air conduction hearing aid.

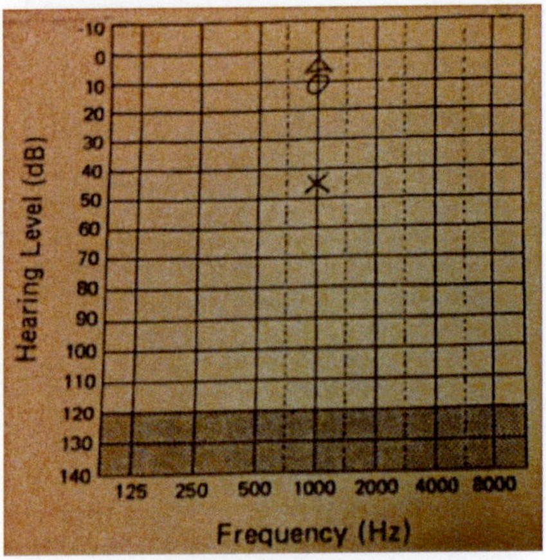

Audiogram 5.6

(J) Masking rule 3 is necessary

(AC testing; test ear is left ear, therefore need to mask the right ear)

- **Rule 3. *Air conduction testing*:** Masking where the bone conduction threshold of the better ear is greater than 40 dB or more than the air conduction of the worse hearing ear.
- With earphones, 40 dB is considered the interaural attenuation, i.e, the amount a signal is decreased in travelling through air from the test ear to the nontest ear, although it may be less for low frequencies and more for higher frequencies. With ear inserts, the interaural attenuation is 55dB. For bone conduction, the interaural attenuation is taken as 0dB because bone conducts sound very effectively.
- For rule 3 of masking to be invoked, a conduction hearing loss must be present in the better ear.

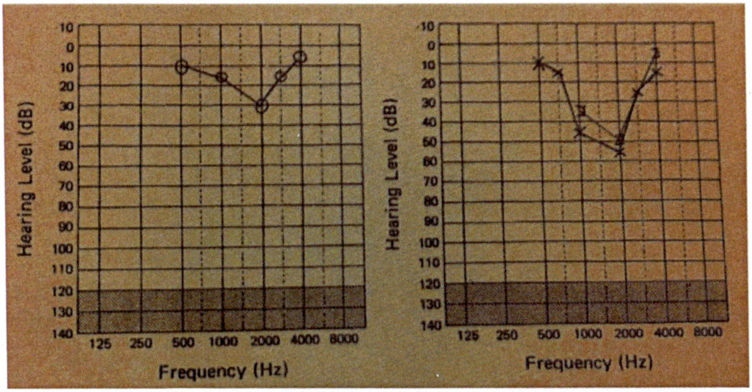

Audiogram 5.7

(C) Congenital hearing loss ('cookie bite' pattern)

Revision Notes

- This audiogram shows bilateral mild to moderate sensorineural hear loss.
- Many children with hearing loss from birth have this cookie bite pattern.
- A child with this hearing may need to use hearing aids as well as assistive listening devices for adequate hearing.
- **Hearing loss rehabilitation**: Air conduction hearing aid.

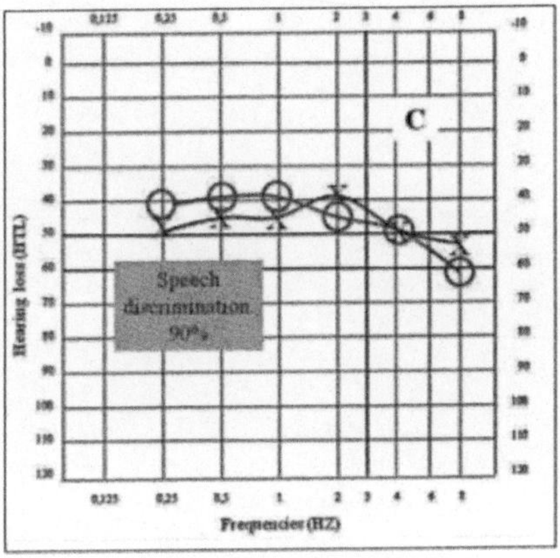

Audiogram 5.8

(S) Strial (metabolic) presbyacusis

Revision Notes

- In strial presbyacusis there is high metabolic activity of the stria vascularis which generates free radicals from oxidative processes. The free radicals cause damage by reacting with intracellular proteins, lipids and DNA.
- Audiogram shows flat bilateral moderate sensorineural hearing loss.
- Speech discrimination is good.
- **Hearing loss rehabilitation**: An air conduction hearing aid.

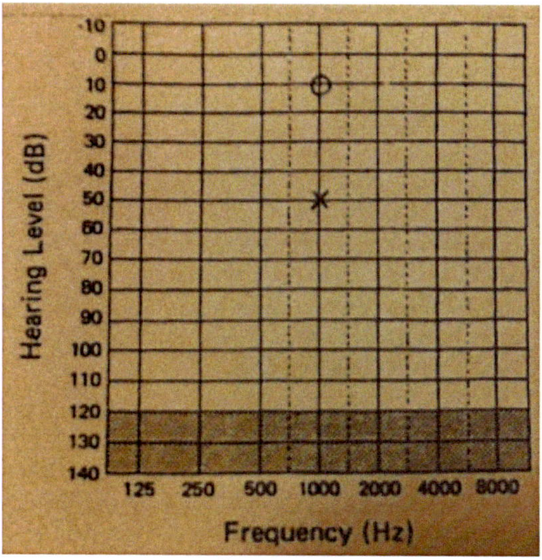

Audiogram 5.9

(H) Masking rule 1 is necessary

(Air conduction testing; test ear is left ear, need to mask the right ear)

Revision Notes

- Rule 1: air conduction testing: masking is needed at any frequency where the difference in air conduction thresholds is 40 dB or more.
- 40 dBHL is the interaural attenuation for supra or circum-aural earphones. If insert earphones are used, the interaural attenuation changes to 55dBHL.

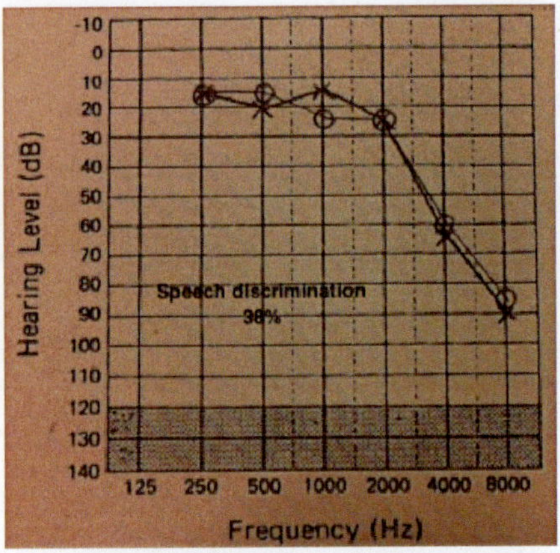

Audiogram 5.10

(L) Mixed presbyacusis

Revision Notes

- Mixed presbyacusis is a combination of different types of presbyacusis eg sensory and neural.
- Audiogram shows bilateral sensorineural hearing loss similar to that seen in sensory presbyacusis.
- Speech discrimination is poor.
- **Hearing loss rehabilitation**: An air conduction hearing aid.

Speech discrimination Right ear 20% and Left ear 100%

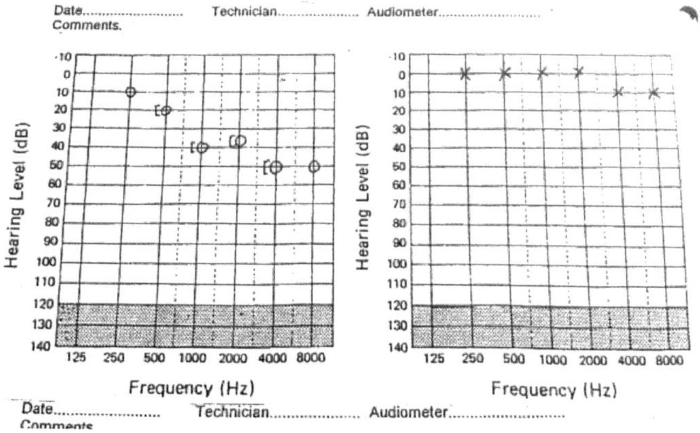

Audiogram 5.11

(A) A retrocochlear lesion

REVISION NOTES

- The audiogram on the left show a moderate sensorineural hearing loss in the right ear.
- When describing audiograms it is very important to state early if one ear is normal (in this case the left ear is normal).
- Because of the poor speech recognition score, the pathology is likely to be retrocochlear, such as a vestibular schwannoma.
- **Hearing loss rehabilitation**: An air conduction hearing aid.

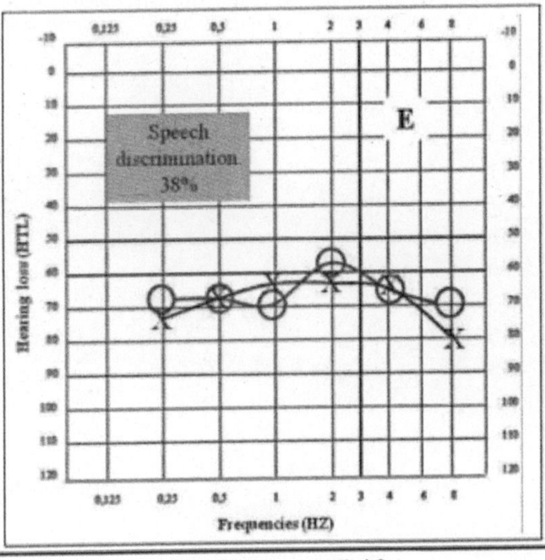

Audiogram 5.12

(F) Intermediate presbyacusis

Revision Notes

- No gross pathological changes is seen in the cochlea.
- Mechanism is thought to be at cellular level, ie, damage to cell metabolism, decline in hair cell synapse and chemical changes in endolymph.
- Audiogram is flat similar to that seen in strial presbyacusis but the difference lies in the speech discrimination, which is poor in this case.
- **Hearing loss rehabilitation**: An air conduction hearing aid.

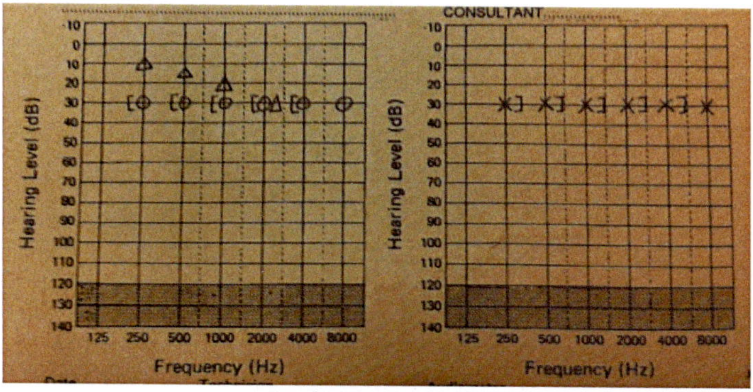

Audiogram 5.13

(P) Occlusion effect

Revision Notes

- Unmasked BC thresholds are better than masked BC.
- There is no true CHL.
- This artifact could be avoided by testing unmasked BC without the masking earphone on the contra-lateral ear (see Figure 5.13).

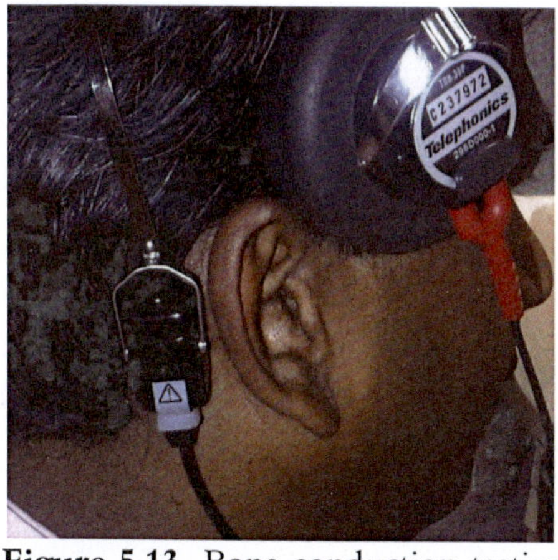

Figure 5.13 Bone conduction testing of the right ear, left ear is being masked.

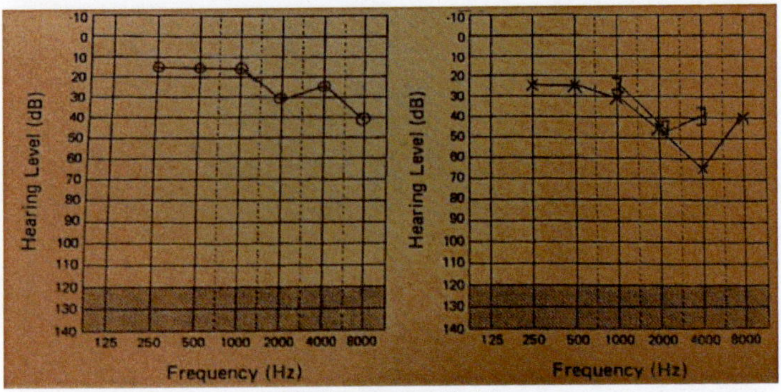

Audiogram 5.14

(N) Noise-induced hearing loss (NIHL)

Revision Notes

- Noise Induced Hearing Loss (NIHL) usually affects both ears equally
- The audiogram shown is from a right handed rifle shooter hence why the NIHL is unilateral (the left ear is more susceptible because the handle of the rifle protects the right ear).
- NIHL is usually associated with a SNHL dip in the high frequency that is worst at 4kH, but may also occur at 3 and 6kH; later it may spread to the low frequencies.
- NIHL is the consequence of over stimulation of the outer hair cells and supporting hair cells.
- NIHL may occur from one-time exposure to excessive sound pressure such as a bomb blast.
- Chronic exposure to sound levels over 80dBA can cause permanent NIHL from the combination of sound intensity and duration of exposure.
- Note that every increase of 3 dB Sound Pressure Level (SPL) results in doubling of intensity, which means that hearing loss can occur at a swifter rate.
- Occupations linked to NIHL include mining, construction, transportation, military and musicians.

- NIHL can be prevented by using ear protection, such as ear plugs and ear muffs.
- In Europe, employees working at least 8 hours per day should be provided hearing protection at noise levels greater than 80dB A; mandatory protection is necessary over 85dB A.
- **Hearing loss rehabilitation**: An air conduction hearing aid

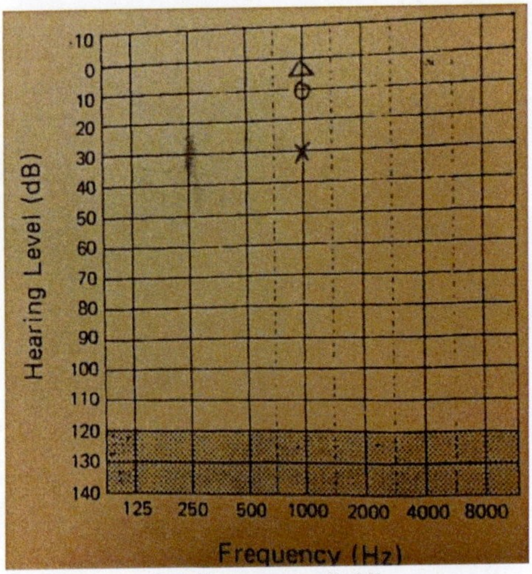

Audiogram 5.15

(I) Masking rule 2 is necessary

(bone conduction testing: test ear is left ear, therefore need to mask right ear)

Revision Notes

- **Rule 2**: ***Bone conduction testing***: Masking is needed at any frequency where the bone conduction threshold is greater than the air conduction threshold by 10 dB or more.
- In the UK, unmasked bone conduction thresholds are indicated by a triangle whilst masked bone conduction thresholds are indicate open brackets.
- Masking noise is always given through air conduction (never through bone conduction); therefore a patent ear canal is necessary.

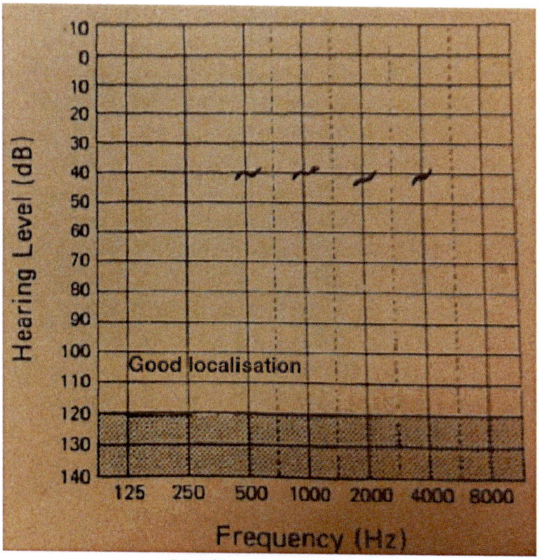

Audiogram 5.16

(E) Free field testing (eg VRE)

Revision Notes

- Here the test sound is given through ear and therefore both ears are tested simultaneously.
- Localization of the sound on the left hand side or on the right hand side suggests equal thresholds on both sides.

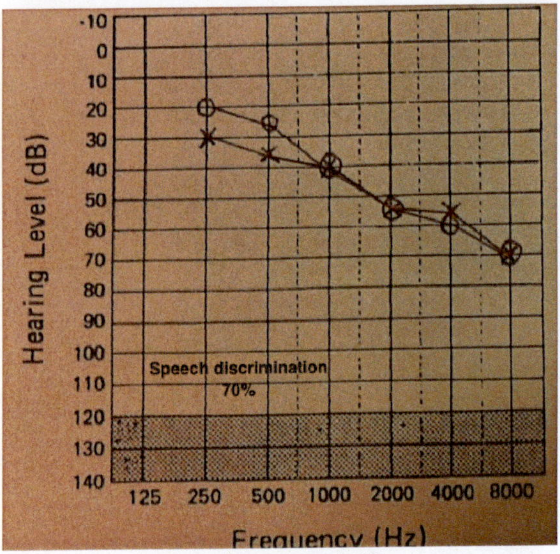

Audiogram 5.17

(B) Cochlear conductive presbyacusis

Revision Notes

- Cochlear conductive presbyacusis results from anatomical alterations of the basilar membrane and spiral ligament while the organ of corti and cochlear neurons are relatively normal.
- The audiogram shows a downward sloping sensory neural hearing loss if the basal turn of the cochlea is affected.
- If the apical part of the cochlea is affected, the audiogram shows bilateral upward sloping sensory neural hearing loss.
- Speech discrimination is good.
- **Hearing loss rehabilitation**: An air conduction hearing aid

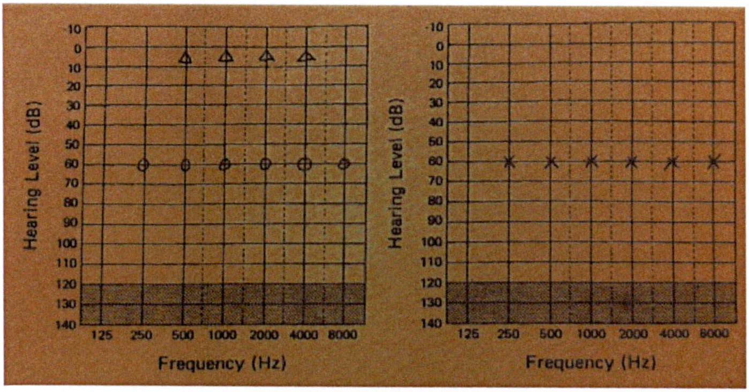

Audiogram 5.18

(G) Masking dilemma

Revision Notes

- Masking dilemma occurs when the noise presented to the non-test ear crosses over to test ear and interferes with the threshold measurements.
- Masking dilemma is present when there is bilateral large CHL (AB=60db) eg in bilateral canal atresia.
- Individual ear thresholds may be determined with auditory brainstem response testing (assessing wave 1 and 2 rather than wave 5)

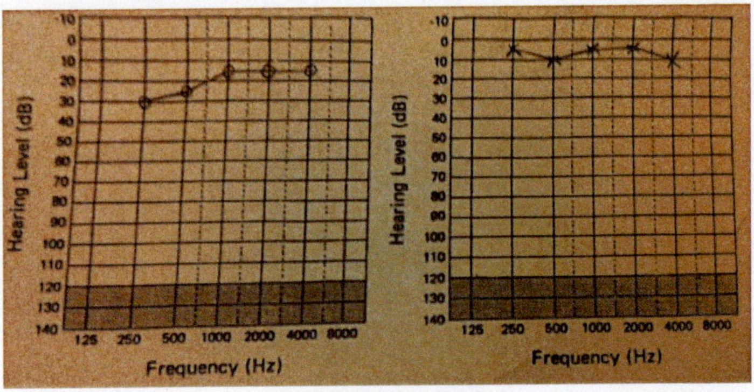

Audiogram 5.19

(K) Meniere's syndrome or hydrops, right ear

Revision Notes

- Low frequency fluctuating hearing loss is typical of Meniere's syndrome.
- Initially the hearing loss may be reversible but later permanent (burnt out Meniere).
- **Hearing loss rehabilitation**: initially an air conduction hearing aid; in cases of end stage Meniere's syndrome, where air conduction hearing aids are inadequate, one may consider assessment for cochlear implants.

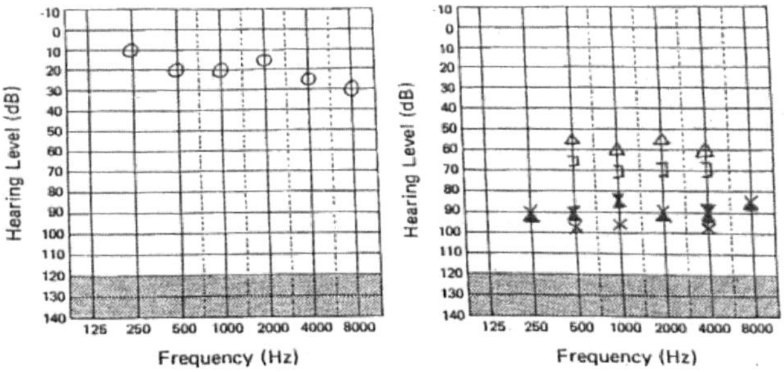

Audiogram 5.20

(O) Non-organic hearing loss

Revision Notes

- The audiogram of the right ear shows air conduction thresholds with average thresholds of about 20dBHL.
- The audiogram of the left ear shows unmasked bone conduction, masked bone conduction, unmasked air conduction and masked air conduction.
- According to the Rules of Masking, the unmasked bone and air conductions should be much higher on the graph because the interaural attenuation for bone conduction is taken as zero and that for air conduction is 40 dBHL (with head-phones). For instance at 250 Hz the left unmasked bone conduction should be 10dBHL (instead of 60dBHL) because the right ear would pick up the bone conducted sound. Similarly at 250Hz the unmasked air conduction on the left side should be approximately 50dBHL (instead of 90dBHL).
- The joined up shaded symbols represent shadow curve* (individual points are called shadow points).
- The most likely diagnosis is therefore non-organic hearing loss (NOHL).
- Stenger's tuning fork test is useful to identify malingering patients in the clinic. Two tuning forks of

the same frequency are used on both ears simultaneously. It the hearing loss is real, the subject will hear the sound in the good ear and report it. However if the hearing is feigned, the subject will hear the sound louder in the 'bad ear' but denies hearing it.

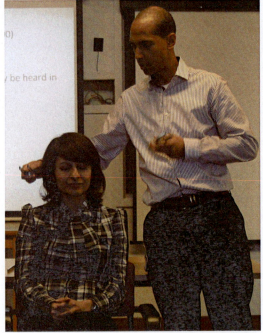

Figure 5.20 Stenger's tuning fork test being performed (actress Miss Mallick, assessor Julian Gaskin).

- Generally a battery of tests are required to confirm the diagnosis but the gold standard is cortical evoked response audiometry. This measures the electrical response to a sound stimulus in the auditory cortex but is strongly influenced by patient's conscious level, therefore requires their co-operation.
- For summary of voice tests and tuning fork tests see Tables 5.20a and b.

- A route of escape without causing embarrassment to the patient is important in the management of patient with non-organic hearing loss.

Shadow curve

- Is obtained when air conduction thresholds recorded for the test ear actually represent the responses of the non-test ear.
- This means that the deaf ear will appear to have responses 40dBHL or more than the threshold of the non-test ear (assuming earphones are used).
- Masking will eliminate the shadow curve and reveal the true responses for the test ear.

Top tips

i. A battery of audiological tests is normally needed before a firm diagnosis is made (so don't act on just one result).
ii. If the patient has ear canals, always try an air conduction hearing aid first.
iii. In a post lingual patient, if hearing aids are inadequate, consider cochlear implant (s).

Table 5.20a Tuning fork tests to identify the malingerer (by Julian Gaskin, FRCS (ORL-HNS)

TUNING FORK TESTS	DESCRIPTION
Stenger test (Stenger 1900)	• ***Principle*** – Sound presented in both ears will only be heard in the ear where the sound is louder • ***Test*** – 2 tuning forks of same frequency used – Eyes closed/blindfolded – 1st tuning fork to good ear at 15cm (heard), then removed – 2nd tuning fork to deaf ear at 5cm (not heard), not removed – Re-introduce 1st tuning fork to good ear at 15cm (heard if not a malingerer) • ***Malingerer Response*** – Denys hearing any sound as can only hear sound in feigned 'deaf' ear
Teal test	• ***Principle*** – Conductive hearing • ***Test*** – Vibrating tuning fork to mastoid of 'deaf' ear (heard) – Patient blind-folded and advised test to be repeated – Non-vibrating tuning fork to 'deaf' ear and simultaneously vibrating tuning fork near EAC of

	same ear (not heard if not a malingerer) • ***Malingerer Response*** – Will claim to hear sound as will assume through bone conduction when it is actually through air conduction
Chimani Moos test	• ***Principle*** – Variation of Weber test • ***Test*** – Tuning fork place on vertex – Heard in good ear – EAC occluded in good ear (heard in good ear still) • ***Malingerer Response*** – Deny hearing any sound at all

Table 5.20b Voice tests to identify the malingerer (by Julian Gaskin, FRCS (ORL-HNS).

VOICE TESTS	DESCRIPTION
Lombard	• ***Principle*** – Person will raise voice in speaking in noisy environment • ***Test*** – Patient asked to read text aloud without stopping – Noise introduced into good ear (ie. Barany box) – Patient's voice will get louder • ***Malingerer Response*** – Will continue to read at even tone
Hummel double conservation test	• ***Principle*** – 2 different voices introduced into either ear will create confusion • ***Test*** – A question is asked into one ear and a different question asked into the other – If deaf in one ear there will be no confusion • ***Malingerer Response*** – Confusion or no response
Erhardt test (loud voice test)	• ***Principle*** – Occlusion of the EAC causes attenuation of 30dB • ***Test*** – Good ear is occluded with a finger – Sound projected into that ear – Normally, the patient will be able to hear the dampened sound

	• ***Malingerer Response*** – Denies hearing *any* sound at all, even when sound increased
Delayed speech feedback test	• ***Principle*** – Delayed sound introduced into the other ear will create confusion • ***Test*** – Patient asked to read text aloud without stopping – His voice is recorded and played back via headphones with 2ms delay into deaf ear • ***Malingerer Response*** – Confusion, change reading pattern (stammer, slow, raise voice)

Section 2

Manned (Interactive) Stations

Chapter 6

History Taking

6.1 Introduction

You will be asked to take a history (i.e. gather information) from a patient during the DOHNS OSCE examination. This may take the form of an abbreviated or a full history.

Before you start taking a history, it is vital that you gel hands, greet the patient, introduce yourself and ask for permission to take a history. This is also relevant when it comes to examining a patient. For the latter you will also have to ask about tenderness before you start examining any patient.

6.2 Full History

Generally, a full adult history is similar to that learnt in medical school, i.e.: age, occupation, presenting complaining, history of presenting complaint, systems review, past medical history, drug history (including allergy), and family history followed by a summary. For a paediatric patient it is important to include immunization history as well as pre-natal, birth and post-natal history. Systems review should always start with an ENT area not covered in the presenting complaint. Thus, if the presenting complaint pertains to the ear, it is best to then asked about the nose and then the throat before asking about the heart, lungs, GI system etc. Similarly if the presenting complaint involves the nose, it is best to continue with the ears and then the throat and so on. One of the most important aspects of history taking is to elicit the main concern of the patient for each presenting complaint (Table 6.1). A fool proof way to capture this information is to ask at the end of information gathering if there is anything else you should know or that is of particular concern.

	Presenting complaint	Main concern
1	Anosmia	Losing job as a chef
2	Dizziness	Worried about a brain tumour
3	Hoarseness	Worried about cancer
4	Single sided deafness	Employment with uniform jobs
5	Unilateral tonsillar enlargement	Worried about cancer
6	Lump in the throat	Worried about cancer

Table 6.1 Some common presenting complaints and patient concerns.

6.3 Targeted History

A targeted history is aimed at a specific area such as the ear, nose or throat. We recommend the following:

EAR

If you are asked to take an otological history, we suggest that you ask the following 5 essential questions (mnemonic **HOPES**):

1. **H**earing loss
2. **O**torrhoea (discharge)
3. **P**ain or pressure (fullness in ear)
4. **E**quilibrium disturbance (vertigo)
5. **S**ounds in the ear (tinnitus)

NOSE

An abbreviated rhinological history consists of asking seven questions (mnemonic **ROPES IS**):

1. **R**hinorhoea
2. **O**bstruction
3. **P**ain or pressure
4. **E**pistaxis
5. **S**mell disturbance
6. **I**tching
7. **S**neezing

THROAT

An abbreviated head and neck history also consists of asking seven questions (mnemonic **THROATS**):

1. **T**enderness (e.g. odynophagia, otalgia)
2. **H**oarseness
3. **R**eflux symptoms (including cough and blood stained saliva)
4. **O**bstruction (dysphagia)
5. **A**irway (difficulty breathing)
6. **T**emperature
7. **S**weats and weight loss (B-symptoms)

Examples of taking a full history are given below.

6.4. Dizziness

Instructions:

Take a history from this patient who is complaining of dizziness.

Here again a full history is needed rather than an abbreviated history. We recommend that you start with asking age and occupation. A brief chat about occupation may help to break the ice of the artificial situation. One should then move on swiftly to the presenting complaint (DIZZINESS) and history of the presenting complaint.

This should be followed by systems review, past medical history, drug history, family history and social history. It is vitally important to elicit the main concerns of the patient (Table. 1) and to show empathy.

Essential information to gather in the history

Presenting Complaint (and defining the main symptom)

Patients often find it difficult to describe their sensations. Vertigo must be differentiated from other types of dizziness such as fainting, light headedness (i.e. feeling of faintness), oscillopsia (i.e. vision instability with head movement), claustrophobia or even some peripheral (musculoskeletal) disequilibrium/imbalance (i.e. an inability to maintain the centre of gravity). The latter often causes the patient to feel unsteady or as if about to fall, the causes of which maybe sensory or motor. Often however this will not be very clear from the patient and the history will need to be correlated with the clinical findings.

Clarifying details of vertigo

If the complaint is thought to be true vertigo, its frequency (i.e. episodic versus continuous), duration if episodic (in seconds, minutes, hours, days or constant) and circumstances need to be elicited. Are there any precipitating factors (e.g. rapid neck movements, loud noises, Valsalva manoeuvre, getting out of bed/a chair, stress). One should specifically ask if the patient gets dizzy when rolling in bed, as that is typical of BPPV. Loud noise induced dizziness (i.e. Tullio phenomenon) is associated with dehiscence of the anterior semicircular canal. Vertigo induced by Valsalva manoeuvre increases middle ear pressure may be indicative of a perilymph fistula or Chiari malformation. One should also specifically ask whether the patient gets dizzy or lightheaded for a few seconds when he or she gets up from bed or a chair. This may indicate dysautonomia or postural hypotension. Constant dizziness may be indicative of a more central cause

Associated symptoms

Vertigo is most commonly associated with nausea or even vomiting. It is important also to ask about other otological symptoms such as hearing loss, tinnitus, otorrhea, facial weakness and aural fullness during the dizzy attack. Because migraines may be accompanied by vertigo, one should enquire about associated headaches, visual symptoms/aura and photophobia (i.e. are you light sensitive during your dizzy spell?). It is worth asking the patient also whether they lose any consciousness with dizziness as that would point out to a cardiovascular cause (e.g. complete heart block).

Past Medical History

Are there any diagnoses related to vestibular pathology, previous ear surgery or head trauma? Is there any history of panic attacks or agoraphobia? It is important to also enquire about non-ENT related past medical history by specifically asking about any cardiovascular, metabolic (i.e. diabetes), musculoskeletal or ocular disease.

Drug History

Is the patient on any vestibulotoxic drugs that may cause bilateral vestibular end–organ damage (e.g. aminoglycosides, diuretics, co-trimoxazole, metronidazole)?

Social History

Ask about alcohol intake as that could aggravate the symptoms. Could also ask about any recent or past life events leading to excessive stress.

Family History
A positive family history of a balance disorder may contribute to the diagnosis, especially in Meniere's disease, neurofibromatosis, migraine and a wide endolymphatic duct.

Closing question
Is there anything else you think I should know or that is bothering you? Now the patient may say he/she is worried about a brain tumour.

6.5 Hoarseness

Instructions:
Take a history from this patient who is complaining of hoarseness
Here a full history is needed rather than an abbreviated history. We recommend that you start by asking about age and occupation. A brief chat about occupation may help to break the ice of the artificial situation. One should then move on swiftly to the presenting complaint (hoarse voice) and history of the presenting complaint. This should then be followed by systems review, past medical history, drug history, family history and social history. It is vitally important to elicit the main concerns of the patient and to show empathy.

Essential information to gather from the history
Ask about onset and pattern of symptom.
Initially a distinction needs to be made between acute and chronic hoarseness. Acute and severe symptoms may be due to bleeding into the vocal cord. A history of vocal abuse may indicate vocal strain. The pattern of the symptom also needs to be determined. Progressive (i.e. becoming gradually worse over the course of a day or generally worse over a given timeframe) and episodic (i.e. episodes of self-limiting

hoarseness on a background of a normal voice) hoarseness need to be determined.

Ask about any recent upper respiratory tract illness.
It is common to get hoarseness secondary to an upper respiratory tract infection that spreads to the larynx and vocal cords.

Need to specifically ask for dysphagia, referred otalgia weight loss and any other oral/oropharyngeal pain.
Any positive answers may indicate a malignancy and therefore should be taken extremely seriously.

A social history covering alcohol intake and smoking is essential.
These are the two major social risk factors for head and neck malignancies. Moreover lung cancer may present with a vocal cord palsy if there is involvement of the recurrent laryngeal nerve. Smoking could also lead to Reinke's oedema, a form of chronic laryngitis that presents with a chronic progressive low-pitched hoarse voice.

Assess patient's voice usage in terms of social and occupational settings.
The patient's occupation (e.g. lecturer, professional singer), social settings (e.g. family with many young children) and hobbies (e.g. singing, attending many sport events) should be looked into as they could all contribute to hoarseness secondary to voice abuse.

Ask about risk factors for laryngopharyngeal reflux (LPR).
A history of heartburn may indicate LPR, however, this is complemented by the completion of a validated assessment instrument [i.e. Reflux Symptom Index (RSI)] and laryngoscopic findings. A score of >13 indicates LPR.

Ask about chest disease.
Any chest disease, because of its interference with respiratory physiological variables can lead to a weak breathy voice. Moreover conditions that cause a chronic cough may lead to vocal cord inflammation or trauma. The chronic use of high-dose steroid inhalers may also contribute to hoarseness in terms of fungal infections, generalised inflammation and mucosal atrophy. Finally, an enquiry into any cardiothoracic surgery may be needed as damage to the left recurrent laryngeal nerve is possible.

Ask about thyroid disease/thyroid surgery.
Hypothyroidism can lead to a hoarse voice but rarely as the sole symptom. Thyroid surgery can also lead to hoarseness by means of recurrent laryngeal nerve damage.

Ask about neurological symptoms.
An enquiry into neurological disease is needed as a few neurological conditions can lead to hoarseness either by leading to vocal cord palsy or as a secondary manifestation of the disease on other aspects of speech production. Moreover, a stroke can lead to ipsilateral vocal cord palsy.

Ask about history of trauma.
Often there may be a history of blunt trauma to the neck. The resultant dysphonia could be due to neck swelling, laryngeal cartilage dislocation or even a fracture. In addition previous intubation could also lead to hoarseness via direct trauma to the vocal cords.

Revision Notes
Hoarseness is a vague term that refers to a change in voice quality ranging from a harsh to a weak breathy voice. It should be used when the pathological source is deemed to be laryngeal, leading to abnormal vocal cord vibration. Hoarseness is a common problem that is frequently

encountered in general ENT clinics. It may have an impact on the quality of life of patients and may also be the presenting complaint of an underlying malignancy. Most cases however are benign, nonetheless, a thorough assessment is required to make the correct diagnosis and offer the appropriate treatment.

In this station on the DOHNS exam, you will not be asked to examine the actor/actress with a hoarse voice. However in clinical practice the following are the essential points to cover in a hoarse patient:

1. *Objective assessment of dysphonia.*
   This is achieved with the GRBAS assessment tool that scores from 0 (normal) to 4 (severe) the various parameters of Grade (severity), Roughness, Breathiness, Asthenia and Strain. This is a very useful measure as it can be used as a baseline when assessing the patient's progress at subsequent appointments.
2. *Examination of the oropharynx.*
   Looking for any evidence of oral disease or a postnasal drip.
3. *Examination of the neck.*
   Look for any scars, examine the thyroid gland and palpate for any cervical lymphadenopathy.
4. *Flexible endoscopic examination of the nose, pharynx and larynx.*

Looking for any signs of rhinosinusitis that could lead to a postnasal drip and hence cause the hoarseness. One should also be looking for any malignancy or other vocal cord lesions. It is important also to look for any inflammatory changes and vocal cord palsy during phonation. The degree of glottic closure needs to be assessed too (also in relation to any identified lesion). In the elderly it is not uncommon to get slackening and bowing of the vocal cords due to muscle atrophy. Nonetheless such impairment can be functional, with marked antero-posterior or lateral compression of the true vocal cords with false vocal cord hyperfunction being characteristic of muscle tension dysphonia. A summary of the aetiology of hoarseness is given in Table 6.2.

Acute laryngitis (<3weeks)	Upper respiratory infection (viral, bacterial), Chemical/environmental irritants, Vocal cord abuse.
Chronic laryngitis (>3weeks)	Smoking, Vocal cord abuse, Gastroesophageal reflux, Postnasal drip (i.e. rhinosinusitis).
Organic benign laryngeal pathology	Vocal fold polyps, Vocal fold nodules, Laryngeal papillomatosis, Laryngeal ulcers, granulomas, Laryngocoele
Malignant disease	Laryngeal cancer, Thyroid cancer, Oesophageal cancer, Lung cancer
Iatrogenic/trauma	thyroid surgery, cervical spine surgery, oesophageal surgery.
Functional involvement	Muscle tension dysphonia.
Systemic	Hypothyroidism, Sarcoidosis, Rheumatoid arthritis, Systemic Lupus Erythematosus, Wegener's granulomatosis, Amyloidosis.
Neurological	Parkinson's disease, Motor neuron disease, Multiple sclerosis, Myasthenia gravis, Spasmodic dysphonia.

Table 6.2 Aetiology of hoarseness.

A Quality of Life assessment with validated questionnaire.
Three validated questionnaires are generally used for this purpose. The Voice Handicap Index (VHI) is the most commonly used. Others include the Voice Symptom Scale (VoiSS) and the Vocal Performance Questionnaire (VPQ).

Treatment options in a nutshell

1. *Vocal hygiene advice (for benign, non-organic disease):*
   Adequate hydration of the pharynx/larynx; avoidance of vocal strain; decrease irritant exposure (ideally smoking cessation and decrease of alcohol intake); reduction of caffeine intake
2. *Treatment of laryngopharyngeal reflux:*
   Dietary advice (e.g. avoidance of spicy food and eating late at night); medical management (i.e. proton pump inhibitors and/or Gaviscon); surgical management if refractory reflux but this is very rare
3. *Voice therapy:*
   For both organic and non-organic causes of dysphonia. Indirect voice therapy (i.e. relaxation techniques and psychological counselling) may be beneficial in some cases.
4. *Referral to specialist voice clinic:*
   For a more detailed assessment when all the above have failed.
5. *Phonosurgery:*
   Any malignant disease should be managed separately by a head and neck department and will not be covered here. In terms of benign disease, surgery is indicated when conservative management has failed. An example includes the excision of vocal cord nodules and polyps. With respect to laryngeal papillomatosis, surgery is often the first line treatment with or without anti-viral therapy. Reinkes oedema can be managed by aspirating some fluid and trimming of redundant mucosa. Unilateral vocal cord palsies may be managed by

injection of the vocalis muscle of the affected side with material that will allow for glottic closure with the aid of the normally functioning vocal cord. This can also be achieved by medialisation thyroplasty.

6.6 Anosmia

Instructions:

Take a history from this patient who is complaining of anosmia.

Altered olfaction is common (prevalence increases exponentially with age, representing 40% of all problems in adults over 65 years of age- US figures) and invariably causes flavour loss, which most patients perceive as taste dysfunction. True taste loss is relatively rare and usually not an age related phenomenon.

Essential information to gather from the history

Presenting Complaint:

Start with an opening question such as 'I understand you have been having some trouble with your sense of smell, is that true? How does this affect you? ...Allow patient freedom to voice out functional (such as appetite, mental state) and real life implications (impact on occupation, hobbies etc).

Then qualify the presenting symptom: onset, duration, progression and fluctuation.

Elicit key features of the presenting complaint such as: unusual smells (olfactory and auditory hallucinations - association with epilepsy); recent prodromal illness (still the commonest cause of anosmia); head trauma (acquired olfactory pathway defect); benign and malignant sinonasal symptoms and laterality (nasal polyposis, allergic rhinitis, and sinonasal neoplasms are all possible causes); associated neurological symptoms consistent with raised intracranial pressure (an intracranial neoplasm as a causative factor)

Past Medical History:
Are there any history of systemic diseases such as diabetes, hypothyroidism

Neurodegenerative conditions such as Parkinson's and Alzheimer's dementia can have olfactory manifestations

Any previous sinonasal surgery that could be a contributing factor or indicative of significant sinonasal disease

Drug History:
Various groups of drugs can cause alteration in the functioning of the olfactory pathway such as chemotherapy agents, cardiac drugs, antibiotics etc
Do not forget drug allergies!

Family History:
Various inherited conditions can lead to anosmia, the underlying pathophysiology being dictated by the condition. These include nasal polyposis, allergic rhinitis. Cystic Fibrosis, Kallman's syndrome.

Social History:
History of exposure to noxious substances such as nickel, nicotine and relevant antigens e.g. cat dander in cases of allergic rhinitis

Closing question:
Re-focus the encounter on the patient's **I**deas, **C**oncerns (patient may then reveal occupational identity as being a Chef in a restaurant) and **E**xpectations in the closing scene as anosmia is more of a quality of life defining symptom.

Revision Notes

An understanding of the olfactory pathway is crucial in order to identify the level of the problem (local versus central) and delineate the likely etiologies (Table.6.3) behind the anosmia complaint.

The smell receptors reside in the olfactory neuroepithelium of the nasal septum, superior turbinate and the roof between the two. They are connected by the olfactory nerve to the olfactory bulb via the cribriform plate. These ultimately project to the olfactory cortex in the subventricular zone.

Likewise, it is also important to clarify during the history taking process the degree of olfactory dysfunction. Anosmia is the complete loss of the sense of smell. Most patients would report a reduction in their smell ability i.e. hysposmia. Cacosmia is the interpretation of normal smell as being foul or unpleasant. Dysosmia is a distorted smell perception.

Obstructive
Nasal polyposis,* deviated nasal septum,* intranasal tumour
Sensory
Viral infection,* chronic sinusitis,* allergic rhinitis,* cigarette smoke,* toxic chemical exposure, drugs
Neural
Head injury,* Alzheimer's disease, Parkinson's disease, hypothyroidism, intracranial tumour
*Most common causes

Table 6.3 Possible causes of olfactory dysfunction.

Physical examination should focus on the head and neck with assessment of cranial nerves and other sensorimotor function as appropriate. Endoscopic examination of the nasal cavity will exclude conductive causes such as nasal polyposis but also sensory causes such as allergic rhinitis. Head and neck imaging is warranted only if sinonasal or intracranial pathology is suspected.

Objective measures of smell function are available for office use (Table.6.4).The University of Pennsylvania Smell Identification Test (UPSIT) is a commercially available standardized scratch and sniff test consisting of 40 microencapsulated odorants. Scores may be particularly useful in longitudinal serial examinations to determine if a patient's performance is constant or deteriorating over time compared to age- and gender-matched adults.

Odor stix

- Used to evaluate gross perception of olfaction
- Commercially available odor-producing magic marker-like pen.
- Wave approximately 3 to 6 inches in front of patient's nose

Twelve-inch alcohol test

- Used to evaluate gross perception of olfaction.
- Open an isopropyl alcohol packet and wave it approximately 12 inches in front of patient's nose

Scratch and sniff cards

- Used to evaluate gross sensation of olfaction.
- Commercially available three-odorant card.

UPSIT (University of Pennsylvania Smell Identification Test)

- Used to quantitate olfactory loss (anosmia, hyposmia) and adjusts for age and gender of the patient
- Commercially available test of 40 scratch and sniff odors
- Delivered by forced choice testing

- High test-retest reliability

Table 6.4 Clinical evaluation of olfactory function.

Treatment options:

- Identification of the organ based etiology as per history and examination (e.g. nasal polyp, hypothyroidism, drug associated).
- Medical management e.g. allergic rhinitis
- Surgical management e.g. those cases with obstructive pathology
- Patient counseling is paramount as anosmia has health and safety implications: use of additional smoke detectors in the living room; avoidance of dwellings with natural gas; use of additional food spoilage precautions and finally use of flavor enhancing agents in foods

6.7. Sudden Hearing Loss

Instructions:

Take a history from this patient who is complaining of single sided deafness.

Hearing loss is the most prevalent sensory deficit reported by patients.Hearing loss can be conductive, sensorineural of mixed origin. The most common type of hearing loss in adults is sensorineural.

Essential information to gather from the history

Presenting Complaint:

Start by ascertaining the pattern of hearing loss: is it unilateral or bilateral; progressive or stepwise; sudden or gradual onset

Then identify any other associated otological symptoms such as: tinnitus; aural fullness; vertigo; imbalance; otalgia and otorrhoea

Past Medical History:

Any previous history of ear infections, noise exposure, head injury, otic -barotrauma, intracranial or otological surgery

Enquire about the general health looking for systemic causes of hearing loss such as diabetes, metabolic, autoimmune or vascular

Drug History:

Ask specifically about ototoxic agents such as antibiotics (aminoglycosides), antimalarials drugs, anti-inflammatories, chemotherapy agents and diuretics.

Family History:

Any family history of hearing loss or otological tumours

Social History:

History of foreign travel: lyme disease

Previous history of STIs: HIV / Syphilis can be responsible for acute sensorineural hearing loss

Closing question:

Re-focus the encounter on the patient's Ideas, Concerns and Expectations. Remember that hearing loss is a disability that can affect employability in fields such as military or aviation industry.

Revision Notes

Sensorineural hearing loss (SNHL) equates to a lesion at the cochlear level or in neural transmission to the brain. The causation of SNHL is quite varied (Table 6.5) with the more common reasons being presbyacusis, noise induced hearing loss, Meniere's disease, drug induced and infectious causes.

Hereditary and developmental
Infection*
Immune disorders
Neurological
Neoplasms*
Ototoxins*
Systemic
Trauma*
Vascular/ haematological
Idiopathic*
* Indicates a more common/important condition

Table 6.5 Causes of sensori-neural hearing loss.

Asymmetrical sensorineural hearing loss (ASNHL) is defined as binaural difference in bone conduction thresholds of >10 dB at two consecutive frequencies or >15 dB at one frequency (0.25–8.0 kHz).

The approach to the patient with assymetrical hearing loss is based on the history and clinical examination (otoscopy, head and neck, cranial nerves and postnasal space).

Adjunctive tests are used to clarify the type and degree of hearing loss (audiology – pure tone audiometry, auditory brainstem response, electrocochleography), identify a possible anatomical cause (imaging – MRI/CT depending on the pathology being investigated) or secure the diagnosis of a possible systemic cause (haematology, biochemistry, serology - antibody testing, fasting blood sugar, erythrocyte sedimentation rate etc.).

Treatment options:

- Identification of the aetiopathology as guided by the history and examination
- Conservative e.g. in cases of noise induced hearing loss and certain cases of vestibular schwannoma. However the resulting disability can be corrected with behind the ear hearing aids, cross-aids and bone anchoring hearing aids
- Medical management e.g. in idiopathic sudden onset sensorineural hearing loss (steroids, hyperbaric oxygen) and in cases of Meniere's (low salt diet, diuretics, betahistine).
- Surgical management e.g. in some cases of Meniere's disease (endolymphatic sac surgery, labyrinthectomy, vestibular nerve section) and vestibular shwannoma (microsurgery, hearing preservation approaches)

6.7. Chronic Cough

Instructions:

Take a history from a patient with a persistent cough.

Overview

Ask about the following:

- Heartburn and regurgitation, globus sensation. Gastro-oesophageal reflux accounts for many cases of cough (but may be otherwise silent in 43 – 75%).
- Change in voice, difficulty swallowing. Cough may occur alongside functional dysphonia resulting from voice misuse and chronic laryngitis. Also consider the possibility of a laryngeal or pharyngeal malignancy.

- Fever or malaise, productive cough, haemoptysis. Cough is a common feature of acute upper and lower respiratory infections, so is usually self-limiting. It may also occur in TB, sarcoidosis and lung cancer.
- Oedema e.g. swollen ankles, paroxysmal nocturnal dyspnoea. Consider left ventricular failure.
- Wheezing, shortness of breath. Consider cough-variant asthma (often nocturnal), and chronic bronchitis.
- Facial discomfort, nasal symptoms, postnasal drip, allergies e.g. hay fever. Consider infective, allergic and intrinsic rhino-sinusitis.
- Smoking and drugs, in particular ACE inhibitors.

Treatment

Initially treatment is often empirical:

- Conservative measures to reduce laryngeal irritation e.g. improved hydration, stopping smoking, reduced vocal load.
- Anti-reflux treatment: weight loss, sleeping with the head elevated, proton pump inhibitors
- Rhino-sinusitis: nasal steroid sprays, anti-histamines if allergy is suspected, and antibiotics if infection is suspected.
- Asthma: bronchodilators and steroid inhalers.
- Replace an ACE inhibitor with an angiotensin II blocker.

1. Laryngeal disease: chronic laryngitis, gastro-oesophageal reflux, vocal cord dysfunction, laryngeal sensory neuropathy, carcinoma.
2. Chest disease: asthma, chronic bronchitis, TB, sarcoid, pulmonary oedema, malignancy.
3. Rhino-sinusitis: infective, allergic, intrinsic.

Table 6.6 *Aetiology of chronic cough.*

Chapter 7

Communication

7.1 Introduction

The communication stations assess your approach and manner towards a patient. However every candidate still needs the basic clinical knowledge in order to perform well at the station. In this section your communication skills are usually put to the test through breaking bad news, discussing management options or explaining procedures. There is usually an actor or an actress present as shown in Figure7.1.

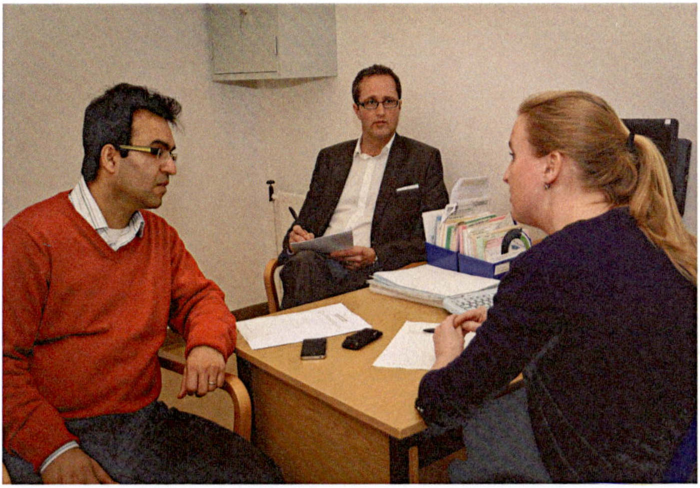

Figure 7.1 Communication station with an examiner (Mr Clifton) and an actor (Mr Kumar).

Top Tips for candidates:

- Greet the patient, confirm their name and introduce yourself to build on the doctor-patient relationship from the onset.

- Ascertain the patient's prior knowledge and understanding of what has gone on and the aim for the consultation.
- Give information in manageable chunks whilst checking for patient understanding with explanations tailored towards the patient. Avoid using jargon and ask the patient what other information they would find useful. Use language that the patient understands, give important information first and repeat or emphasise on these aspects. Drawings / diagrams can be useful.
- Respond to cues from the patient through empathy. There will always be a situation in the exam where you need to look out for a patient's anxieties or worries which need to be addressed.
- Always ask about the patient's ideas, concerns and expectations. Remember the importance of non-verbal behaviours - body language, eye contact and facial expression.
- Confirming points and summarising helps to prove that you are listening to the patient. This may also help the patient remember an important point they forgot to mention!
- Silences or pauses in conversation can be a useful tool. It allows the patient to digest information but in an exam setting can give the candidate an opportunity to consolidate their own thoughts and plan for the next step in the consultation. This is also the case when summarising.
- By summarising and conveying a plan at the end of the consultation, this reassures the patient and gives hope to the patient that their problem is being addressed and that progress is being made.

STAGES	DESCRIPTION
Introduction	Gives full name and role • 'I'm Sam Cho and I'm a junior ENT Surgeon' Confirms patient's identity and preferred mode of address • 'Is it okay if I call you Mrs Jones?' (rather than using patient's first name without permission) Outlines the purpose of the discussion and obtains consent • 'Is it okay if I talk with you for 10 minutes before I talk to the examiner?'
Information gathering	Uses open questions early on • 'Can you tell me what brought you to clinic today?' Assesses patient's prior understanding • 'Have you had this procedure before?' or • 'Can you tell me what you understand about…' Makes empathic statements in response to concerns • 'I understand this must be frightening for you', • 'I can see that you're concerned about the procedure' • 'How else can I help you that might ease your concern?' Uses signposts or transition statements • 'I'd like to ask you some questions about your family and home life'

	• 'Now we've talked about your pain, I'd like to ask you some questions about how your health has generally been' Actively listens to the patient (acknowledges and responds to what patient says) Identifies patient's ideas about his condition Interacts appropriately with patient through eye contact and non-verbal skills throughout Summarises (either interim summary or closing summary)
Information giving	Explains what the procedure will involve Gives information in manageable chunks and checks intermittently that the patient has understood Empowers patient to ask questions Checks patient's understanding of the information given Uses terms the patient understands (avoids medical terminology/jargon or explains it if used)
Closure	Uses skills important in closing the interview • 'Have you got any questions that you'd like to ask me?' • 'Is there anything else that you think I should know?' • 'Do you have any other concerns?'

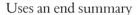

	Uses an end summary • 'If I can just summarise what we've discussed....' Offers leaflets/further contact advice Says what will happen next • 'If you wait here, the Consultant will see you as soon as possible' Treats patient courteously and maintains patient's dignity throughout. Gives a fluent and systematic report to the examiner (where asked)

Table 7.1 Typical instructions given to assessors of Communication skills stations.

7.2 Breaking Bad News: Cancer Diagnosis

Instructions:

Explain to a 60 year old patient, who is a heavy smoker and drinker, that his ML results show T1a vocal cord tumour.

It is best to tackle this scenario in a step-wise approach as there can be many points to cover in a limited amount of time. A common method is to use **SPIKES**:

1. Step 1: **SETTING** up the Interview – ask patient If they want someone with them, avoiding physical barriers between you and the patient, appropriate body language and eye contact
2. Step 2: Assess the patient's **PERCEPTION** – use open ended question to ascertain the patient's understanding of the situation and insight into the potential outcomes – 'what do you understand about what has happened so far'

3. Step 3: Obtaining the patient's **INVITATION** – getting an idea of how much detail the patient wants regarding information
4. Step 4: Giving **KNOWLEDGE** to the patient – warning the patient of bad news, give the information to the patient in language that they can understand in small chunks and keep checking that they understand what you are saying.
5. Step 5: Addressing the patient's **EMOTIONS** – these may vary from silence, crying, anger or shock. By showing empathy it provides support to the patient in a difficult setting.
6. Step 6: **STRATEGY** and **SUMMARY** – gain permission from the patient if they feel ready to discuss treatment options, understand specific patient goals.

Baile W, Buckman R et al. SPIKES - a six step protocol for delivering bad news. *Oncologist* 2000; 5[4]: 302-311. Available online via *theoncologist.alphamedpress.org.*

What you should do

- Greet the patient and ask their name whilst introducing yourself and role. Encourage inviting a relative or friend or give the option of the presence of a nurse.
- Assess the patients prior knowledge by asking an open question such as "what do you understand about what has happened so far" and also assessing how much detail the patient is comfortable with. You can then confirm the focus of the consultation, such as in this case collecting results.
- When breaking the news it is useful to give a warning shot such as "I'm afraid it's not good news". Be clear when giving the news and try to avoid jargon. A pause or period of silence is useful as it gives time for the patient to react and collect their thoughts. You can then give further information through small amounts of

information and checking the patient understands as you go along.

- Address any specific concerns the patient may have or questions they may have. You can use empathy through both verbal ("I can understand that this is a lot to take in and I'm sorry to have broken this news to you today") and non-verbal (tone of voice, posture, facial expression).
- Encouraging questions from the patient may help to alleviate any initial worries. It may be useful to address possible treatment options if the patient allows. Explaining that their case would be discussed at a local meeting to recommend best treatment but would likely involve radiotherapy may be sufficient information at the time.
- Summarising and closure of the consultation is important and arrangements for follow up should be confirmed before the patient leaves.

7.3 Laryngectomy and voice rehabilitation

Instructions:

Explain to an actor that his father has a recurrence of laryngeal cancer and will require a laryngectomy, include options for voice rehabilitation.

- Whilst keeping in mind the advice above there are many important aspects to cover. It is useful to ask the father what he has been told so far. He may already be aware of the recurrence of cancer and so discussing this would not be a shock. However if you are talking about a laryngectomy and the father was not aware of the new diagnosis, it could prove to be disastrous!
- You should initially first check the relatives understanding of a laryngectomy. First explain that a laryngectomy is an operation to remove the voice box and in this case in order to remove the cancer. The voice

box is at the top of the windpipe and is involved in breathing and producing voice.

- By removing the voice box this would affect these two functions. When the voice box is removed a hole in the neck (a stoma) is made and the windpipe is brought to the surface and breathing would occur through this. The patient would now not breathe through the mouth as before but through the stoma.
- The patient will also not be able to talk as before but there are ways to re-create a voice through different methods. A common method is by using tracheo-oesophageal speech. This involves the placement of a valve at the back of the stoma through the windpipe and gullet which lies behind. This allows air flow to be diverted in to the gullet causing it to vibrate and produce sound. Another option is an electrolarynx which is a device that can be applied to the side of the chin to produce vibrations and allow speech. Some patients use just oesophageal speech which is a technique where sounds are created purely through the oesophagus or gullet and does not require a prosthesis. The important message to get across is that there are options to help with communication after the removal of the voice box.
- It may be suitable to mention that initially after the operation they will be fed on a liquid diet through a tube going in through the nose in to the stomach. Then after usually a week after everything has healed they can start on a soft diet and built up thereafter.
- This is of course a lot of information for someone to take in and it is vital to give information in small sections and check for understanding. Diagrams can also be very useful. You could re-iterate this by saying at a suitable point "I know this is a lot to take in but if you have any questions or are unclear about anything then please ask".

- It is also important to give reassurance. They will have support on the ward initially through the medical team, specialist nurses, physiotherapists and speech therapists. It will take time to manage their stoma but they will receive training and also in the community if needed.

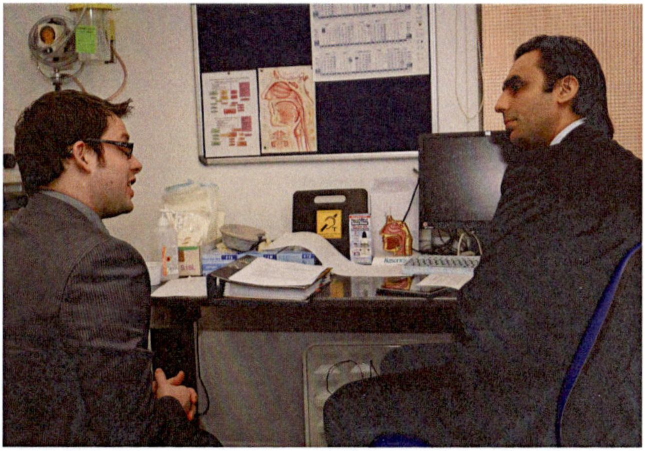

Figure 7.2 Communication skills station with the assessor (Mr Argiris) acting as the son of a patient with cancer.

7.4 Epistaxis

Instructions:

Explain to this 70 year-old patient that is getting recurrent episodes of epistaxis (idiopathic) and all the management options.

- Introduction and confirm purpose of consultation as usual when beginning any station.
- Confirm the patient's knowledge of what has happened up to the point of the consultation.
- Explain that the lining in the nose is fragile and if a blood vessel breaks this can cause a nose bleed.
- This can occur after a recent infection or after injury, but often can occur unexpectedly.

- Some people might be more prone to nosebleeds if they are on medications that thin the blood such as aspirin and warfarin, or if they have high blood pressure, or drink a lot of alcohol.
- There are different ways in which to treat nose bleeds depending on the severity. Nose bleeds are most common at the front of the nose which are easier to treat but can also come from the area at the back of the nose.
- Often minor nose bleeds can be dealt with applying pressure to the area.
- If this doesn't work then the area in the nose causing the bleeding can be sealed off using a chemical silver nitrate stick whilst using a numbing spray. This then forms a scab around the bleeding area. Antiseptic cream can then be used around the area for the next couple of weeks as the area heals.
- A similar method involves using diathermy across a bleeding vessel whilst using a telescope in the nose to visualise where the bleeding is coming from. Diathermy stops the bleeding by passing a weak electric current across the area to seal the vessel.
- Sometimes however if the bleeding is severe, the nose is packed in order to control the bleeding. There are different types of nasal packing that can be used at the front and back of the nose. The most common used is a sponge like pack that expands when placed in the nose when in contact with blood. If the bleeding is coming from the back of the nose then a balloon packing may need to be used (i.e. posterior packing).
- In severe cases, such as in your case, some patients may continue to bleed despite the above measures. In these instances surgery is then an option as a last resort to stop the bleeding. The nose is supplied by different arteries and most commonly the sphenopalatine is involved in nose bleeds. An operation involves using a telescope in

the nose to identify this blood vessel and applying a clip on it to stop the bleeding. This is known as sphenopalatine artery ligation.

- In some cases when nose bleeds are a result of physical injury to the nose, another artery commonly involved is the anterior ethmoid. If this artery needs to be clipped, then an operation would involve a cut in the skin between the eye and nose to find this artery in order to apply a clip to it.
- Make sure to summarise and clarify the details with the patient as you go along, ensuring patient's understanding.

7.5 Benign Parasysmal Positional Vertigo (BPPV)

Instructions:

Explain to this 38 year-old patient the new diagnosis of BPPV.

Basic communication skills need to be applied here as explained in the introduction. Further condition-specific details that need to be communicated are shown below:

- It is one of the most common causes of vertigo which is the sensation of the room spinning.
- Commonly can get brief episodes of vertigo caused by changes in head position.
- Often no specific underlying cause (i.e. trigger) for BPPV can be found. Sometimes it is associated with a minor to severe blow to the head. It is rarely serious but it can increase the chance of falls.
- It is important to reassure the patient about the benign nature of the condition.
- Patients are often very anxious irrespective of knowing that this condition is benign. It is therefore important to ask about any particular worrying concerns they may have and address these tactfully.

- A simplified description of the pathophysiology is needed in such a station by describing initially the basic anatomy of the ear.
- The ear consists of outer, middle and inner divisions and this problem involves the inner ear. It includes three loop-shaped structures (semi-circular canals) that contain fluid and fine hair-like sensors that monitor the rotation of your head.
- The inner ear senses certain head movements by utilizing certain calcium crystals that are placed separately from the semi-circular canals. For a variety of reasons, some of these move from where they should be to one of the canals, causing it to become sensitive to head position changes it would normally not respond to. The result of this is the unpleasant sensation of vertigo.
- In BPPV, the vertiginous episodes last seconds to minutes, even though patients subjectively feel it goes for much longer.
- The attacks usually disappear with time and the majority of patients who experience episodes of vertigo will recover within a few weeks or month of the onset of the symptoms.
- The condition is diagnosed with a very simple manouevre called the Dix-Hallpike test. It needs some degree of neck movement and patient cooperation. Its purpose is to trigger an attack of vertigo while looking at the eyes that effectively confirms the diagnosis.
- Once the condition is confirmed it can be treated instantaneously with a further set of manuvres called the Epley's manoeuvre. The head is moved in certain directions in order to realign the crystals. Each position is held for about 30 seconds or after the vertigo or abnormal eye movement (i.e. nystagmus) stops.
- It is advised that the patient does not drive after these manuevres. In addition the patients should be made

aware that she will experience some degree of disequilibrium for a few hours but that should settle. It also helps if the patient avoids lying flat following the treatment.

- Rarely as a last choice surgery can be an option to help symptoms. This involves surgery to the inner ear by either blocking one of the semicircular canals or disconnecting the nerves involved in balance.
- You can also give lifestyle advice. Balance problems can lead to falls and potential injury. General advice includes the use of good lighting when getting up at night, sitting down immediately when vertigo/dizziness ensues, and walking with aids if there is a risk of falling.
- Sudden vertigo attacks can lead to serious harm if the patient is driving at the time. The DVLA therefore needs to be informed of such cases. It is very likely in such circumstances that the patient is disallowed from driving.

7.6 Tonsillitis: information gathering and information giving

Instructions:

Take a history from this 18 year-old lady that has presented to your clinic with recurrent episodes of sore throat (tonsillitis), explaining also any relevant management options

The candidate should have recognized at this point that the station is examining both information gathering and information giving skills. A general introduction is needed as described in the introduction (section 7.1)

Information gathering

- An opening question is needed to ascertain what has been troubling the patient (e.g. 'Can you please tell me what has brought you to the clinic today?')

- Being clear from the onset that this station is a case of recurrent tonsillitis, the candidate should continue by taking a focused history.
- To achieve this, one should be familiar with the Scottish Intercollegiate Guidance Network (SIGN) guidelines on the management of sore throats and indications for tonsillectomy.
- Further data gathering should therefore focus on:
  - o Confirming that all sore throats are due to tonsillitis. (N.B. this is often not straight forward but for the purpose of the assessment, confirmation that all of these infections have been diagnosed by her GP and attributed to tonsillitis should suffice)
  - o Extent of symptoms. This should include the presence of pyrexia, vomiting or nausea, dysphagia (fluids and/or solids) and any previous hospital admissions. It should also be asked whether the patient ever had a quinsy (peritonsillar abscess) as this would alter the management (N.B. two quinsies are an indication for tonsillitis). Adults might also present with two associated symptoms, including change in the quality of voice and food impaction within the tonsils.
  - o Overall disability. The candidate needs to assess how disabling the recurrent tonsillitis is as it should prevent normal functioning. This can be addressed by asking the patient how many days off work/university she has taken.
  - o Frequency of tonsillitis. This is a crucial aspect of the SIGN guidance even though in real life it is not always straight forward. In order to be listed for a tonsillectomy, other that fulfilling the criteria set above, the patient should have had seven or more documented and treated episodes in the preceding year *or* five or more episodes in each of the previous

two years *or* three or more episodes in each of the preceding three years

- As this patient is potentially a surgical candidate a full (but brief) history is needed (PMH, DH and allergies, SH, FH, systems review)
- All basic communication skills as described in the introduction should be applied.

Information giving

- Even though there are situations where a tonsillectomy may be appropriate outside of these criteria (e.g. severe sleep disturbance, possible malignancy etc), in the context of a DOHNS OSCE, the patient will either clearly fulfill the criteria or not.
- If the candidate did not fulfill the SIGN guidelines, a wait and watch approach should be suggested.
- If the candidate fulfills the SIGN guidelines, a tonsillectomy can be offered (which is the case here).
- It is good practice to summarise all key findings to the patient, setting the scene for the second part of the station (i.e. the information giving).
- The management options will have to be discussed openly covering the pros and cons of each.
- This will allow for the patient to make the ultimate decision, therefore giving the patient autonomy.
- A wait and watch approach could be used on the one hand. This would effectively mean that there is no surgical risk and the patient may stop experiencing tonsillitis (even though this cannot be guaranteed). The patient however could possibly continue experiencing recurrent sore throats and be treated with regular painkillers and antibiotics (i.e. symptomatic treatment).
- Surgery on the other hand would be indicated here and the issues of a tonsillectomy would need to be discussed.

- It should be re-instated that the purpose of the procedure would be to treat the tonsillitis by removing the tonsils.
- Other important aspects that have to be discussed with respect to the surgery are:
  - o Procedure routinely done as a day case (with possibility of overnight stay)
  - o Being a sensitive area there will be a degree of discomfort/pain that becomes worse by post-op day 3 before it gets better
  - o Need to stress importance of regular painkillers for at least a week
  - o Nausea and vomiting are also not uncommon, even though usually anaesthetically induced
  - o Infection of the tonsil beds can occur and a course of antibiotics may be needed
  - o Bleeding has to be discussed in some detail in order to educate the patient as it can be potentially quite serious. Bleeding rates vary but the commonly quoted figure is 2%. Bleeding can be reactionary (in immediate post-operative period) and surgery is usually needed quickly to arrest the bleed. Secondary haemorrhage that can happen up to a week post-operatively is more common and is often attributed to infection. The patient should be made aware that if she notices blood at any point, she should seek medical advice by coming to A&E. It should also be stressed that surgery is not always needed in these cases and that an overnight hospital admission for observation is the more common course.
  - o Damage to teeth and lips. Because of the way the procedure is carried out (use of the Boyle-Davis gag etc) damage to teeth and lips – even though very rare – can happen. Reassurance is needed here.
  - o It is good practice to tell the patient that because of waiting list and other managerial constraints, patients

are placed on a general pool and therefore the surgeon might be another member of the team.

- At this point the consultation is approaching to closure (N.B. refer to introduction section).
- The patient must be asked if she has any questions first. Following that she must be asked what management option she wants to proceed with.
- If it's the surgical option, you need to let her know that you are putting her name on the waiting list but she should feel free to contact the department if she has any questions or even cancel if she changes her mind. The candidate could provide her with procedure leaflets and thank the patient.
- If the patient does not want surgery or wants to think about it alternative arrangements need to be made. A leaflet can still be provided.

Chapter 8

Clinical Examinations

8.1 Introduction

During the OSCE Examination, you will be asked to examine a few patients, so time spent practicing will pay dividends. In any clinical examination, it is not just about spotting the signs or making a diagnosis. The examiners will be looking at the candidate's bedside manner (i.e. doctor-patient interaction), structure of the clinical examination (i.e. organised and methodical approach), confidence and finally his/her ability to determine whether the patient has any pathology or not and conveying that information in a clear succinct manner.

At the outset of all clinical examinations, one should always use alcohol gel on hands, greet the patient, introduce oneself, ask for permission to examine and finally ask about any tenderness or pain (in summary: gel, greet, introduce, permission, pain or tenderness).

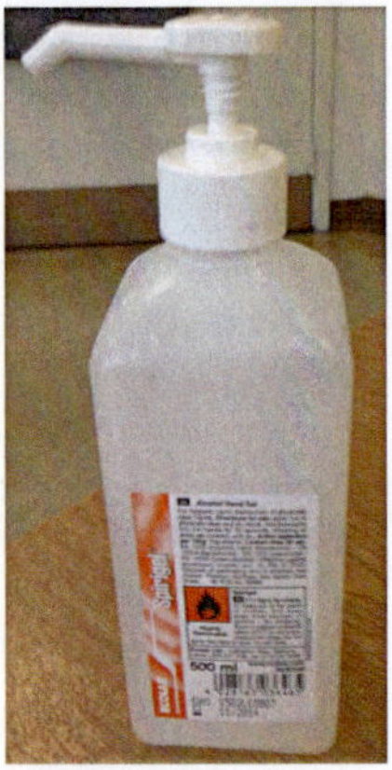

Figure 8.1 Alcohol gel used in the UK (will be present in the manned station of the examination).

We also recommend that you collect all the relevant instruments and lay them out on the side table before you start examining the patient. In this way you will avoid forgetting any specific manoeuvre such as the spatula misting test. It is difficult to learn clinical examination by reading text. Here the key points pertaining to each clinical examination in are highlighted in note format. Some common mistakes will also be pointed out.

The first important point to note is that the surgeon normally sits on a chair with wheels (Figure 1a) whilst the patient either sits on either a specially designed ENT chair (Figure 1b) or on a non-wheely one (Figure 1c). Secondly, when examining a patient, it is also necessary for the surgeon to sit with his/her legs at the side of the patient's closed legs (Figure 1.d).

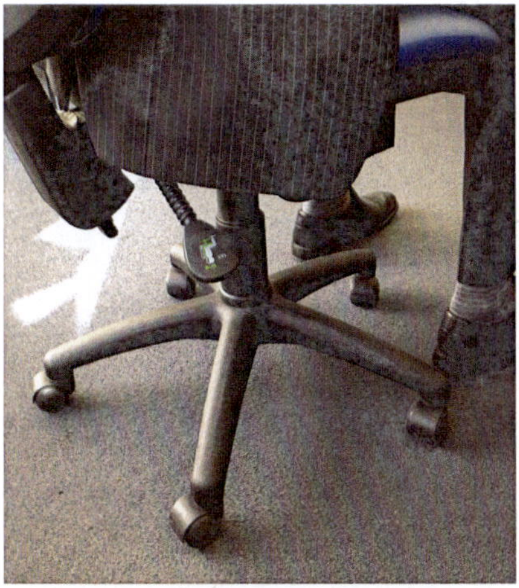

Figure 8.2a The surgeon gets the chair with wheels for clinical examination and consultation.

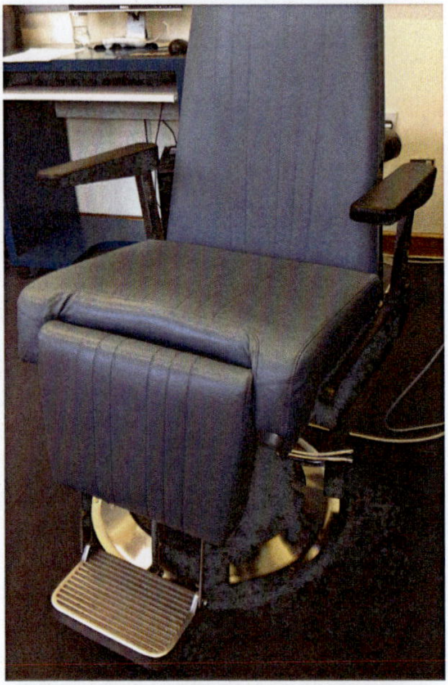

Figure 8.2b A bespoke ENT examining chair for patients.

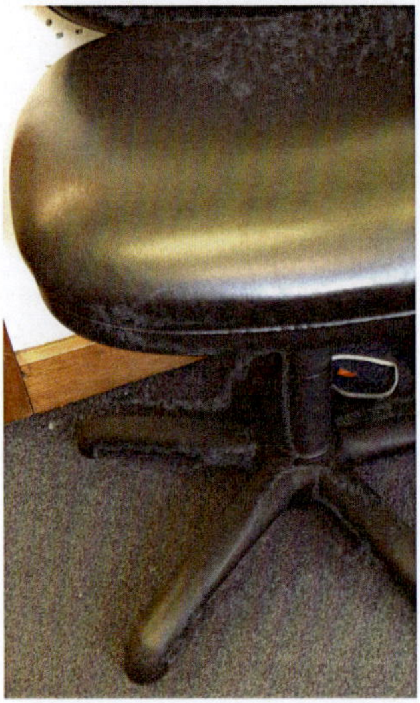

Figure 8.2c A non-wheelie chair suitable for examining patients, if an ENT chair is not available.

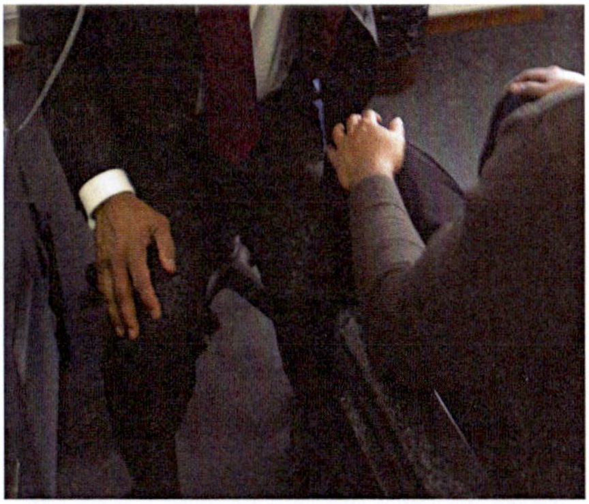

Figure 8.2d Correct position of the legs of the patient and doctor before examination (not straddling the patient).

8.2 Ear Examination

- Alcohol gel
- Introduction
- Greet patient
- Ask for permission
- Ask about any pain or tenderness

Inspection

- Pinna, external auditory meatus (EAM), mastoid
- Symmetry, scars, swelling, erythema, discharge

Otoscopy

- External auditory canal
- Tympanic membrane:
  MIPC structured approach
  1. **M**alleus
  2. **I**ntact (Pars tensa, pars flaccida)
  3. **P**osition of drum
  4. **C**olour e.g. grey, dull, pink, white (tympanosclerosis)
     These points are illustrated in Figure 1

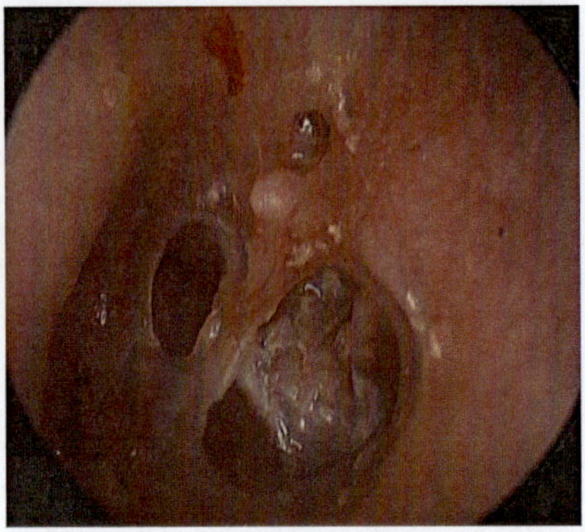

Figure 8.3 Clinical photograph of a left tympanic membrane showing malleus, perforations, retraction of *pars flaccida* and *pars tensa* (with incudostapial joint visible) and thin pale tympanic membrane.

Fistula test

- Pressure applied to tragus for 2-3 seconds
- Can be performed with pneumatic otoscope
- Positive test: Deviation of eyes away from examined side; nystagmus towards the diseased side.

Hearing tests

1) Tuning fork tests: Select 512Hz
   - *Rinne's:* AC>BC - positive test (normal / SNHL)
     BC>AC - negative test (CHL ≥ 20dB / severe SNHL)
   - *Weber's*: central i.e. normal
     lateralises to affected ear with CHL >10dB
     lateralises to normal ear with SNHL

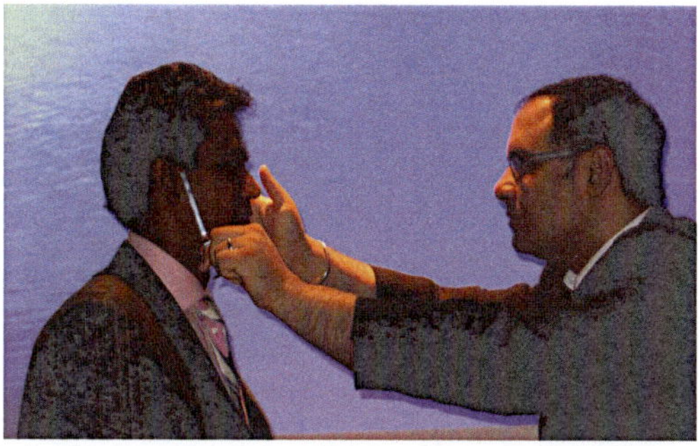

Figure 8.4a Demonstrating Rinne's tuning fork test.

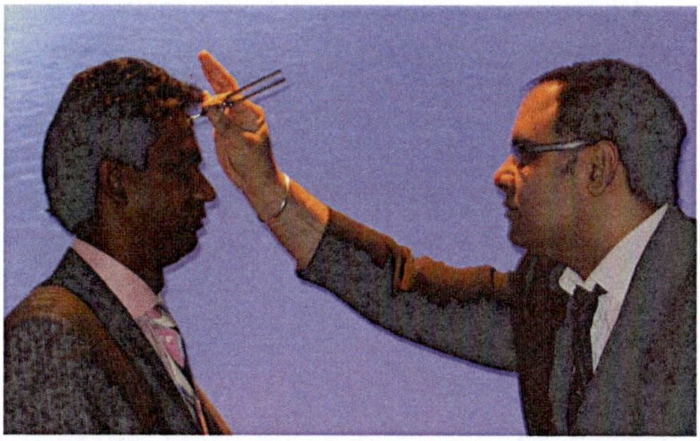

Figure 8.4b Demonstrating Weber's tuning fork test.

RINNE'S	WEBER'S	INTERPRETATION
Positive bilaterally (AC>BC)	Central	Normal or bilateral SNHL (presbyacusis)
Negative on right, positive on left	Louder in right ear	CHL right ear
Negative on left, positive on right	Louder in right ear	Profound SNHL left ear ('dead' ear)
Positive bilaterally (AC>BC)	Louder right ear	SNHL left or small CHL right

Right unequivocal (AC=BC); left positive	Louder in right ear	CHL right

Table 8.1 Interpretation of tuning fork tests.

2) Free field speech testing: Use a letter and number (eg A4 or B7)

- 60 cm from the ear
- Test with whispered, conversational then loud voice.
- Mask opposite ear with tragal rub
- Ask patient to repeat words; stop when >50% correct
- If patient can hear a whisper at 60cm, then hearing threshold >30dB

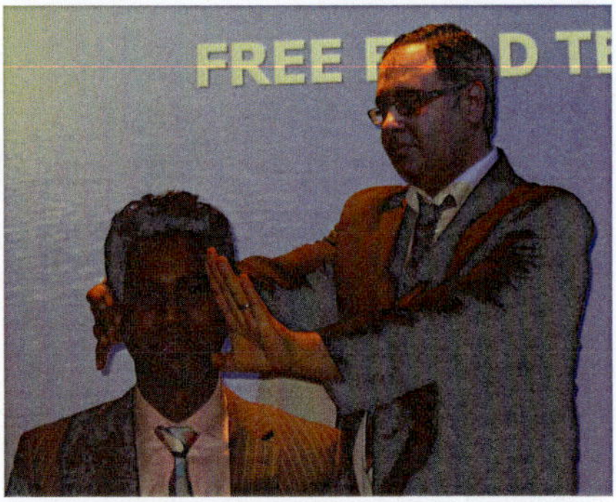

Figure 8.5 Demonstrating free field testing.

Flexible nasoendoscopy

- Examine post-nasal space and Eustachian tube orifices

Facial nerve

- House-Brackmann grading
- Cranial nerve examination

To complete the examination, request a pure tone audiogram and tympanogram

* Remember the five 'Fs':
1) Fistula test
2) Free field speech test
3) Forks (tuning)
4) Facial nerve
5) Flexible nasendoscopy

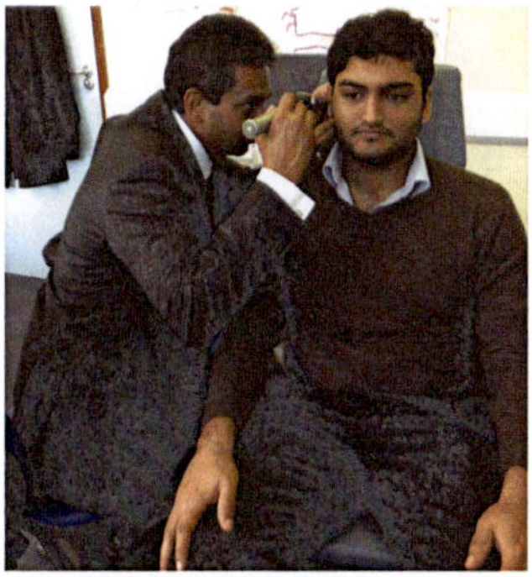

Figure 8.6a Correct position to examine the ear with an auroscope, ie, sit comfortably so that you are at the same level as the patient (note the correct way to hold the auroscope).

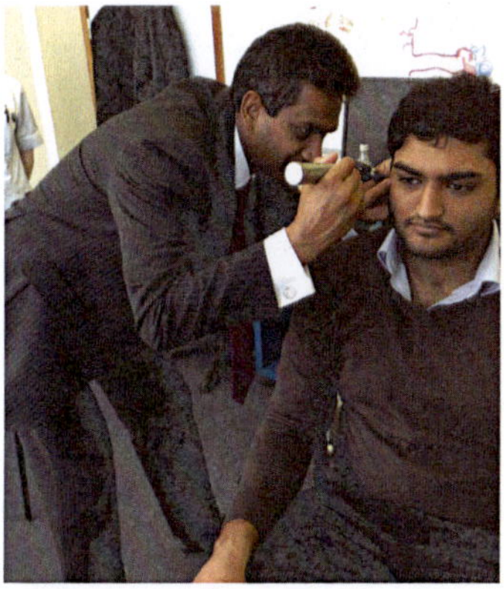

Figure 8.6b Incorrect position to examine the ear

8.3 Nose Examination

- Alcohol gel
- Introduction
- Greet
- Ask for permission
- Ask about any pain or tenderness
- Headlight

Inspection

- Symmetry
- Scars
- Erythema
- External nasal anatomy defects: Dorsal hump, tip ptosis, saddle deformity, lateral deviation

Anatomy

- Lift nasal tip: Assess vestibule and caudal end of septum
- Anterior rhinoscopy: Using Thudichum's speculum
  - Septal deviation, perforation
  - Nasal mucosa
  - Turbinates
  - Polyps

Function

- Patency of nasal airway:
  - Inflow: look for alar collapse
  - Outflow: check misting size and pattern on a cold Lack's tongue depressor

Flexible nasoendoscopy

- Posterior septum
- Turbinates
- Nasopharynx, adenoidal pad
- Eustachian tube orifices
- Fossae of Rosenmüller

Neck

- Palpate neck for lymphadenopathy (submandibular, deep cervical)

Olfactory function

- Ask about sense of smell
- Olfactory testing kit (eg UPSIT)

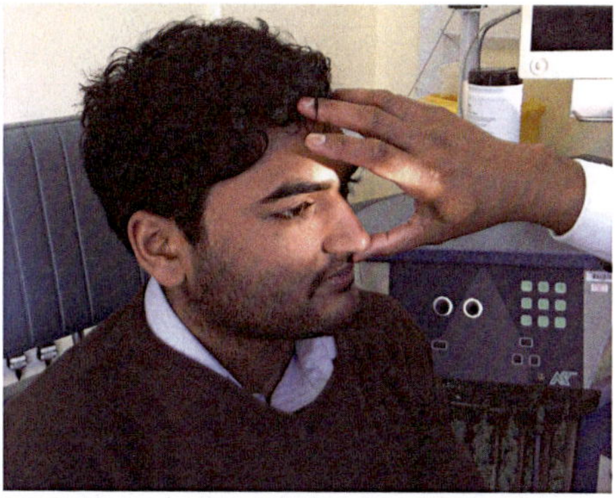

Figure 8.7a Correct way to check for right nasal **inflow** and right alar collapse.

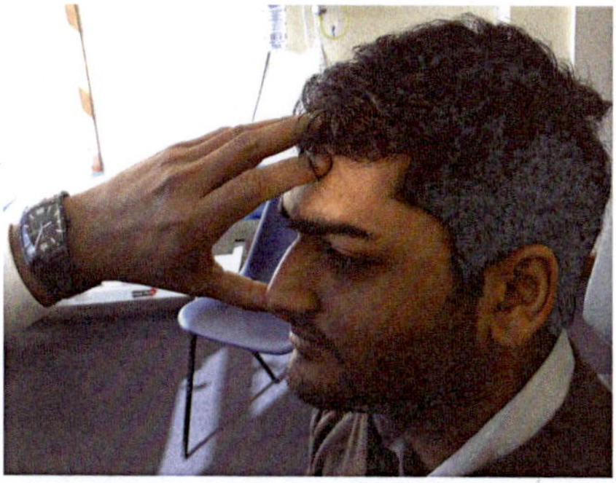

Figure 8.7b Correct way to check left nasal **inflow** and left alar collapse.

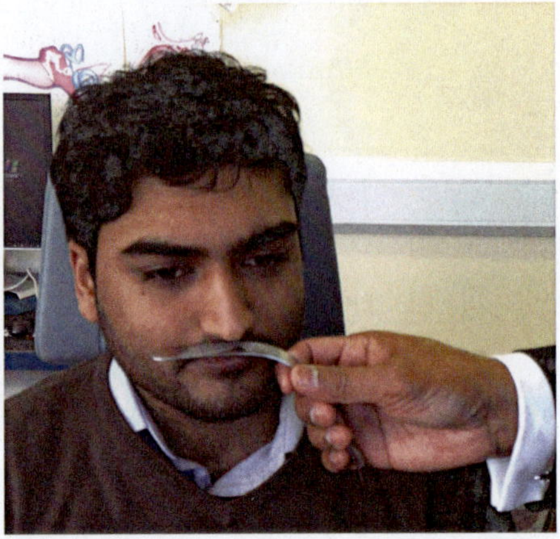

Figure 8.7c Misting test using a Lack spatula (to test for outflow from the nose).

8.4 Oral Examination

- Alcohol gel
- Introduction
- Greet
- Ask for permission
- Ask about any pain or tenderness
- Headlight

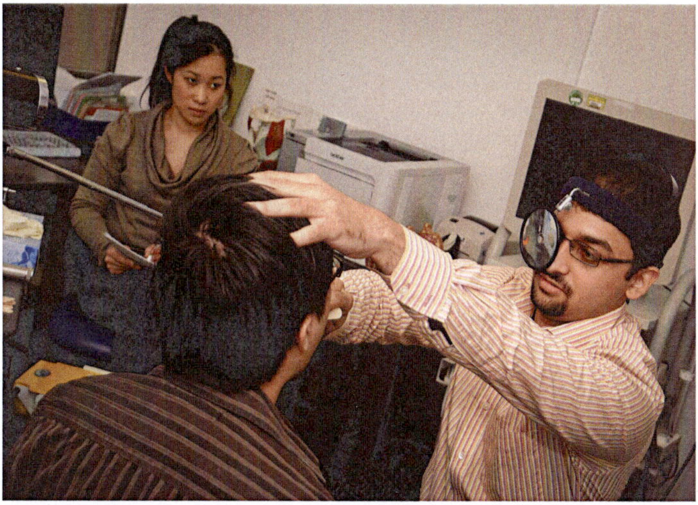

Figure 8.8 Oral examination at DOHNS OSCE Course.

Inspection

- Scars, asymmetry, tracheostomy
- Examine oral cavity using two Lack's tongue depressors:
  - Buccal mucosa
  - Stensen's duct
  - Floor of mouth
  - Wharton's duct
  - Dentition
  - Examine tonsils, uvula and posterior pharyngeal wall using one Lack's tongue depressor

Palpation

- Bimanual palpation of parotid and submandibular glands

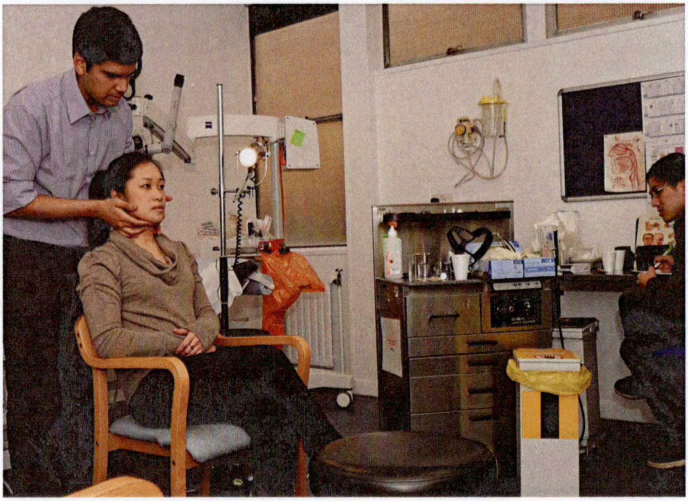

Figure 8.9 Palpating the submandibular gland on ENTTZAR DOHNS OSCE Course.

Flexible nasoendoscopy

- Postnasal space
- Base of tongue
- Epiglottis
- Valleculae
- Larynx
- Vocal cords
- Arytenoids
- Ventricular folds
- Piriform fossae

Speech

- Ask patient to count to five
- Assess for hoarseness, 'breathy' speech

8.5 Neck Examination

- Alcohol gel
- Greet
- Introduction
- Ask for permission to examine
- Ask about any tenderness or pain
- Expose neck to clavicles
- Glass of water

Inspection

- From front and side (Figure 8.8)
- Scars, asymmetry, skin changes, tracheostomy
- If neck lump visible, does it move?
    - o On swallowing
    - o On tongue protrusion

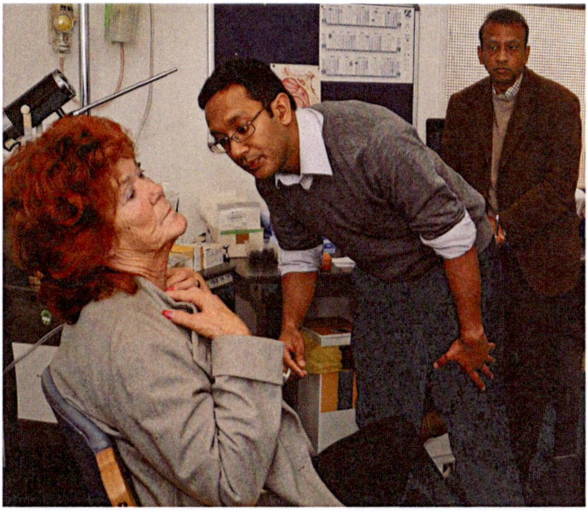

Figure 8.8 Careful inspection under examination conditions on ENTTZAR FRCS Course (Mr Kothari ENT Consultant, Mr Pal FRCS Gold Medalist).

Palpation

- Stand behind patient (Figure 8.9)
- Ask to relax neck muscles
- Use gentle, sweeping movements
- Palpate groups of lymph nodes:
  - o Start at suprasternal notch
  - o Midline to trachea, thyroid, larynx
  - o (Do not palpate both sides simultaneously!)
  - o Submental triangles
  - o Submandibular and jugulodigastric nodes
  - o Deep cervical chain (sternocleidomastoid posteriorly displaced)
  - o Supraclavicular nodes
  - o Posterior border of SCM to parotid gland, pre-auricular nodes
  - o Post-auricular and occipital nodes
- If there is a palpable lump, assess: Size, site, shape, skin, surface, tenderness, transillumination, temperature, consistency, attached to underlying structure, mobile, pulsatile, fixed, irreducible, reducible,extra lumps such as lymphadenopathy.
- For a parotid (or submandibular) lump:
  - o Perform bimanual palpation.
  - o Examine facial nerve function
- For a thyroid lump, examine the thyroid gland

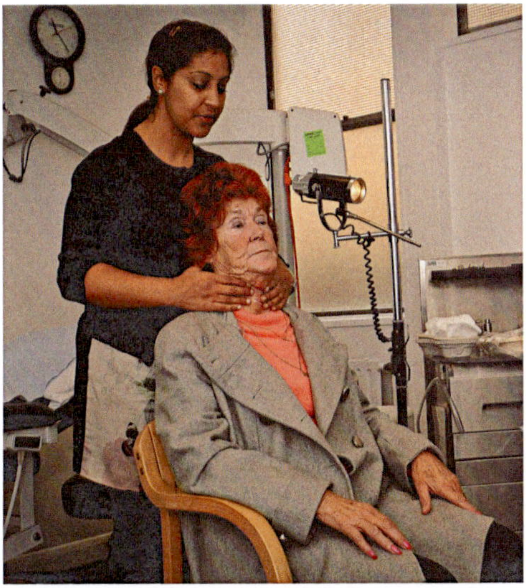

Figure 8.9 ***Correct*** position to palpate the neck, ie, Surgeon is standing behind the patient.

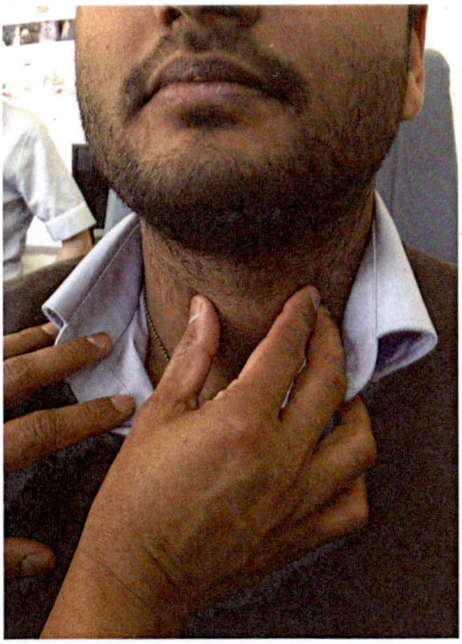

Figure 8.10 ***Incorrect*** position to palpate the neck (Surgeon is in front of patient).

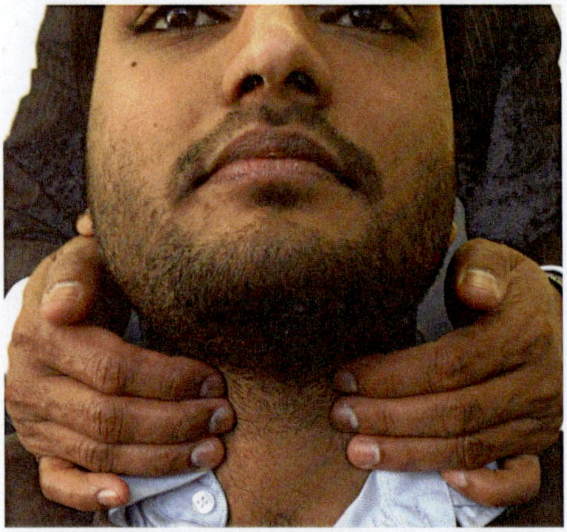

Figure 8.11 ***Incorrect*** way to palpate the neck (i.e. using nails)

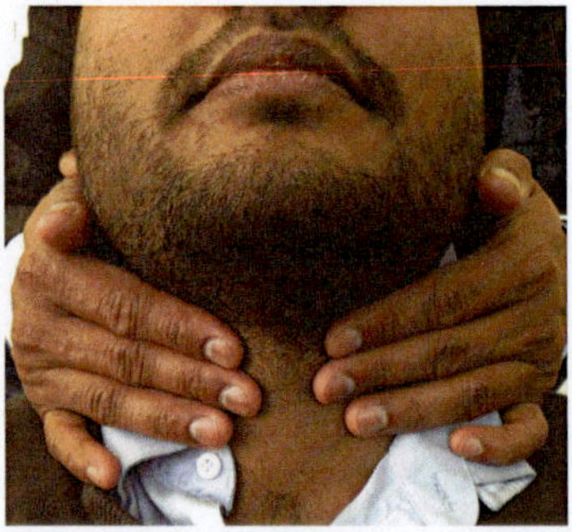

Figure 8.12 ***Correct*** way to palpate the neck (i.e. using soft part of distal phalanges)

8.6 Thyroid examination

Inspection

- Restlessness, sweaty, skin texture, hair.
- Hands (sweating, palmar erythema, **tremor,** thyroid acropachy)
- Pulse (AF, tachycardia)
- Eyes (Lid retraction, lid lag, exopthalmos, chemosis, proptosis)

- Ask patient to count to 10, to assess for hoarseness

Palpation

- Reassess movement with swallowing (water) and tongue protrusion whilst palpating
- Palpate thyroid lobes and isthmus
- Tracheal deviation
- Cervical lymphadenopathy

Percussion

- Percuss over sternum for possible retrosternal extension

Auscultation

- Auscultate for thyroid bruit

Flexible nasoendoscopy

- Assess vocal cord movements
- To complete the examination, assess ankle reflexes, and for pre-tibial myxoedema and proximal myopathy.

Chapter 9

Outpatients Skills

9.1 Flexible nasendoscopy (FNE)

This is a vital outpatient skill for all ENT surgeons to master and it is repeatedly tested in the DOHNS examination. One will have to demonstrate confidence, good handling of the instrument and excellenbt communication skills with the patient actor. The station usually has an actor for the explanation of procedure and a manikin for demonstrating the procedure.

Procedure

As with all procedures, nasal endoscopy has 3 separate components:

I. pre-procedural steps
II. procedure *per se*
III. post-procedural care.

Pre-procedural steps

Verbal consent should be carried out ensuring patients are adequately prepared, warning them of potential complications: sneezing, coughing, gagging, and "tearing" from the eyes. The procedure is usually carried out without premedication. However some patients may request a local anaesthetic spray such as Xylocaine (Figure 9.1). If the nasal mucosa is sensitive or very swollen then a 0.5% phenylephrine and 5% lidocaine spray can be used to decongest and anaesthetize the area respectively. Ensure you have checked for allergies and allow 5 minutes if used. The patient should be sat upright against a chair, so as to prevent them from leaning away. The flexible endoscope is usually available only as one size in most centers (4mm). Other equipment that will be required:

- Tissue for patient to wipe tears and nose
- Lubricating gel (Figure 9.2)
- Antifog solution (an alcohol pad can be used alternatively, Figure 9.3)
- Light source +/- monitor

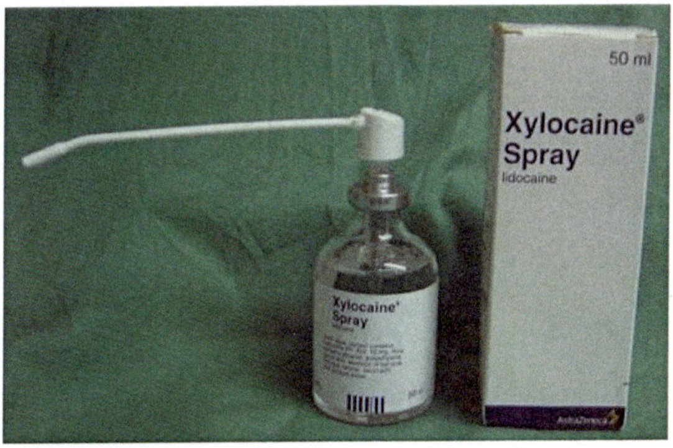

Figure 9.1 Xylocaine spray for numbing the nose.

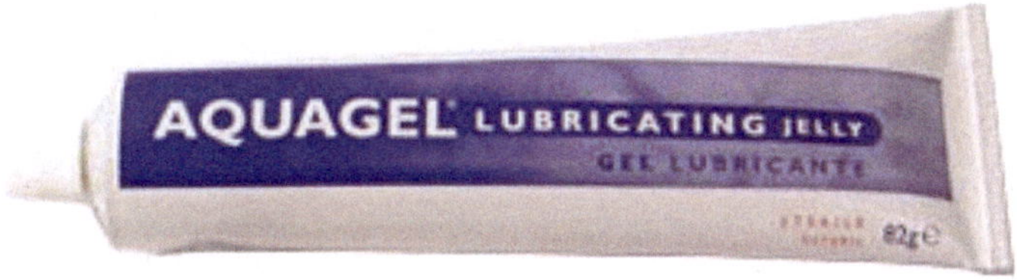

Figure 9.2 Gel for lubricating the flexible nasendoscopy.

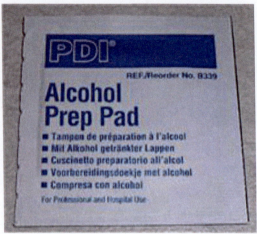

Figure 9.3 Alcohol pad may be used as an anti-misting agent (saliva of the patient is an alternative).

The procedure

Once everything has been explained and you have allowed the local to work the actual procedure should follow the sequence below. This examination is based on a patient with laryngeal pathology. Clearly if one is assessing the PNS or nasal pathology, the scope needs to be passed through both nostrils and the rigid scope may be more appropriate (see rigid endoscopic examination below). The steps for flexible nasoendoscopy can be considered as follows:

- When holding the scope, ensure you are happy with the focus and lighting
- Put some lubricant and ask the patient to stick out their tongue in order to moist the front part of the scope
- Whichever finger you have learned to control the scope (i.e. index or thumb) just stick to that so you do not confuse yourself. Both are acceptable
- Pass the scope about 1-2cm just beyond each vestibule to identify the better nasal passage (Figure 9.4)

- While inserting it ask the patient to remain calm and breath from his mouth
- Pass the scope through the floor of the nasal cavity
- Examine eustachian tube orifices, fossae of Rosenmuller and posterior pharyngeal wall
- Once in the PNS curve the scope inferiorly and as you push it further down straighten it out again
- You may then ask the patient to start breathing from the nose
- Once at the tongue ask the patient to stick it out, examining posterior aspects of tonsils, tongue base, epiglottis and valeculla
- Advance further to laryngopharynx (you can ask patient to also extend chin to open airway further)
- Obstruct patient's nose with your fingers and perform a Valsalva manoeuvre while looking at the pyriform fossae. Turning the patient's head to the left/right will open up right/left pyriform fossa further.
- Inspect the rest of the larynx, including the false vocal cords, true vocal cords, arytenoid cartilages, aryepiglottic folds, anterior and posterior commisures and ventricles
- Ask the patient to take a deep breath in and out looking for vocal fold abduction.
- Assess vocal cord adduction by asking to patient to say "eee"
- Ask the patient to count to 5 looking for vocal fold movement
- Progress scope as far down as possible to get a glimpse of the subglottis
- Remove scope and hand over to nurse for cleaning or state you would clean yourself
- You then document in the notes your findings.

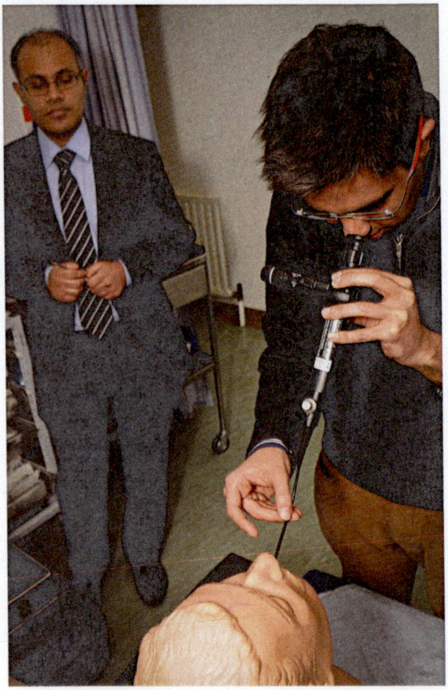

Figure 9.4 DO-HNS Candidate performing flexible nasendoscopy on a manikin on ENTTZAR OSCE course (Mr Hiten Joshi, Examiner)

Useful manoeuvres during flexible nasendoscopy
Extend chin to open airway
Turning the patients head to left/right will open up right/left piriform fossa, respectively.
Sticking out tongue to assess tongue base and vallecullae
Performing valsalva to open up ventricles

Table 9.1 Tips to aid visualization during flexible nasendoscopy.

Scoring events	Marks		
Explains procedure	0	1	2
Obtains verbal consent	0	1	2
Considers use of topical anaesthesia	0	1	2
Give patient tissue to clean eyes and nose afterwards	0	1	2
Performs anterior rhinoscopy to choose side	0	1	2
Lubricates scope and use saliva or alcohol as anti-fog agent	0	1	2
Inserts and advance scope gently along inferior meatus	0	1	2
Makes systematic assessment of anatomical features	0	1	2
Withdraws scope carefully without hurting patient	0	1	2
Document findings accurately	0	1	2

Table 9.2 An example of the marking scheme.

Documentation

At this point the candidate should not fall into the trap of simply drawing a larynx. The patient's details should be clearly written on the top. The time and date should also be recorded. The details of the medical interaction (both positive and negative findings) should be written legibly, with the aid of diagrams (Figure 9.5) if possible and in the presence of the sticker indicating the use of the nasendoscope. It is probably best to document findings in a systematic order, as encountered in turn during the examination.

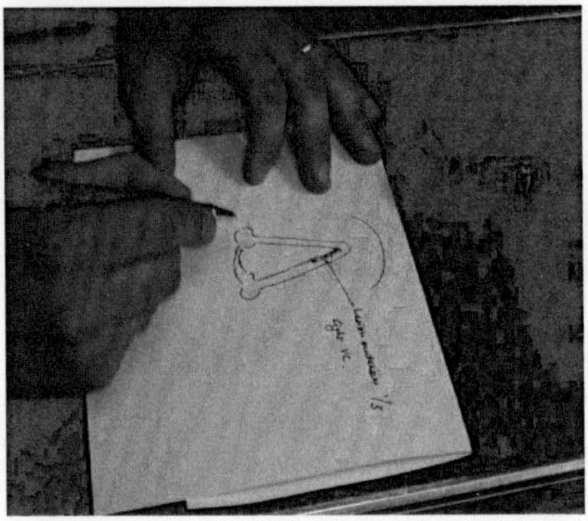

Figure 9.5 Documentation of findings.

9.2 Rigid nasendoscopy

Endoscopic examination of the nasal cavity is best performed with a rigid endoscope (Figure 9.6) for two main reasons: (1) the optics are better than with a flexible scope and (2) one hand is free do perform other functions, such as, suctioning or cautery.

A 4mm 0° scope (Figure 9.5) is usually selected first and three separate passes of the scope in to each nasal cavity are made. With the patient's head kept slightly flexed, for the **first pass** the scope is passed along the nasal floor towards the nasopharynx. The inferior turbinate and inferior meatus are examined first. The scope is then advanced further posteriorly to the nasopharynx where the eustachian tube orifices, fossa of Rosenmüller, soft palate motility and posterior pharyngeal wall are inspected. For the **second pass** the scope is passed between the middle and inferior turbinates. This is to examine the middle meatus, fontanelles and to assess for accessory maxillary ostia. A Freer's elevator can be used to gently medialise the middle turbinate in order to visualize the middle meatus. In the **third pass**, the scope should then be passed medially and posteriorly to the middle turbinate in order to examine the sphenoethmoidal recess which is located medial to the middle and superior turbinates.

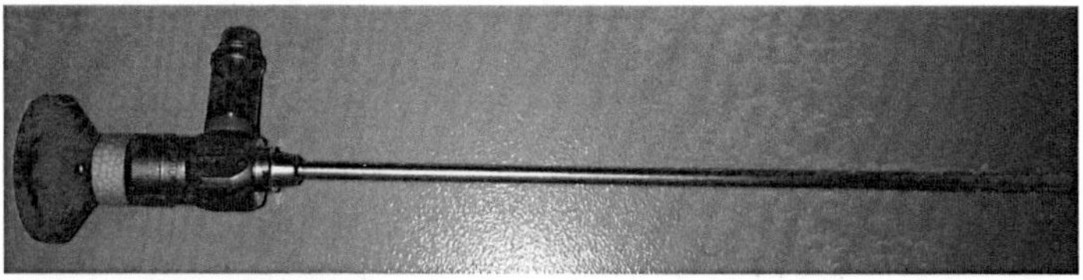

Figure 9.6 Hopkin's rigid endoscope (4mm zero degree) used for rigid nasendoscopy.

Post-procedure Care

Once the examination is complete, one should explain both the positive and negative findings to the patients in order to help alleviate any anxiety. Future management plans should also be discussed. If it is possible to take photos during the examinations then these should be placed in the notes for future reference. If topical anaesthetic has been used, then the patient should be warned not to eat or drink any hot items for approximately one hour post-procedure to prevent burn injuries.

Chapter 10

Informed Consent

10.1 Introduction

The consent station assesses your knowledge of common ENT operations and your communication skills. Consent literally means *to give permission.* However poor communication between the doctor and patient often leads to a complaint and even litigation. Patients who feel that they have part of the consent process and have some control over the final decision are less likely to complain. In surgery, we seek valid informed consent from a patient before any surgical procedure. In order to be valid, the decision needs to be made:

(i) Voluntarily
This means without pressure (time or coercion)

(ii) By a competent patient
This is a patient who is able to *understand* the information, *retain* it and *weigh* the balance of risks and benefits in order to come to a *particular decision.* This has to then be *communicated* to the medical team by the patient. Adults are assumed to be competent unless proven otherwise.

(iii) With sufficient information provided
This requires disclosure of the necessary information and options for the patient to make an autonomous decision. You must use appropriate language and ensure adequate comprehension of the information provided during the meeting.

Therefore consent is a process, not merely obtaining a signature on a form. The consent form also constitutes a part of your evidentiary documentation that a consultation and a dialogue have occurred.

In the UK there are 4 different types of consent forms (Table 10.1). The patient actor in the examination will be an adult with capacity. Therefore, it is up to you to make sure points (I) and (III) are adequately fulfilled for valid informed consent.

What will you have to do in your station?

(i) Introduce yourself

- Use your full name and role
- Check the patients name and age
- Explain what you intend to do

(ii) Gather information

Explore the patient's ideas, concerns and expectations (ICE) about

- Their condition
- The management options

(iii) Give information

Use the information you gathered to guide what you say in this section but generally cover:

- **C**ondition
- **O**ptions (i.e. no action, conservative, surgical)
- **N**amed option (include operation name, site, peri-operative course)
- **S**ide effects: benefits and risks
- **E**xtra procedures (e.g. drain, transfusion)
- **N**amed surgeon responsible
- **T**eaching and training
- **S**econd opinion

(iv) Closure

- Summarise/ check understanding

- Anything else patient wishes to discuss?
- Patient information leaflet
- Signature
- Contact (should they have any queries)

Top Tips

- Listen to the patient's verbal cues
- Watch the patient's body language
- Use non-jargon language appropriate to the patient
- Read patient information leaflets from ENT UK to see the level at which to pitch your information
- Practice!

Consent Form	Application
1	**For a competent adult**. ***NB*** *'This form documents the patient's agreement to go ahead with the investigation or treatment you have proposed. It is not a legal waiver – if patients for example, do not receive enough information on which to base their decision, then the consent may not be valid, even though the form has been signed.'* (Figure 10.1)
2	For an adult with parental responsibility consenting on behalf of a child (Figure 10.2)
3	When no impairment of consciousness is involved (Figure 10.3)
4	For an adult lacking capacity (Figure 10.4)

Table 10.1. Consent forms used in the UK.

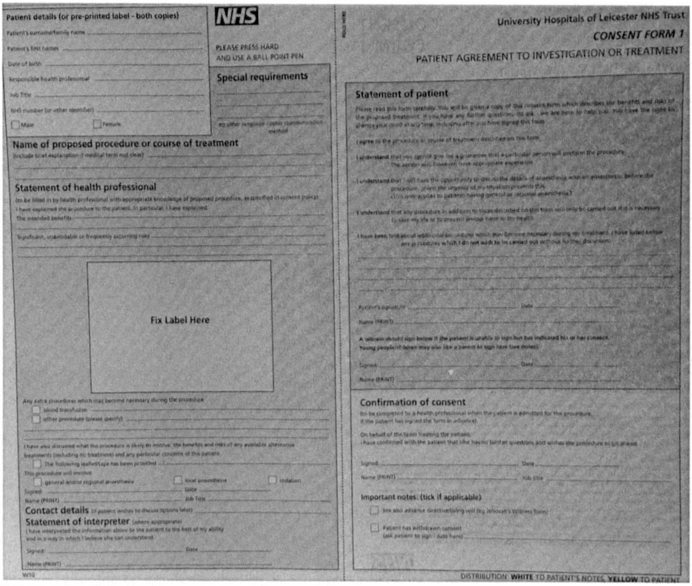
Patient details (or pre-printed label - both copies)
NHS
PLEASE PRESS HARD
AND USE A BALL POINT PEN
Special requirements
Name of proposed procedure or course of treatment
Statement of health professional
Fix Label Here
Contact details
Statement of interpreter
University Hospitals of Leicester NHS Trust
CONSENT FORM 1
PATIENT AGREEMENT TO INVESTIGATION OR TREATMENT
Statement of patient
Confirmation of consent
Important notes: (tick if applicable)
DISTRIBUTION: WHITE TO PATIENT'S NOTES, YELLOW TO PATIENT

Figure 10.1 Consent Form 1.

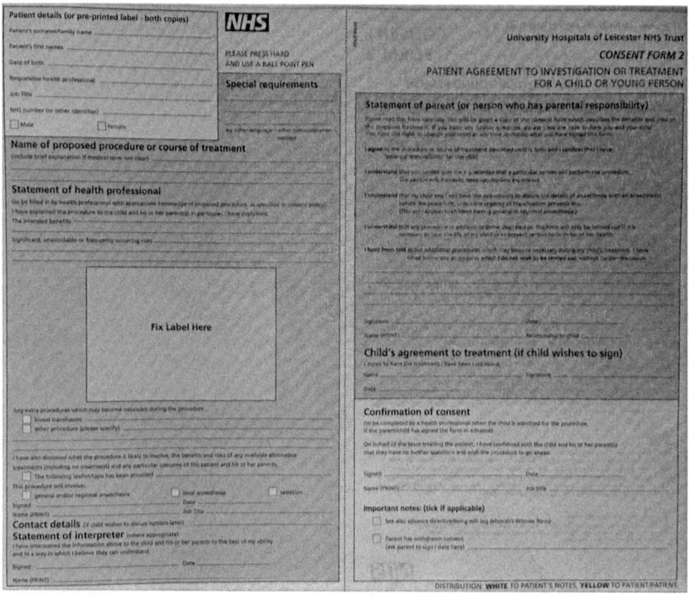
Patient details (or pre-printed label - both copies)
NHS
PLEASE PRESS HARD
AND USE A BALL POINT PEN
Special requirements
Name of proposed procedure or course of treatment
Statement of health professional
Fix Label Here
Contact details
Statement of interpreter
University Hospitals of Leicester NHS Trust
CONSENT FORM 2
PATIENT AGREEMENT TO INVESTIGATION OR TREATMENT
FOR A CHILD OR YOUNG PERSON
Statement of parent (or person who has parental responsibility)
Child's agreement to treatment (if child wishes to sign)
Confirmation of consent
Important notes: (tick if applicable)
DISTRIBUTION: WHITE TO PATIENT'S NOTES, YELLOW TO PATIENT/PATIENT

Figure 10.2 Consent Form 2.

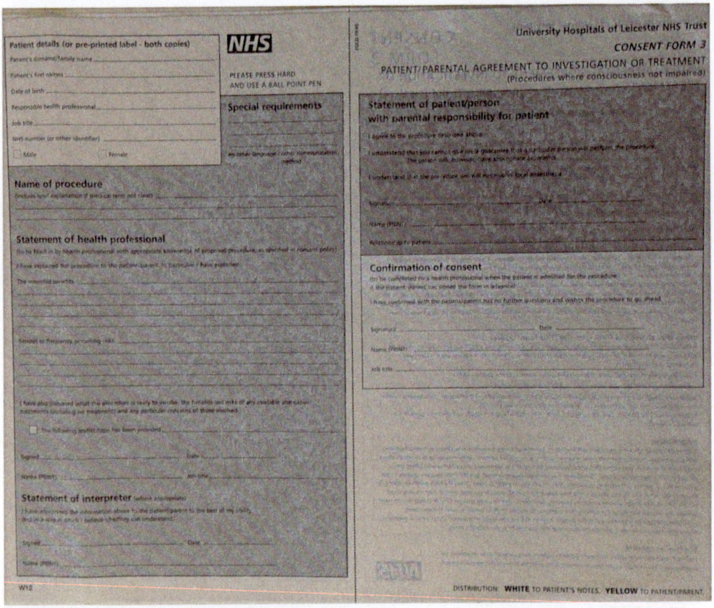
Patient details (or pre-printed label - both copies)

NHS

PLEASE PRESS HARD
AND USE A BALL POINT PEN

Special requirements

Name of procedure

Statement of health professional

Statement of interpreter

W12

University Hospitals of Leicester NHS Trust

CONSENT FORM 3

PATIENT/PARENTAL AGREEMENT TO INVESTIGATION OR TREATMENT
(Procedures where consciousness not impaired)

Statement of patient/person
with parental responsibility for patient

Confirmation of consent

DISTRIBUTION: WHITE TO PATIENT'S NOTES. YELLOW TO PATIENT/PARENT.

Figure 10.3 Consent Form 3.

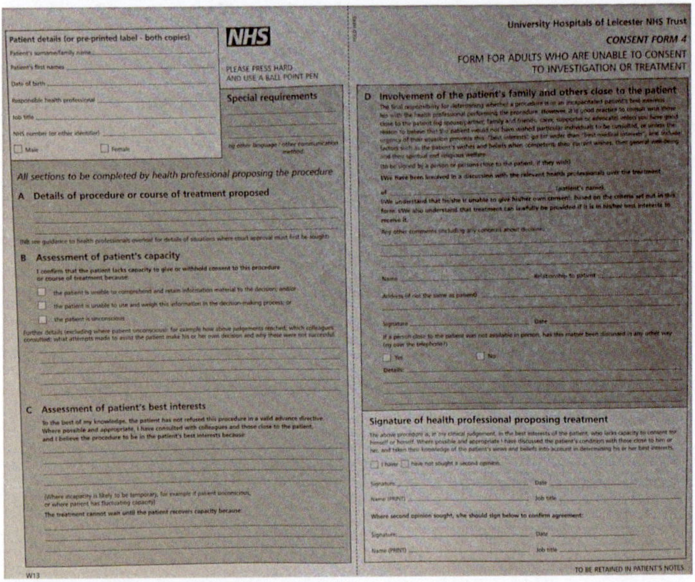
Patient details (or pre-printed label - both copies)

NHS

PLEASE PRESS HARD
AND USE A BALL POINT PEN

Special requirements

All sections to be completed by health professional proposing the procedure

A Details of procedure or course of treatment proposed

B Assessment of patient's capacity

C Assessment of patient's best interests

W13

University Hospitals of Leicester NHS Trust

CONSENT FORM 4

FORM FOR ADULTS WHO ARE UNABLE TO CONSENT
TO INVESTIGATION OR TREATMENT

D Involvement of the patient's family and others close to the patient

Signature of health professional proposing treatment

TO BE RETAINED IN PATIENT'S NOTES

Figure 10.4 Consent Form 4.

Consenting in action

At this stage it is worth highlighting the key points pertaining to informed consent using common operations, such as, superficial parotidectomy, myringoplasty, septoplasty and adenotonsillectomy. In the examination there will be an assessor and an actor as shown in Figure 10.1.

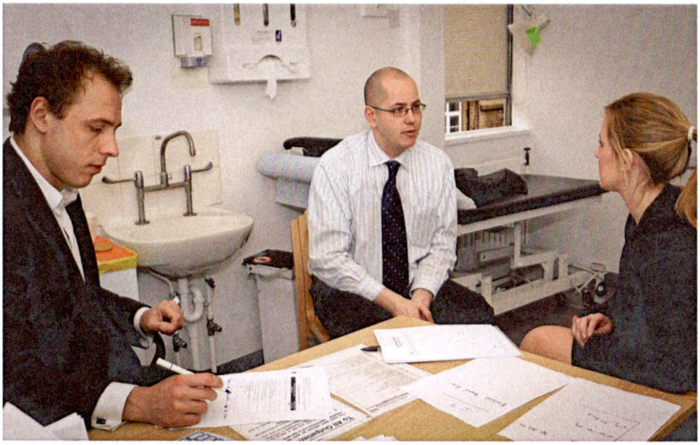

Figure 10.1. Typical arrangement for taking informed consent during an examination (Assessor Mr Hamilton and actor Mr Zotonski).

10.2 Superficial parotidectomy

Operation:	Superficial parotidectomy
Options:	Conservative (but risk of tumour growth and cancerous changes). Surgery
Surgery:	Incision (demonstrate modified Blair or face lift incisions) Identification of the important structures eg nerve that moves the face

Remove the outer portion of the gland and preserve nerve to the face; nerve monitor will be used.
Close with absorbable (6.0 vicyl rapide) or fine non-absorbable sutures (GP to remove in 5-7 days).

Side effects: Bleeding, haematoma, infection, facial nerve palsy (temporary marginal mandibular nerve palsy 10%, complete 1-2%), Frey's syndrome (up to 80%), ear lobule numbness, seroma, salivary fistula, further surgery, scar.
Post-op: May have a drain *in situ* for 24-48 hours
Signatures: Surgeon and patient or parent

10.3 Myringoplasty

Operation: Left myringoplasty to close hole in ear drum and make ear water-tight.
Options: Conservative (no change in symptomology)
Medical: treat infection with antibiotics, advice on water precaution, consider hearing aid.
Surgery to make ear water-tight (preferred option)

Surgery: Myringoplasty
Incision behind/ in front of ear or through canal
The hole is patched using your own tissue (eg sheet around the muscle called fascia
Or perichrondrium)
Packing and head bandage.

Side effects: Scar, infection, graft failure (20-30%), loss of hearing, tinnitus, dizziness, facial paralysis (local anaesthetic), change in taste, allergic reaction to dressing.
Post-op: Head bandage and dressing over-night.
Signatures: Surgeon and patient or parent

10.4 Septoplasty

Operation: Septoplasty
Options: Conservative (no change in symptomology)
Medical: no role unless concurrent rhinitis
Surgery (preferred option)

Surgery: Operation to straighten middle partition wall of the nose and improve breathing through nose
Incision inside the nostril
Nasal lining lifted
Septum manipulated +/-cartilage/bone excision
Nasal lining returned and stitched in place (absorbable suture)

Side effects: Bleeding, infection, nasal deformity (saddle nose), septal perforation, adhesions, numbness to the upper front teeth
Post-op: Nasal packs for 4 hours
Signatures: Surgeon and patient or parent

10.5 Adenotonsillectomy

Operation: Adenotonsillectomy
Options: Conservative
Surgery (preferred option)

Surgery: Removal of adenoid and tonsils.

	Instruments are passed through the mouth Adenoids reduced Tonsils removed Bleeding stopped
Side effects:	Risks: Bleeding (go to nearest A&E, may be life threatening), infection, pain, damage to lips/ teeth/ gums.
Post -op:	Encourage eating and drinking Take analgesia regularly No red coloured drinks (eg ribena) for first 24 hours (may be confused with ingested blood).
Signatures:	Surgeon and patient or parent.

Appendix

Table 1 Inventory of OSCE STATIONS

Station No.	Clinical Subject
1	Periorbital cellulitis
2	Inhaled foreign body
3	Acute otitis media
4	Inactive squamous chronic otitis media (COM)
5	Septal perforation
6	Nystagmus
7	Hereditary haemorrhagic telangiectasia (HHT)
8	Pharyngeal pouch
9	Vocal cord palsy
10	CT/pansinusitis/FESS complications
11	Button battery
12	Squamous cell carcinoma of tongue
13	Squamous cell carcimoma of larynx
14	Tympanometry
15	Tonsillitis and complications
16	Attic cholesteatoma
17	Skull base foramen
18	Sudden SNHL
19	Branchial cyst
20	Nerves of larynx
21	Nerves of EAM and pinna
22	Meniere's disease
23	Active mucosal chronic otitis media (COM)
24	Local anaesthesia and calculations
25	ABR, OAE and screening
26	Data interpretation – thyroid biochemistry
27	Hearing aids
28	laryngeal papillomas
29	Enlarged inferior turbinates and rhinorhoea
30	Bilateral acoustic neuromas and NF2

31	Otitis externa
32	Tracheostomy tubes
33	Neck levels, zones and triangles
34	Ramsay Hunt syndrome – chorda tympani
35	Prominent (bat) ear
36	Thyroglossal duct cyst
37	Microtia
38	Otosclerosis
39	Pre-auricular sinus
40	Submandibular calculus
41	Epistaxis
42	Otomycosis
43	Deviated nasal septum
44	BIPP
45	Submandibular gland excision and complications
46	Thyroidectomy
47	Nasopharyngeal carcinoma and TNM staging system
48	Frey's syndrome
49	Deep neck space infection
50	Drooling
51	Acute mastoiditis
52	2nd Branchial arch anomaly
53	Fractured temporal bone
54	Histology temporal bone
55	Superior orbital fissure syndrome
56	Waardenburg syndrome
57	Malignant melanoma
58	Pleomorphic adenoma
59	Epley and BPPV
60	Nasal polyps
61	Congenital HL – Pendred (EVA & Mondini)
62	Vascular anomalies (haemangiomas and vascular malformations).

TNM classification

The TNM system is the commonest method to classification malignant disease and is used internationally. T describes the size (in its greatest dimension) and extent of the primary tumour, N describes the presence or absence and extend of regional lymph nodes, and M describes the presence or absence and extent of distant spread. Table 2.0 shows the general definitions used throughout the TNM classification.

General TNM classification (relevant to all)					
Tumour		Nodes		Metastasis	
TX	Primary tumour cannot be assessed	**NX**	Regional lymph nodes cannot be assessed	**MX**	Distant metastasis cannot be assessed
T0	No evidence of primary tumour	**N0**	No regional lymph node metastasis	**M0**	No distant metastasis
Tis	Carcinoma *in situ*			**M1**	Distant metastasis

Table 2 TNM General Definitions

It is important to understand the difference between the **TNM classification** and the **STAGE** of the disease. For instance, a **T1N1M0** laryngeal cancer is **Stage III** disease, which has a poorer prognosis than **Stage I** disease (**T1N0M0**) and so on. For further details on stage grouping and its relationship with the TNM classification, please refer to page 57 and Table 13.2.

All of the following TNM classifications are adapted from:

Sobin LH, Gospodarowicz, Wittekind C (eds). TNM Classification of Malignant Tumours.
7th edn. Oxford, Wiley-Blackwell, 2009.

Table 3a TNM Supraglottic cancer.
It is worth noting that laryngeal cancer includes tumour of the supraglottis, glottis and subglottis.

TNM classification for supraglottic cancer					
Tumour		Nodes		Metastasis	
T0	No evidence of primary tumour	**N0**	No regional lymph node metastasis	**M0**	No distant metastasis
Tis	Carcinoma *in situ*	**N1**	Single ipsilateral lymph node, 3 cm or less in greatest dimension	**M1**	Distant metastasis
T1	Tumour limited to one subsite of supraglottis (false cord, arythenoid, suprahyoid epiglottis, infrahyoid epiglottis or arythenoid fold) with normal vocal cord movements.	**N2 a**	Single ipsilateral lymph node, more than 3 cm but not more than 6 cm in greatest dimension		
T2	Tumour invades mucosa of more than one adjacent subsite of supraglottis or glottis or region outside the supraglottis (eg mucosa of the tongue base, vallecula, medial wall of the piriform sinus) with normal vocal cord	**N2 b**	Multiple ipsilateral lymph nodes, none more than 6 cm in greatest dimension		

	movements.				
T3	Tumour limited to the with vocal cord fixation and/or invades any of the following: postcricoid area, pre-epiglottic tissues, paraglottic space, and/or with invasion of the inner cortex of the thyroid cartilage	**N2 c**	Bilateral or contralateral lymph nodes, none more than 6 cm in greatest dimension.		
T4 a	Tumour invases through the thyroid cartilage and/or tissues beyond the larynx, eg. Trachea, soft tissue of the neck including extrinsic muscle of tongue(genioglossus, hyoglossus, palatoglossus and styloglossus, strap muscles, thyroid, oesophagus.	**N3**	Node more than 6 cm in greatest dimension		
T4 b	Tumour invades prevertebral space, mediastinal structure or encases carotid artery.				

Table 3b TNM Glottic cancer.

TNM classification for glottic cancer					
Tumour		Nodes		Metastasis	
T1 a	Tumour limited to one vocal cord with normal vocal cord mobility	**N1**	Single ipsilateral lymph node, 3 cm or less in greatest dimension	**M0**	No Distant metastasis
T1 b	Tumour involves both vocal cords with normal vocal cord mobility	**N2a**	Single ipsilateral lymph node, more than 3 cm but not more than 6 cm in greatest dimension	**M1**	Distant metastasis
T2 a	Tumour extends to supraglottis and/or subglottis with normal vocal cord mobility	**N2 b**	Multiple ipsilateral lymph nodes, none more than 6 cm in greatest dimension		
T2 b	Tumour extends to supraglottis and/or subglottis with impaired vocal cord mobility	**N2c**	Bilateral or contralateral lymph nodes, none more than 6 cm in greatest dimension.		
T3	Tumour associated with no vocal cord mobility and/or invades paraglottic space, inner cortex of thyroid cartilage.	**N3**	Node more than 6 cm in greatest dimension		
T4 a	Tumour invades both cortex of the thyroid cartilage or invades tissue beyond the larynx				

	eg trachea, soft tissue of the neck including deep/extrinsic muscle of tongue (genioglossus,hyoglossus, palatoglossus and styloglossus, strap muscles, thyroid, oesophagus.				
T4 b	Tumour invades prevertebral space, mediastinal structures, or encases carotid artery.				

Table 3c TNM Subglottic cancer.

TNM classification for subglottic cancer					
Tumour		Nodes		Metastasis	
T1	Tumour limited to subglottis	**N1**	Single ipsilateral lymph node, 3 cm or less in greatest dimension	**M0**	No Distant metastasis
T2	Tumour extends to vocal cords with normal or impaired mobility	**N2 a**	Single ipsilateral lymph node, more than 3 cm but not more than 6 cm in greatest dimension	**M1**	Distant metastasis
T3	Tumour limited to larynx with vocal cord immobility	**N2 b**	Multiple ipsilateral lymph nodes, none more than 6 cm in greatest dimension		
T4a	Tumour invades through cricoid or thyroid cartilage and/or invade soft tissue beyond thelarynx, eg trachea, soft tissue of the neck including deep/extrinsic muscle of tongue (genioglossus,hyo glossus, palatoglossus and styloglossus, strap muscles, thyroid, oesophagus.	**N2 c**	Bilateral or contralateral lymph nodes, none more than 6 cm in greatest dimension.		
T4b	Tumour invades prevertebral space, mediastinal structures, or encases carotid artery.	**N3**	Node more than 6 cm in greatest dimension		

Table 4 TNM Oral cavity cancer.
This includes mucosal surface of the lip, buccal mucosa, retromolar triangle, alveolus, hard palate, anterior two-thirds of tongue and floor of mouth.

TNM classification for oral cavity cancer					
Tumour		**Nodes**		**Metastasis**	
T0	No evidence of primary tumour	**N0**	No regional lymph node metastasis	**M0**	No distant metastasis
Tis	Carcinoma *in situ*	**N1**	Metastasis in a single ipsilateral lymph node, 3 cm or less in greatest dimension	**M1**	Distant metastasis
T1	Tumour 2 cm or less in greatest dimension	**N2a**	Metastasis in a single ipsilateral lymph node, more than 3 cm but not more than 6 cm in greatest dimension		
T2	Tumour more than 2 cm but not more than 4 cm in greatest dimension	**N2b**	Metastasis in multiple ipsilateral lymph nodes, none more than 6 cm in greatest dimension		
T3	Tumour more than 4 cm in greatest dimension.	**N2c**	Metastasis in bilateral or contralateral lymph nodes, none more than 6 cm in greatest dimension		
T4 a (lip)	Tumour invades through cortical bone, inferior alveolar nerve,	**N3**	Metastasis in a lymph node more than 6 cm in greatest		

	floor of mouth, or skin (chin or nose). *Note: Superficial erosion alone of bone/tooth socket by gingival primary is not sufficient to classify a tumour as T4.*		dimension		
T4 b (oral cavity)	Tumour invades through cortical bone, into deep/extrinsic muscle of tongue (genioglossus, hyoglossus, palatoglossus, and styloglossus), maxillary sinus, or skin of face.				
T4c (lip and oral cavity)	Tumourinvades masticator space, pterygoid plates, or skull base; or encases internal carotid artery.				

Table 5 TNM Nasopharyngeal cancer.

TNM classification for nasopharyngeal cancer					
Tumour		**Nodes**		**Metastasis**	
T0	No evidence of primary tumour	**N0**	No regional lymph node metastasis	**M0**	No distant metastasis
TIs	Carcinoma *in situ*	**N1**	Unilateral metastasis in lymph node(s) 6 cm or less in greatest dimension, above the supraclavicular fossa	**M1**	Distant metastasis
T1	Tumour confined to the nasopharynx, or tumor extends to oropharynx and/or nasal cavity without parapharyngeal extension	**N2**	Bilateral metastasis in lymph node(s) or 6 cm or less in greatest dimension, above the supraclavicular fossa.		
T2	Tumour with parapharyngeal extension	**N3**	Metastasis in a lymph node(s): N3a - greater than 6 cm in dimension. N3b - extension to the supraclavicular fossa.		
T3	Tumour involves bony structures of skull base and/or paranasal sinuses				
T4	Tumour with intracranial extension and/or involvement of				

	cranial nerves, hypopharynx, orbit, or with extension to the infratemporal fossa/masticator space				

Table 6 TNM Oropharyngeal cancer.
Oropharyngeal cancer involves tumours of the tonsils, tongue base and soft palate

TNM classification for oropharyngeal cancer					
Tumour		Nodes		Metastasis	
T1	Tumour 2 cm or less in greatest dimension	**N1**	Single ipsilateral lymph node, 3 cm or less in greatest dimension	**M0**	No distant metastasis
T2	Tumour more than 2 cm but not more than 4 cm in greatest dimension	**N2 a**	Single ipsilateral lymph node, more than 3 cm but not more than 6 cm in greatest dimension	**M1**	Distant metastasis
T3	Tumour more than 4 cm in greatest dimension	**N2 b**	Multiple ipsilateral lymph nodes, none more than 6 cm in greatest dimension		
T4 a	Tumour invades any of the following: larynx, deep/extrinsic muscle of tongue, medial pterygoid, hard palate or mandible	**N2 c**	Metastasis in bilateral or contralateral lymph nodes, none more than 6 cm in greatest dimension		
T4 b	Tumour invades any of the following: lateral pterygoid muscles, pterygoid plates, lateral nasopharynx or skull base, or encases the carotid artery.	**N3**	Node more than 6 cm in greatest dimension		

Table 7 TNM Hypopharyngeal cancer.
Hypopharyngeal cancer includes tumours of the post-cricoid region, piriform sinus and posterior pharyngeal wall.

TNM classification for hypopharyngeal Cancer					
Tumour		Nodes		Metastasis	
T0	No evidence of primary tumour	**N0**	No regional lymph node metastasis	**M0**	No distant metastasis
T1	The tumour is limited to one subsite of the hypopharynx and is 2 cm or less at its greatest dimension	**N2 a**	Metastasis in a single ipsilateral lymph node (>3 cm but < 6 cm at its greatest dimension).	**M1**	Distant metastasis
T2	The tumour involves more than one subsite of the hypopharynx or an adjacent site or is larger than 2 cm but not larger than 4 cm at its greatest diameter without fixation of the hemilarynx.	**N2 b**	Metastasis in multiple ipsilateral lymph nodes (none >6 cm at greatest dimension) N2c - Metastasis in bilateral or contralateral lymph nodes (none >6 cm at greatest dimension)		
T3	The tumour is larger than 4 cm at its greatest dimension or involves fixation of the hemilarynx.	**N3**	Metastasis is found in a lymph node larger than 6 cm at its greatest dimension.		
T4 a	Tumour invades the thyroid/cricoid cartilage, hyoid bone, thyroid gland, oesophagus, or central compartment soft				

	tissues, including prelaryngeal strap muscles and subcutaneous fat.				
T4 b	T4b - Tumour invades the prevertebral fascia, encases the carotid artery, or involves mediastinal structures.				

Table 8 TNM Nasal cavity and ethmoid sinuses.

TNM classification for nasal cavity and ethmoid sinuses cancer					
Tumour		Nodes		Metastasis	
T1	Tumour restricted to one subsite of the nasal cavity (septum, floor, lateral wall or vestibule) or ethmoid sinus, with or without bony erosion	**N1**	Single ipsilateral node 3 cm or less	**MX**	Distant metastasis cannot be assessed
T2	Tumour involves 2 subsites or extends to involve an adjacent site within the nasoethmoidal complex, with or without bony erosion.	**N2a**	Single ipsilateral node greater than 3cm but less than 6cm in greatest dimension.	**M0**	No distant metastasis.
T3	Tumour invades the medial wall or floor of orbit, maxillary sinus, palate or cribiform plate.	**N2b**	Multiple ipsilateral nodes no more than 6cm in greatest dimension.	**M1**	Distant metastasis
T4a	Tumour invades any of the following: anterior orbital contents, skin of nose or cheek, pterygoid plates, sphenoid or frontal sinuses,	**N2c**	Bilateral or contralateral node less than 6cm in greatest dimension.		

	extension into anterior cranial fossa				
T4b	Tumour invades any of the following: orbital apex, dura, brain, middle cranial fossa, nasopharynx, clivus or cranial nerves other than maxillary division of trigeminal nerve	**N3**	Node 6cm in greatest dimension or larger.		

Table 9 TNM Maxillary sinus cancer.

TNM classification for maxillary sinus cancer					
Tumour		Nodes		Metastasis	
T1	Tumour limited to the mucosa with no erosion or destruction of bone.	**N1**	Single ipsilateral node 3 cm or less	**MX**	Distant metastasis cannot be assessed
T2	Tumour erodes bone and extends into hard palate and/or middle nasal meatus, except extension to posterior wall of maxillary sinus and pterygoid plates.	**N2a**	Single ipsilateral node greater than 3cm but less than 6cm in greatest diamension.	**M0**	No distant metastasis
T3	Tumour invades any of the following: bone of posterior wall of maxillary sinus, subcutaneous tissue, floor or medial wall of orbit, pterygoid fossa, ethmoid sinuses.	**N2b**	Multiple ipsilateral nodes no more than 6cm in greatest diameter.	**M1**	Distant metastasis
T4a	Tumour invades any of the following: anterior orbital contents, skin of cheek, pterygoid plates, infratemporal fossa, cribiform plate, sphenoid or frontal sinuses.	**N2c**	Bilateral or contralateral node less than 6cm in greatest diameter		

T4b	Tumour invades any of the following: orbital apex, dura, brain, middle fossa dura, nasopharynx, clivus or cranial nerves other than maxillary division of trigeminal nerve.	**N3**	Node 6cm or greater in dimension		

Table 10 TNM Thyroid gland cancer.

Multifocal tumours of all histological types are designated 'm' (the largest determines the classification, eg, T3(m).

TNM classification for thyroid cancer					
Tumour		Nodes		Metastasis	
T0	No evidence of primary tumour.	**N0**	No spread to nearby lymph nodes.	**M0**	No distant metastasis
T1 a	Tumour < 1 cm in greatest diamension and limited to the thyroid	**N1a**	Spread to level VI (pretracheal, paratracheal and prelaryngeal and Delphian nodes).	**M1**	Distant metastasis
T1 b	Tumour >1 cm but <2 cm in greatest diamension and limited to the thyroid	**N1b**	Spread to other cervical lymph nodes and retropharyngeal or superior mediastinal.		
T2	Tumour is more than 2 cm but no more than 4 cm and limited to the thyroid gland				
T3	Tumour is greater than 4 cm or it has begun to invade surrounding tissue.				
T4 a	Tumour extends beyond the thyroid capsule into nearby				

	tissues of the neck, such as the larynx, trachea, oesophagus or the recurrent laryngeal nerve.				
T4 b	Tumour has grown beyond of the thyroid, invades the prevertebral fascia, mediastinial vessels or encases the carotid artery.				

Table 11 TNM Salivary glands cancer.

TNM classification for salivary gland cancer					
Tumour		Nodes		Metastasis	
T1	Tumour 2cm or less without extraparenchymal extension	**N1**	Single ipsilateral node 3cm or less	**MX**	Distant metastasis cannot be assessed
T2	Tumour more than 2 cm but not more than 4cm without extraparenchymal extension	**N2a**	Single ipsilateral node greater than 3cm but less than 6cm in greatest dimension	**M0**	No distant metastasis
T3	Tumour more than 4cm and/or tumour with extraparenchymal extension	**N2b**	Multiple ipsilateral nodes no more than 6cm in greatest dimension	**M1**	Distant metastasis
T4a	Tumour invades skin, mandible, ear canal or facial nerve.	**N2c**	Bilateral or contralateral nodes less than 6cm in greatest dimension		
T4b	Tumour invades base of skull, pterygoid plates or encases the carotid artery	**N3**	Node greater than 6cm in greatest dimension		

Table 12 Mucosal malignant melanomas.
Mucosal melanomas are very aggressive tumours and therefore T1 and T2 are omitted from the classification.

TNM classification for mucosal malignant melanomas					
Tumour		Nodes		Metastasis	
T3	Limited to epithelium/submucosal/mucosal disease	**N0**	No regional nodal metastasis	**MX**	Distant metastasis cannot be assessed
T4a	Invading deep soft tissue, cartilage bone or overlying skin	**N1**	Regional nodal metastasis	**M0**	No distant metastasis
T4b	Invading brain, dura, skull base, lower cranial nerves, masticator space, carotid artery, prevertebral space, mediastinal structures			**M1**	Distant metastasis

Request from the Authors

There is always room for improvement and therefore we would be very grateful for your constructive feedback and comments on the content of this book. Please send your feedback via email to info@enttzar.co.uk or ricardopersaud@yahoo.co.uk. You may also wish to review this book on Amazon. Your comments are important to us as we think about improvements for the 2nd edition.

Many thanks

RP, SC, AT, KA & HP

www.enttzar.co.uk